P9-DEB-500

Contributors

Audrey Knippa, MS, MPH, RN, CNE
Nursing Education Coordinator and
  Content Project Leader

Sheryl Sommer, PhD, MSN, RN
Director, Nursing Curriculum and
  Education Services

Brenda Ball, MEd, BSN, RN
Nursing Education Specialist

Lois Churchill, MN, RN
Nursing Education Specialist

Carrie B. Elkins, DHSc, MSN, PHCNS, BC
Nursing Education Specialist

Mary Jane Janowski, MA, BSN, RN
Nursing Resource Specialist

Karin Roberts, PhD, MSN, RN, CNE
Nursing Education Coordinator

Mendy G. Wright, DNP, MSN, RN
Nursing Education Specialist

Derek Prater, MS Journalism
Lead Product Developer and Editorial Project Leader

Erika A. Archer, BS Education, Foreign Language
Product Developer

Johanna Barnes, BA Journalism
Product Developer

Chris Crawford, BS Journalism
Product Developer

Hilary E. Groninger, BS Journalism
Product Developer

Megan E. Herre, BS Journalism
Product Developer

Amanda Lehman, BA English
Product Developer

Joanna Shindler, BA Journalism
Product Developer

Brant L. Stacy, BS Journalism, BA English
Product Developer

Consultants

Fleurdeliza T. Cuyco, BSN

Lisa M. Easterby, MSN, RN, CNE

Beth E. Schultz, MSN, RN

INTELLECTUAL PROPERTY NOTICE

IMPORTANT NOTICE TO THE READER

USER'S GUIDE

Welcome to the Assessment Technologies Institute® RN Maternal Newborn Nursing Review Module Edition 8.0. The mission of ATI's Content Mastery Series® review modules is to provide user-friendly compendiums of nursing knowledge that will:

- Help you locate important information quickly.

- Assist in your remediation efforts.

- Provide exercises for applying your nursing knowledge.

- Facilitate your entry into the nursing profession as a newly licensed RN.

Organization

This review module is organized into units covering antepartum, intrapartum, postpartum, and newborn nursing care. Chapters within these units conform to one of three organizing principles for presenting the content:

- Nursing concepts

- Procedures

- Complications of pregnancy

Nursing concepts chapters begin with an overview describing the central concept and its relevance to nursing. Subordinate themes are covered in outline form to demonstrate relationships and present the information in a clear, succinct manner.

Procedures chapters include an overview describing the procedure(s) covered in the chapter. These chapters will provide you with nursing knowledge relevant to each procedure, including indications, interpretations of findings, client outcomes, nursing actions, and complications.

Complications of pregnancy chapters include an overview describing the complication, followed by risk factors. These chapters will cover assessment, including subjective and objective data, and collaborative care, including nursing care, medications, health promotion, and client outcomes.

Application Exercises

Questions are provided at the end of each chapter so you can practice applying your knowledge. The Application Exercises include both NCLEX-style questions, such as multiple-choice and multiple-select items, and questions that ask you to apply your knowledge in other formats, such as short-answer and matching items. After the Application Exercises, an answer key is provided, along with rationales for the answers.

NCLEX® Connections

To prepare for the NCLEX-RN, it is important for you to understand how the content in this review module is connected to the NCLEX-RN test plan. You can find information on the detailed test plan at the National Council of State Boards of Nursing's Web site: https://www.ncsbn.org/. When reviewing content in this review module, regularly ask yourself, "How does this content fit into the test plan, and what types of questions related to this content should I expect?"

To help you in this process, we've included NCLEX Connections at the beginning of each unit and with each question in the Application Exercises Answer Keys. The NCLEX Connections at the beginning of each unit will point out areas of the detailed test plan that relate to the content within that unit. The NCLEX Connections attached to the Application Exercises Answer Keys will demonstrate how each exercise fits within the detailed content outline.

These NCLEX Connections will help you understand how the detailed content outline is organized, starting with major client needs categories and subcategories and followed by related content areas and tasks. The major client needs categories are:

- Safe and Effective Care Environment
  - Management of Care
  - Safety and Infection Control
- Health Promotion and Maintenance
- Psychosocial Integrity
- Physiological Integrity
  - Basic Care and Comfort
  - Pharmacological and Parenteral Therapies
  - Reduction of Risk Potential
  - Physiological Adaptation

An NCLEX Connection might, for example, alert you that content within a unit is related to:

- Health Promotion and Maintenance
  - Ante/Intra/Postpartum and Newborn Care
    - Assess client psychosocial response to pregnancy.

Icons

Icons are used throughout the review module to draw your attention to particular areas. Keep an eye out for these icons:

 This icon indicates an Overview, or introduction, to a particular subject matter. Descriptions and categories will typically be found in an Overview.

 This icon is used for the Application Exercises and the Application Exercises Answer Keys.

 This icon is used for NCLEX connections.

This icon is used for content related to safety. When you see this icon, take note of safety concerns or steps that nurses can take to ensure client safety and a safe environment.

This icon indicates that a media supplement, such as a graphic, an animation, or a video, is available. If you have an electronic copy of the review module, this icon will appear alongside clickable links to media supplements. If you have a hardcopy version of the review module, visit www.atitesting.com for details on how to access these features.

Feedback

ATI welcomes feedback regarding this review module. Please provide comments to: comments@ atitesting.com.

Table of Contents

UNIT 1: ANTEPARTUM NURSING CARE

- Human Reproduction

- Low-Risk, Uncomplicated Pregnancy: Changes During Pregnancy

- Complications of Pregnancy

NCLEX® CONNECTIONS

When reviewing the chapters in this unit, keep in mind the relevant sections of the NCLEX® outline, in particular:

CLIENT NEEDS: HEALTH PROMOTION AND MAINTENANCE

Relevant topics/tasks include:

- Ante/Intra/Postpartum and Newborn Care
  - Provide prenatal care and education.
- Developmental Stages and Transitions
  - Identify expected body image changes associated with the client's developmental age.
- Lifestyle Choices
  - Assess the client's need/desire for contraception.

CLIENT NEEDS: REDUCTION OF RISK POTENTIAL

Relevant topics/tasks include:

- Diagnostic Tests
  - Monitor the results of maternal and fetal diagnostic tests.
- Potential for Complications of Diagnostic Tests/Treatments/Procedures
  - Monitor the client for signs of bleeding.
- System Specific Assessment
  - Perform focused assessment and reassessment.

CLIENT NEEDS: BASIC CARE AND COMFORT

Relevant topics/tasks include:

- Nonpharmacological Comfort Interventions
  - Assess the client's need for alternative and/or complementary therapy.

CLIENT NEEDS: PHYSIOLOGICAL ADAPTATION

Relevant topics/tasks include:

- Alterations in Body Systems
  - Identify signs of potential prenatal complications.

UNIT 1	ANTEPARTUM NURSING CARE
Section	Human Reproduction
Chapter 1	Contraception

Overview

- Contraception refers to strategies or devices used to reduce the risk of fertilization or implantation in an attempt to prevent pregnancy.

- A nurse should assess a client's need/desire for contraception. In addition, a thorough discussion of benefits, risks, and alternatives of each method should be discussed.

- A client's preference for contraception should be considered. The decision may be individual. Methods of contraception include natural-family planning, barrier, hormonal, and intrauterine methods, as well as surgical procedures.

- Sexual partners often make a joint decision regarding a desired preference (vasectomy or tubal ligation). Postpartum discharge instructions should include the discussion of future contraceptive plans.

- Expected outcomes for family planning methods consist of preventing pregnancy until a desired time.

- Nurses should support clients in making the decision that is best for their individualized situations.

Natural-Family Planning Methods

ABSTINENCE	
Definition	• Abstaining from having sexual intercourse eliminates the possibility of sperm entering a woman's vagina.
Client Instructions	• Refrain from sexual intercourse. This method can be associated with saying "no," but can also incorporate saying "yes" to other gratifying sexual activities such as affectionate touching, communication, holding hands, kissing, massage, and oral and manual stimulation.
Advantages	• Most effective method of birth control. • Abstinence during fertile periods (rhythm method) can be used, but requires an understanding of the menstrual cycle and fertility awareness. • Can eliminate the risk of STDs if there is no genitalia contact.

ABSTINENCE	
Disadvantages	• Requires self-control
Risks/possible complications/ contraindications	• If complete abstinence is maintained there are no risks.

COITUS INTERRUPTUS (WITHDRAWAL)	
Definition	• Man withdraws penis from vagina prior to ejaculation.
Client Instructions	• Be aware of fluids leaking from the penis.
Advantages	• Possible choice for monogamous couples with no other option for birth control, such as those opposed to birth control due to religious conviction.
Disadvantages	• Most ineffective method of contraception. • No protection against STDs.
Risks/possible complications/ contraindications	• Depends on a man's ability to control ejaculation. Adolescent boys frequently lack control to make this an effective method. • Leakage of fluid that contains spermatozoa prior to ejaculation can be deposited in vagina. • Risk of pregnancy

CALENDAR METHOD (RHYTHM METHOD)	
Definition	• A woman records her menstrual cycle by calculating her fertile period based on the assumption that ovulation occurs about 14 days before the onset of her next menstrual cycle, and avoids intercourse during that period. Also, taken into account is the timing of intercourse with this method, because sperm are viable for 48 to 120 hr and the ovum is viable for 24 hr.

Client Instructions	• Accurately record the number of days in each cycle counting from the first day of menses for a period of at least 6 cycles.
	• The start of the fertile period is figured by subtracting 18 days from the number of days in the woman's shortest cycle.
	• The end of the fertile period is established by subtracting 11 days from the number of days of the longest cycle. For example:
	  ○ Shortest cycle, 26 – 18 = 8th day
	  ○ Longest cycle, 30 – 11 = 19th day
	  ○ Fertile period is days 8 through 19.
	• Refrain from intercourse during these days to avoid conception.

CALENDAR METHOD (RHYTHM METHOD)	
Advantages	• Most useful when combined with basal body temperature or cervical mucus method. • Inexpensive
Disadvantages	• Not a very reliable technique. • Requires accurate record keeping. • Requires compliance by both partners in regards to abstinence during fertile periods.
Risks/possible complications/ contraindications	• Various factors can affect and change the time of ovulation and cause unpredictable menstrual cycles. • Risk of pregnancy.

BASAL BODY TEMPERATURE (BBT)	
Definition	• Temperature can drop slightly after the time of ovulation. This can be used to facilitate conception or be used as a natural contraceptive.
Client Instructions	• A woman is instructed to measure oral temperature prior to getting out of bed each morning to monitor ovulation.
Advantages	• Inexpensive, convenient, and no side effects
Disadvantages	• BBT reliability can be influenced by many variables that can cause inaccurate interpretation of temperature changes, such as stress, fatigue, illness, alcohol, and warmth or coolness of sleeping environment.
Risks/possible complications/ contraindications	• Risk of pregnancy

BILLINGS METHOD (CERVICAL MUCUS METHOD)	
Definition	• Fertility awareness method based on ovulation. Ovulation occurs approximately 14 days prior to the next menstrual cycle, which is when a woman is fertile. Following ovulation, the cervical mucus becomes thin and flexible under the influence of estrogen and progesterone to allow for sperm viability and motility. The ability for the mucus to stretch between the fingers is greatest during ovulation. This is referred to as spinnbarkeit sign.
Client Instructions	• Engage in good hand hygiene prior to and following assessment. • Begin examining mucus from the last day of the menstrual cycle. • Mucus is obtained from the vaginal introitus. It is not necessary to reach into the vagina to the cervix. • Do not douche prior to assessment.

BILLINGS METHOD (CERVICAL MUCUS METHOD)	
Advantages	• A woman can become knowledgeable in recognizing her own mucus characteristics at ovulation and self-evaluation can be very accurate. • Self-evaluation of cervical mucus can also be diagnostically helpful in determining the start of ovulation while breastfeeding, in noting the commencement of menopause, and in planning a desired pregnancy.
Disadvantages	• Some women may be uncomfortable with touching their genitals and mucus and therefore, will find this method objectionable.
Risks/possible complications/ contraindications	• Assessment of cervical mucus characteristics may be inaccurate if mucus is mixed with semen, blood, contraceptive foams, or discharge from infections. • Risk of pregnancy

Barrier Methods

CONDOMS	
Definition	• A thin flexible sheath worn on the penis during intercourse to prevent semen from entering the uterus.
Client Instructions	• A man places a condom on his erect penis, leaving an empty space at the tip for a sperm reservoir. • Following ejaculation, a man withdraws his penis from the woman's vagina while holding the rim of the condom to prevent any semen spillage to the woman's vulva or vaginal area. • May be used in conjunction with spermicidal gel or cream to increase effectiveness.
Advantages	• Protects against STDs and involves the male in the birth control method.
Disadvantages	• High rate of noncompliance • May reduce spontaneity of intercourse. • The penis must be erect to apply a condom. • If the penis is withdrawn while still erect, this can interfere with sexual intercourse.
Risks/possible complications/ contraindications	• Condoms can rupture or leak, thus potentially resulting in an unwanted pregnancy. • Condoms have a one-time usage, which creates a replacement cost. • Condoms made of latex should not be worn by those who are sensitive or allergic to latex. • Only water-soluble lubricants should be used with latex condoms to avoid condom breakage.

DIAPHRAGM AND SPERMICIDE

Definition	• A dome-shaped cup with a flexible rim made of latex or rubber that fits snugly over the cervix with spermicidal cream or gel placed into the dome and around the rim.
Client Instructions	• A female client should be fitted with a diaphragm properly by a primary care provider. • A client must be refitted by the primary care provider every 2 years, if there is a 7 kg (15 lb) weight change, full-term pregnancy, or second-term abortion. • Requires proper insertion and removal. Prior to coitus, the diaphragm is inserted vaginally over the cervix with spermicidal jelly or cream that is applied to the cervical side of the dome and around the rim. The diaphragm must remain in place for at least 6 hr after coitus. • More spermicide must be reapplied with each act of coitus. • A client should empty her bladder prior to insertion of the diaphragm.
Advantages	• This barrier method eliminates surgery and gives a woman more control over contraception.
Disadvantages	• Diaphragms are inconvenient, interfere with spontaneity, and require reapplication with spermicidal gel, cream, or foam with each act of coitus to be effective. • Requires a prescription and a visit to a health care provider. • Must be inserted correctly to be effective.
Risks/possible complications/ contraindications	• Diaphragm is not recommended for clients who have a history of toxic shock syndrome (TSS) or frequent, recurrent urinary tract infections. • Increased risk of acquiring TSS. • TSS is caused by a bacterial infection. Signs and symptoms include high fever, a faint feeling and drop in blood pressure, watery diarrhea, headache, and muscle aches. • Proper hand hygiene aids in prevention of TSS as well as removing diaphragm promptly at 6 hr following coitus. • Diaphragms made of latex should not be worn by those who are sensitive or allergic to latex.

Hormonal Methods

COMBINED ORAL CONTRACEPTIVES	
Definition	• Hormonal contraception containing estrogen and progestin, which acts by suppressing ovulation, thickening the cervical mucus to block semen, and altering the uterine decidua to prevent implantation.
Client Instructions	• Medication that requires a prescription and follow-up appointments with the primary care provider. • Medication requires consistent and proper use to be effective. • A client is instructed in observing for side effects and danger signs of medication. Signs include chest pain, shortness of breath, leg pain from a possible clot, headache, or eye problems from a cerebrovascular accident, or hypertension. • In the event of a client missing a dose, the nurse should instruct the client that if 1 pill is missed, take 1 as soon as possible; if 2 or 3 pills are missed, instruct the client to follow the manufacturer's instructions. Instruct the client on the use of alternative forms of contraception or abstinence to prevent pregnancy until regular dosing is resumed.
Advantages	• Highly effective if taken correctly and consistently. • Medication can alleviate dysmenorrhea by decreasing menstrual flow and menstrual cramps. • Reduces acne.
Disadvantages	• Oral contraceptives do not protect against STDs. • Birth control pills can increase the risk of thromboses, breast tenderness, scant or missed menstruation, stroke, nausea, headaches, and hormone-dependent cancers. • Exacerbates conditions affected by fluid retention such as migraine, epilepsy, asthma, kidney, or heart disease.
Risks/possible complications/ contraindications	• Women with a history of blood clots, cerebrovascular accident, cardiac problems, breast or estrogen-related cancers, pregnancy, or smoking (if over 35 years of age), are advised not to take oral contraceptive medications. • Oral contraceptive effectiveness decreases when taking medications that affect liver enzymes such as anticonvulsants and some antibiotics.

MINIPILL	
Definition	• Oral progestins that provide the same action as combined oral contraceptives.
Client Instructions	• A client should take the pill at the same time daily to ensure effectiveness secondary to a low dose of progestin. • A client cannot miss a pill. • A client may need another form of birth control during the first month of use to prevent pregnancy.
Advantages	• The minipill has fewer side effects when compared to a combination of oral birth control pills. • Considered safe to take while breastfeeding.
Disadvantages	• Less effective in suppressing ovulation than combined oral contraceptives. • Pill increases occurrence of ovarian cysts. • Pill does not protect against STDs. • Users frequently report breakthrough, irregular, vaginal bleeding, and decreased libido. • Increases appetite
Risks/possible complications/ contraindications	• Oral contraceptive effectiveness decreases when taking medications that affect liver enzymes such as anticonvulsants and some antibiotics.

EMERGENCY ORAL CONTRACEPTIVE	
Definition	• Morning after pill that prevents fertilization from taking place.
Client Instructions	• Pill is taken within 72 hr after unprotected coitus. • A primary care provider will recommend an over-the-counter antiemetic to be taken 1 hr prior to each dose to counteract the side effects of nausea that can occur with high doses of estrogen and progestin. • Advise a woman to be evaluated for pregnancy, if menstruation does not begin within 21 days. • The nurse should provide a client with counseling about contraception and modification sexual behaviors that are risky. • Is considered a form of "Emergency Birth Control."
Advantages	• Pill is not taken on a regular basis. • Can be obtained without a prescription by women 17 years and older.

EMERGENCY ORAL CONTRACEPTIVE	
Disadvantages	• Nausea, heavier than normal menstrual bleeding, lower abdominal pain, fatigue, and headache • Does not provide long-term contraception. • Does not terminate an established pregnancy. • Does not protect against STDs.
Risks/possible complications/ contraindications	• Contraindicated if a client is pregnant or has undiagnosed abnormal vaginal bleeding. • If menstruation does not start within 1 week of expected date, a client may be pregnant.

TRANSDERMAL CONTRACEPTIVE PATCH	
Definition	• Contains norelgestromin (progesterone) and ethinyl estradiol, which is delivered at continuous levels through the skin into subcutaneous tissue.
Client Instructions	• A client applies the patch to dry skin overlying subcutaneous tissue of the buttock, abdomen, upper arm, or torso, excluding breast area. • Requires patch replacement once a week. • Patch is applied the same day of the week for 3 weeks with no application of the patch on the fourth week.
Advantages	• Maintains consistent blood levels of hormone. • Avoids liver metabolism of medication since it is not absorbed in the gastrointestinal tract. • Decreases risk of forgetting daily pill.
Disadvantages	• Patch does not protect against STDs. • Poses same side effects as oral contraceptives. • Skin reaction may occur from patch application.
Risks/possible complications/ contraindications	• Same as those of oral contraceptives • Avoid applying of patch to skin rashes or lesions.

INJECTABLE PROGESTINS (DEPO-PROVERA)	
Definition	• An intramuscular injection given to a female client every 11 to 13 weeks.
Client Instructions	• Start of injections should be during the first 5 days of a client's menstrual cycle and every 11 to 13 weeks thereafter. • Advise a client to keep follow-up appointments. • A client should maintain an adequate intake of calcium and vitamin D.
Advantages	• Very effective and only requires four injections per year. • Does not impair lactation

INJECTABLE PROGESTINS (DEPO-PROVERA)	
Disadvantages	<ul><li>Can prolong amenorrhea</li><li>Irregular or unpredictable bleeding or spotting.</li><li>Increases the risk of thromboembolism.</li><li>Decreases bone mineral density (loss of calcium).</li><li>Does not protect against STDs.</li><li>Should only be used as a long-term method of birth control (greater than 2 years) if other birth control methods are inadequate.</li></ul>
Risks/possible complications/ contraindications	<ul><li>The nurse should avoid massaging injection site following administration to avoid accelerating medication absorption, which will shorten the duration of its effectiveness.</li></ul>

CONTRACEPTIVE VAGINAL RING (NUVARING)	
Definition	<ul><li>Contains etonogestrel and ethinyl estradiol that is delivered at continuous levels vaginally.</li></ul>
Client Instructions	<ul><li>A client inserts the ring vaginally.</li><li>Requires ring replacement after 3 weeks, and placement of new vaginal ring within 7 days. Insertion should occur on the same day of the week monthly.</li></ul>
Advantages	<ul><li>Vaginal ring does not have to be fitted.</li><li>Decreases the risk of forgetting to take the pill.</li></ul>
Disadvantages	<ul><li>Vaginal ring does not protect against STDs.</li><li>Poses the same side effects as oral contraceptives.</li><li>Some clients report discomfort during intercourse.</li></ul>
Risks/possible complications/ contraindications	<ul><li>Blood clots, hypertension, stroke, heart attack.</li><li>Vaginal irritation, increased vaginal secretions, headache, weight gain, and nausea.</li></ul>

IMPLANTABLE PROGESTIN ETONOGESTREL (IMPLANON)	
Definition	<ul><li>Requires a minor surgical procedure to subdermally implant and remove a single rod containing etonogestrel on the inner side of the upper aspect of the arm.</li></ul>
Client Instructions	<ul><li>Avoid trauma to the area of implantation.</li></ul>
Advantages	<ul><li>Effective continuous contraception for 3 years.</li><li>Reversible</li><li>Can be used by mothers who are breastfeeding after four weeks postpartum.</li></ul>

IMPLANTABLE PROGESTIN ETONOGESTREL (IMPLANON)	
Disadvantages	• Etonogestrel can cause irregular menstrual bleeding. • Etonogestrel does not protect against STDs. • Most common side effect is irregular and unpredictable menstruation. • Headache
Risks/possible complications/ contraindications	• Increased risk of ectopic pregnancy if pregnancy occurs.

INTRAUTERINE DEVICE (IUD)	
Definition	• A chemically active T-shaped device that is inserted through a woman's cervix and placed in the uterus by the primary care provider. Releases a chemical substance that damages sperm in transit to the uterine tubes and prevents fertilization.
Client Instructions	• The device must be monitored monthly by a client after menstruation to assure the presence of the small string that hangs from the device into the upper part of the vagina to rule out migration or expulsion of the device.
Advantages	• An IUD can maintain effectiveness for 1 to 10 years. • Contraception can be reversed. • Does not interfere with spontaneity. • Safe for mothers who are breastfeeding. • It is 99% effective in preventing pregnancy.
Disadvantages	• An IUD can increase the risk of pelvic inflammatory disease, uterine perforation, or ectopic pregnancy. • A client should report to the primary care provider late or abnormal spotting or bleeding, abdominal pain or pain with intercourse, abnormal or foul-smelling vaginal discharge, fever, chills, a change in string length, or if IUD cannot be located. • An IUD does not protect from STDs.
Risks/possible complications/ contraindications	• Contraindicated in women who have not had a least one child or are not in a monogamous relationship. • May cause irregular menstrual bleeding. • A risk of bacterial vaginosis, uterine perforation, or uterine expulsion. • Must be removed in the event of pregnancy.

Transcervical Sterilization

ESSURE	
Definition	• Insertion of small flexible agents through the vagina and cervix into the fallopian tubes. This results in the development of scar tissue in the tubes preventing conception. • Examination must be done after 3 months to ensure fallopian tubes are blocked.
Client Instruction	• Normal activities may be resumed by most clients within 1 day of the procedure.
Advantages	• Quick procedure that requires no general anesthesia. • Nonhormonal means of birth control. • Essure is 99.8% effective in preventing pregnancy. • Rapid return to normal activities of daily living.
Disadvantages	• Not reversible • Not intended for use in the client who is postpartum. • Delay in effectiveness for 3 months. Therefore, an alternative means of birth control should be used until confirmation of blocked fallopian tubes occurs. • Changes in menstrual patterns.
Risks/possible complications/contraindications	• Perforation can occur • Unwanted pregnancy can occur if a client has unprotected sexual intercourse during the first 3 months following the procedure. • Increased risk of ectopic pregnancy, if pregnancy occurs.

Surgical Methods

FEMALE STERILIZATION (BILATERAL TUBAL LIGATION SALPINGECTOMY)	
Definition	• A surgical procedure consisting of severance and/or burning or blocking the fallopian tubes to prevent fertilization.
Procedure	• The cutting, burning, or blocking of the fallopian tubes to prevent the ovum from being fertilized by the sperm.
Advantages	• Permanent contraception • Sexual function is unaffected.
Disadvantages	• A surgical procedure carrying risks related to anesthesia complications, infection, hemorrhage, or trauma. • Considered irreversible in the event that a client desires conception.
Risks/ possible complications/ contraindications	• Risk of ectopic pregnancy if pregnancy occurs.

MALE STERILIZATION (VASECTOMY)	
Definition	• A surgical procedure consisting of ligation and severance of the vas deferens.
Procedure	• The cutting of the vas deferens in the male as a form of permanent sterilization. The nurse should reinforce the need for alternate forms of birth control for approximately 20 ejaculations or 1 week to several months to allow all of the sperm to clear the vas deferens. This will assure complete male infertility.
Client Instruction	• Following the procedure, scrotal support and moderate activity for a couple of days is recommended to reduce discomfort. • Sterility is delayed until the proximal portion of the vas deferens is cleared of all remaining sperm (approximately 20 ejaculations). • Alternate forms of birth control must be used until the vas deferens is cleared of sperm. • Follow up is important for sperm count.
Advantages	• A vasectomy is a permanent contraceptive method. • Procedure is short, safe and simple. • Sexual function is not impaired.
Disadvantages	• Requires surgery • Considered irreversible in the event that a client desires conception.
Risks/ possible complications/ contraindications	• Complications are rare, but may include bleeding, infection, and anesthesia reaction.

View Media Supplement:
- Bilateral Tubal Ligation (Image)
- Vasectomy (Image)

CHAPTER 1: CONTRACEPTION

 Application Exercises

1. Explain why a bilateral tubal ligation is not a good option for a 19-year-old mother?

2. A nurse is instructing a client who has been prescribed oral contraceptives about danger signs. The nurse evaluates that the client understands the teaching regarding side effects when she states the need to report

    A. reduced menstrual flow or amenorrhea.

    B. weight gain or breast tenderness.

    C. chest pain or shortness of breath.

    D. mild hypertension or headaches.

3. A nurse in an obstetrical clinic is providing education about contraception to a 21-year-old client. Which of the following statements by the client requesting information regarding an IUD indicates a need for additional teaching?

    A. "An IUD may increase my risk for an ectopic pregnancy."

    B. "I will wait until I have a child before I can have an IUD."

    C. "I might have irregular bleeding after I get an IUD."

    D. "A change in the string length of my IUD is expected."

4. Which contraceptive method has the potential to decrease a client's bone mineral density?

5. Which of the following should the nurse include when teaching a client about the potential disadvantages of the minipill? (Select all that apply.)

    _____ Amenorrhea

    _____ Irregular vaginal bleeding

    _____ Increased appetite

    _____ Lowered libido

    _____ Ovarian cysts

CHAPTER 1: CONTRACEPTION

 Application Exercises Answer Key

1. Explain why a bilateral tubal ligation is not a good option for a 19-year-old mother?

> **The client is 19 years old and a tubal ligation would not be an option because it is considered a permanent form of sterilization. Most state Medicaid plans will not cover this expense unless the client is older.**

 NCLEX® Connection: Health Promotion and Maintenance, Family Planning.

2. A nurse is instructing a client who has been prescribed oral contraceptives about danger signs. The nurse evaluates that the client understands the teaching regarding side effects when she states the need to report

> A. reduced menstrual flow or amenorrhea.
>
> B. weight gain or breast tenderness.
>
> **C. chest pain or shortness of breath.**
>
> D. mild hypertension or headaches.

> **Chest pain or shortness of breath may be indicative of a pulmonary embolus or myocardial infarction. Options A, B, and D are all common side effects of oral contraceptives that usually subside after a few months of use or can be alleviated by switching to an alternative brand.**

 NCLEX® Connection: Health Promotion and Maintenance, Family Planning.

3. A nurse in an obstetrical clinic is providing education about contraception to a 21-year-old client. Which of the following statements by the client requesting information regarding an IUD indicates a need for additional teaching?

> A. "An IUD may increase my risk for an ectopic pregnancy."
>
> B. "I will wait until I have a child before I can have an IUD."
>
> C. "I might have irregular bleeding after I get an IUD."
>
> **D. "A change in the string length of my IUD is expected."**

> **Any change in the length of the string of the IUD must be reported to the primary care provider. Clients must have at least one child to be a candidate for an IUD. An IUD may cause irregular vaginal bleeding and may increase the risk for an ectopic pregnancy.**

 NCLEX® Connection: Health Promotion and Maintenance, Family Planning.

4. Which contraceptive method has the potential to decrease a client's bone mineral density?

   Depo Provera

   Depo Provera has the potential for causing decreased bone density in clients. It is important to educate the client regarding dietary measures, such as adding calcium and vitamin D to her diet to decrease the likelihood of this occurring.

 NCLEX® Connection: Health Promotion and Maintenance, Family Planning.

5. Which of the following should the nurse include when teaching a client about the potential disadvantages of the minipill? (Select all that apply).

	Amenorrhea
X	**Irregular vaginal bleeding**
X	**Increased appetite**
X	**Lowered libido**
X	**Ovarian cysts**

   The nurse should educate the client regarding potential disadvantages of using the minipill. These include irregular vaginal bleeding, decreased libido, increased appetite, and increased occurrence of ovarian cysts. Amenorrhea is not a disadvantage of the minipill.

 NCLEX® Connection: Health Promotion and Maintenance, Family Planning.

UNIT 1	ANTEPARTUM NURSING CARE
Section	Human Reproduction
Chapter 2	Infertility

Overview

- Infertility is defined as an inability to conceive despite engaging in unprotected sexual intercourse for a period of at least 12 months.

- Common factors associated with infertility may include decreased sperm production, endometriosis, ovulation disorders, and tubal occlusions.

- Partners who experience infertility may experience stress related to:

  ○ Physical inability to conceive.

  ○ Expense.

  ○ Impact on the couple's relationship.

  ○ Lack of family support.

- Infertility procedures, assessments, and genetic counseling may be performed.

Infertility Assessments

- Age – older than 35 years of age may affect fertility.

- Duration of infertility – more than 1 year of coitus without contraceptives.

- Medical history – atypical secondary sexual characteristic such as abnormal body fat distribution or hair growth, which is indicative of an endocrine disorder.

- Surgical history – particularly, pelvic and abdominal procedures.

- Obstetric history – past episodes of spontaneous abortions.

- Gynecologic history – abnormal uterine contours or any history of disorders that may contribute to the formation of scar tissue that can cause blockage of ovum or sperm.

- Sexual history – intercourse frequency, number of partners across the lifespan, and any history of STDs.

- Occupational/environmental exposure risk assessment – exposure to hazardous teratogenic materials in the home or at a place of employment.

- Weight – women who are overweight or underweight.

Infertility Procedures

- Semen collection – a procedure in which semen is collected from the man in a sterile collection device and evaluated and analyzed. In 40% of couples who are infertile, inability to conceive is due to male infertility. Therefore, this infertility test is a preferred starting point in evaluating a couple. It costs less and is less invasive compared to female infertility testing. More than one sample may need to be provided.

- Pelvic examination – assesses for uterine or vaginal anomalies. The nurse should position a client on the exam table and have equipment and supplies prepared for the primary care provider.

- Ultrasonography – a transvaginal or abdominal ultrasound procedure performed to visualize female reproductive organs.

- Hysterosalpingography – radiological procedure that is outpatient where dye is used to assess the patency of the fallopian tubes. The nurse should obtain the client's history of allergies to iodine and seafood.

- Hysteroscopy – a radiographic procedure where the uterus is examined for signs of defect, distortion, or scar tissue that may impair successful impregnation.

- Laparoscopy – a procedure where gas insufflation is used to observe internal organs. This procedure may cause postprocedural pain. General anesthesia is required for this procedure.

Nursing Interventions for Infertility

- Encourage couples to express and discuss their feelings.

- Monitor for side effects associated with medications to treat female and male infertility.

- Advise that the use of medications to treat female infertility may increase the risk of multiple births by more than 25%.

- Provide information regarding assisted reproductive therapies (in vitro fertilization and embryo transfer, intrafallopian gamete transfer, surrogate parenting, and reproductive alternatives such as adoption).

- Make referrals to support groups.

Genetic Counseling

- Genetic counseling may be recommended by the primary care provider if there is a family history of birth defects. The age of the mother may also play a role in this decision: a maternal age less than 16 years old or older than 35 years being a risk factor.

- Identify clients who are in need of genetic counseling. For example, a client who has either a sickle cell trait or sickle cell anemia, or a client older than 35. Make referrals to genetic specialists as necessary.

- Prenatal assessment of genetic disorders (percutaneous umbilical blood sampling, chorionic villus sampling, and amniocentesis) can pose potential risks to the fetus.

- Provide and clarify information pertaining to the risk of or the occurrence of genetic disorders within a family preceding, during, and following a genetic counseling session.

Nursing Interventions for Genetic Counseling

- Assist in the construction of family medical histories of several generations.

- Provide emotional support. Client responses vary and include denial, anger, grief, guilt, and self blame.

- Make referrals to support groups and provide follow up.

CHAPTER 2: INFERTILITY

 Application Exercises

1. A 40-year-old woman who is pregnant for the third time is concerned about the possibility of having a newborn born with Down syndrome. What are the advantages of genetic counseling for this client?

2. A couple arrives at the clinic to discuss how they will begin their infertility assessment. Which of the following statements made by the nurse gives an appropriate understanding of the infertility assessment process?

   A. "Infertility assessments are very expensive and your insurance may not cover the cost."

   B. "It is usually the woman who is 'having trouble,' so the man doesn't have to be involved."

   C. "The man is the easiest to assess and the primary care provider will usually begin there."

   D. "Think about adopting first because there are many babies that need good homes."

3. A nurse in an infertility clinic is providing care to a couple who has been unable to conceive for 18 months. Discuss the assessment questions that the nurse should explore with the couple?

CHAPTER 2: INFERTILITY

 Application Exercises Answer Key

1. A 40-year-old woman who is pregnant for the third time is concerned about the possibility of having a newborn born with Down syndrome. What are the advantages of genetic counseling for this client?

> **A specialist will be available to discuss the concerns of the client. Arrangements can be made to follow up with testing to determine if the client has genetic issues. The client should be informed that the testing requires a chorionic villus sampling or an amniocentesis to make a definite diagnosis. These tests could potentially pose a risk to the fetus.**

NCLEX® Connection: Health Promotion and Maintenance, Family Planning

2. A couple arrives at the clinic to discuss how they will begin their infertility assessment. Which of the following statements made by the nurse gives an appropriate understanding of the infertility assessment process?

   A. "Infertility assessments are very expensive and your insurance may not cover the cost."

   B. "It is usually the woman who is 'having trouble,' so the man doesn't have to be involved."

   C. "The man is the easiest to assess and the primary care provider will usually begin there."

   D. "Think about adopting first because there are many babies that need good homes."

Option C is correct since assessment of the male involves a noninvasive specimen exam. Option A is incorrect because although an infertility assessment can be very expensive, it is inappropriate to say this at this time because this is the couple's initial visit. Option B is incorrect because it is almost evenly divided as to which partner the infertility issue may rest with. However, conceiving a child is a partnership, and both partners should support one another. Option D is incorrect. Adoption may be an option for this couple after they have investigated having their own biological child.

NCLEX® Connection: Reduction of Risk Potential, Diagnostic Tests

3. A nurse in an infertility clinic is providing care to a couple who has been unable to conceive for 18 months. Discuss the assessment questions that the nurse should explore with the couple?

- Age – How old are you?

- Duration of infertility – How long have you been trying to conceive?

- Medical history – Explore medical history of both partners.

- Surgical history – Have you had any pelvic and abdominal surgeries?

- Obstetric history – Have you had any spontaneous abortions?

- Gynecologic history – Question the client about gynecological history and any abnormal findings.

- Sexual history – What is the frequency of your intercourse? How many sexual partners have you had? Have you ever had a history of sexually transmitted infections?

- Occupational/environmental exposure risk assessment – Have you been exposed to hazardous teratogenic materials in the home or at place of employment?

Ⓝ NCLEX® Connection: Health Promotion and Maintenance, Family Planning

UNIT 1	ANTEPARTUM NURSING CARE
Section	Low-Risk, Uncomplicated Pregnancy: Changes During Pregnancy
Chapter 3	Normal Physiological Changes During Pregnancy

Overview

- Recognizing changes during pregnancy is helpful for both a client and a nurse. The nurse and primary care provider will assess these findings during the client's initial prenatal visit.

- Signs of pregnancy are classified into three groups.

  - Presumptive

  - Probable

  - Positive

- Calculating delivery date, number of pregnancies, and evaluating the physiological status of a client who is pregnant will be explored.

Signs of Pregnancy

- Presumptive signs – changes that are experienced by the woman that make her think that she may be pregnant. These changes may be subjective symptoms or objective signs. Signs may also be a result of physiological factors other than pregnancy (peristalsis, pelvic congestion, and tumors).

  - Amenorrhea

  - Fatigue

  - Nausea and vomiting

  - Urinary frequency

  - Breast changes – Darkened areola, enlarged Montgomery's tubules

  - Quickening – slight fluttering movements of the fetus felt by a woman, usually between 16 to 20 weeks of gestation.

  - Uterine enlargement

  - Linea nigra

  - Chloasma (mask of pregnancy)

  - Striae gravidarum

- Probable signs – changes that make the examiner suspect a woman is pregnant (primarily related to physical changes of the uterus). Signs can be caused by physiological factors other than pregnancy (peristalsis, pelvic congestion, tumors).

  o Abdominal enlargement related to changes in uterine size, shape, and position

  o Cervical changes

  o Hegar's sign – softening and compressibility of lower uterus

  o Chadwick's sign – deepened violet-bluish color of vaginal mucosa secondary to increased vascularity of the area

  o Goodell's sign – softening of cervical tip

  o Ballottement – rebound of unengaged fetus

  o Braxton Hicks contractions – false contractions, painless, irregular, and usually relieved by walking

  o Positive pregnancy test

  o Fetal outline felt by examiner

- Positive signs – signs that can only be explained by pregnancy.

  o Fetal heart sounds

  o Visualization of fetus by ultrasound

  o Fetal movement palpated by an experienced examiner

Verifying Possible Pregnancy Using Serum and Urine Pregnancy Testing

- Serum and urine tests provide an accurate assessment for the presence of human chorionic gonadotropin (hCG). hCG production can start as early as the day of implantation and can be detected as early as 7 to 10 days after conception.

- Production of hCG begins with implantation, peaks at about 60 to 70 days of gestation, and then declines until around 80 days of pregnancy, when it begins to gradually increase until term.

- Higher levels of hCG can indicate multifetal pregnancy, ectopic pregnancy, hydatidiform mole (gestational trophoblastic disease), or a genetic abnormality such as Down syndrome. Lower blood levels of hCG may suggest a miscarriage.

- Some medications (anticonvulsants, diuretics, tranquilizers) can cause false-positive or false-negative pregnancy results.

- Urine samples should be first-voided morning specimens.

Calculating Delivery Date and Determining Number of Pregnancies for Pregnant Client

- Nägele's rule – take the first day of the woman's last menstrual cycle, subtract 3 months, and then add 7 days and 1 year.

  o Remember how many days there are in each particular month when adding 7 days.

- McDonald's method – measure uterine fundal height in centimeters from the symphysis pubis to the top of the uterine fundus (between 18 to 30 weeks of gestation). The calculations are as follows:

  ○ Estimate gestational age to be equal to that of the fundal height.

- Gravidity – number of pregnancies.

  ○ Nulligravida – a woman who has never been pregnant.

  ○ Primigravida – a woman in her first pregnancy.

  ○ Multigravida – a woman who has had two or more pregnancies.

  ○ Parity – number of pregnancies in which the fetus or fetuses reach viability (approximately 20 to 24 weeks or fetal weight of more than 500 g [2 lb]) regardless of whether the fetus is born alive or not.

    ▪ Nullipara – no pregnancy beyond the stage of viability.

    ▪ Primipara – has completed one pregnancy to stage of viability.

    ▪ Multipara – has completed two or more pregnancies to stage of viability.

- GTPAL acronym

  ○ Gravidity

  ○ Term births (38 weeks or more)

  ○ Preterm births (from viability up to 37 weeks)

  ○ Abortions/miscarriages (prior to viability)

  ○ Living children

Physiological Status of Pregnant Client

- Reproductive – the uterus will increase in size and change shape and position. Ovulation and menses cease during pregnancy.

- Cardiovascular – cardiac output and blood volume increase (45% to 50% at term) to meet the greater metabolic needs. Heart rate increases during pregnancy.

- Respiratory – maternal oxygen needs increase. During the last trimester, the size of the chest may enlarge, allowing for lung expansion, as the uterus pushes upward. Increased respiratory rate and decreased total lung capacity.

- Musculoskeletal – body alterations and weight increase necessitate an adjustment in posture. Pelvic joints relax.

- Gastrointestinal – nausea and vomiting may occur due to hormonal changes and/or an increase of pressure within the abdominal cavity as the pregnant client's stomach and intestines are displaced within the abdomen. Constipation may occur due to increased transit time of food through the gastrointestinal system and thus, increased water absorption.

- Renal – filtration rate increases during pregnancy secondary to the influence of pregnancy hormones and an increase in blood volume and metabolic demands. The amount of urine produced remains the same. Urinary frequency is common during pregnancy.

- Endocrine – the placenta becomes an endocrine organ that produces large amounts of hCG, progesterone, estrogen, human placental lactogen, and prostaglandins. Hormones are very active during pregnancy and function to maintain pregnancy and prepare the body for delivery.

- Body Image Changes

  o Due to the physical changes as well as the psychological changes that occur during pregnancy, the pregnant woman requires support from her primary care provider and family members.

  o In the first trimester of pregnancy, physiological changes are not very obvious. Many women look forward to the changes so that pregnancy will be more noticeable.

  o During the second trimester there are rapid physical changes. The most obvious is the enlargement of the abdomen and breasts. Skin changes also occur, such as stretch marks and hyperpigmentation of the face (chloasma). The physical changes can also affect a woman's mobility. She may find herself losing her balance and feeling back or leg discomfort and fatigue. All of these factors may lead to a negative body image. The client may make statements of resentment toward the pregnancy and express anxiousness for the pregnancy to be over soon.

- Expected Vital Signs

  o Blood pressure measurements are within the prepregnancy range during the first trimester.

  o Blood pressure decreases 5 to 10 mm Hg for both the diastolic and the systolic during the second trimester.

  o Blood pressure should return to the prepregnancy baseline range after approximately 20 weeks of gestation.

  o Position of the pregnant woman may also affect her blood pressure. In the supine position, blood pressure may appear to be lower due to the weight and pressure of the gravid uterus on the vena cava, which decreases venous blood flow to the heart. Maternal hypotension and fetal hypoxia may occur, which is referred to as supine hypotensive syndrome or supine vena cava syndrome. Signs and symptoms include dizziness, lightheadedness, and pale, clammy skin. Encourage the client to engage in maternal positioning on the left-lateral side, semi-Fowler's position, or, if supine, with a wedge placed under one hip to alleviate pressure to the vena cava.

  o Pulse increases 10 to 15/min around 20 weeks of gestation and remains elevated throughout the remainder of the pregnancy.

  o Respirations increase by 1 to 2/min. Respiratory changes in pregnancy are attributed to the elevation of the diaphragm by as much as 4 cm as well as changes to the chest wall to facilitate increased maternal oxygen demands. Some shortness of breath may be noted.

- Expected Physical Assessment Findings

  - Fetal heart tones are heard at a normal baseline rate of 110 to 160/min with reassuring FHR accelerations noted, which indicates an intact fetal CNS.

  - The client's heart will change in size and shape with resulting cardiac hypertrophy to accommodate increased blood volume and increased cardiac output. Heart sounds during pregnancy also change to accommodate the increase in blood volume with a more distinguishable splitting of S_1 and S_2, with S_3 more easily heard following 20 weeks of gestation. Murmurs may also be auscultated. Heart size and shape will return to normal shortly after delivery.

  - Uterine size changes from a uterine weight of 50 to 1,000 g (0.1 to 3 lb). By 36 weeks of gestation, the top of the uterus and the fundus, will reach the xiphoid process. This may cause the pregnant woman to experience shortness of breath as the uterus pushes against the diaphragm.

  - Cervical changes are obvious because of the color change. The cervix becomes a purplish-blue color that extends into the vagina and labia. This is known as Chadwick's sign. The cervix markedly softens in consistency, which is referred to as Goodell's sign.

  - Breast changes occur due to hormones secreted during pregnancy. The breasts increase in size and the areolas take on a darkened pigmentation.

  - Skin changes

    - Chloasma – mask of pregnancy (pigmentation increases on the face)

    - Linea nigra – dark line of pigmentation from the umbilicus extending to the pubic area

    - Striae gravidarum – stretch marks most notably found on the abdomen and thighs

Nursing Interventions for the Pregnant Client

- Offer acknowledgement and encouragement of the client in the sharing of feelings regarding the pregnancy by providing an atmosphere free of judgment.

- Discuss with the client the expected physiological changes and a possible timeline for a return to the prepregnant state.

- Assist the client in setting goals for the postpartum period in regard to self-care and newborn care.

- Refer the client to counseling if the body image concerns begin to have a negative impact on the pregnancy.

- Provide education about the expected physiological and psychosocial changes. Common discomforts of pregnancy and ways to resolve those discomforts can be reviewed during prenatal visits.

- The client should be encouraged to keep all follow-up appointments and to contact the primary care provider immediately if there is any bleeding, leakage of fluid, or contractions at any time during the pregnancy.

CHAPTER 3: NORMAL PHYSIOLOGICAL CHANGES DURING PREGNANCY

Ⓐ Application Exercises

Scenario: A nurse in an antepartum clinic is caring for a client that presents for a pregnancy test. She states that her last menstrual period was on 12-01-09. The result of the test is positive. She has been pregnant two other times, delivered once at term, has a child that is 2 years old, and has had one miscarriage at 8 weeks.

1. Which of the following is the client's expected date of delivery or confinement?

   A. September 8, 2010

   B. September 11, 2010

   C. October 8, 2010

   D. October 8, 2010

2. Identify the client's obstetrical history using the GTPAL method.

3. A nurse understands that a client is demonstrating probable signs of pregnancy when which of the following signs are observed by a primary care provider? (Select all that apply.)

   _____ Chloasma

   _____ Goodell's sign

   _____ Ballottement

   _____ Chadwick's sign

   _____ Quickening

4. The following are probable and presumptive signs of pregnancy. Match each sign nomenclature with its correct explanation.

   _____ Hegar's sign   A. Mask of pregnancy (pigmentation increases on the face)

   _____ Chadwick's sign   B. Slight fluttering movements of fetus felt by a woman

   _____ Goodell's sign   C. Deepened violet-bluish color of vaginal mucosa secondary to increased vascularity of the area.

   _____ Ballottement   D. Dark line of pigmentation from the umbilicus to the pubic area

   _____ Braxton Hicks   E. Softening and compressibility of the lower uterus

   _____ Quickening   F. Painless, irregular contractions that are usually relieved with walking

   _____ Chloasma   G. Softening of cervical tip

   _____ Linea nigra   H. Stretch marks most often found on the abdomen and thighs

   _____ Striae gravidarum   I. Rebound of unengaged fetus

CHAPTER 3: NORMAL PHYSIOLOGICAL CHANGES DURING PREGNANCY

 Application Exercises Answer Key

Scenario: A nurse in an antepartum clinic is caring for a client that presents for a pregnancy test. She states that her last menstrual period was on 12-01-09. The result of the test is positive. She has been pregnant two other times, delivered once at term, has a child that is 2 years old, and has had one miscarriage at 8 weeks.

1. Which of the following is the client's expected date of delivery or confinement?

   A. September 8, 2010

   B. September 11, 2010

   C. October 8, 2010

   D. October 8, 2010

   12-01-09 minus 3 months, plus 7 days and 1 year = EDC of September 8, 2010.

    NCLEX® Connection: Health Promotion and Maintenance, Ante/Intra/Postpartum and Newborn Care

2. Identify the client's obstetrical history using the GTPAL method.

   G 3 T 1 P 0 A 1 L 1

   G 3 – the client has been pregnant twice and is currently pregnant; T 1 – the client delivered one newborn at term; P 0 – the client has had no preterm deliveries; A 1 – the client has had one miscarriage; L 1 – the client has one living child.

    NCLEX® Connection: Health Promotion and Maintenance, Ante/Intra/Postpartum and Newborn Care

3. A nurse understands that a client is demonstrating probable signs of pregnancy when which of the following signs are observed by a primary care provider? (Select all that apply.)

   _____ A. Chloasma

   __X__ **B. Goodell's sign**

   __X__ **C. Ballottement**

   __X__ **D. Chadwick's sign**

   _____ E. Quickening

   Goodell's sign, ballottement and Chadwick's sign are probable signs of pregnancy.

    NCLEX® Connection: Health Promotion and Maintenance, Ante/Intra/Postpartum and Newborn Care

4. The following are probable and presumptive signs of pregnancy. Match each sign nomenclature with its correct explanation.

__E__	Hegar's sign	A. Mask of pregnancy (pigmentation increases on the face)
__C__	Chadwick's sign	B. Slight fluttering movements of fetus felt by a woman
__G__	Goodell's sign	C. Deepened violet-bluish color of vaginal mucosa secondary to increased vascularity of the area.
__I__	Ballottement	D. Dark line of pigmentation from the umbilicus to the pubic area
__F__	Braxton Hicks	E. Softening and compressibility of the lower uterus
__B__	Quickening	F. Painless, irregular contractions that are usually relieved with walking
__A__	Chloasma	G. Softening of cervical tip
__D__	Linea nigra	H. Stretch marks most often found on the abdomen and thighs
__H__	Striae gravidarum	I. Rebound of unengaged fetus

Ⓝ NCLEX® Connection: Health Promotion and Maintenance, Ante/Intra/Postpartum and Newborn Care

UNIT 1	ANTEPARTUM NURSING CARE
Section	Low-Risk, Uncomplicated Pregnancy: Changes During Pregnancy
Chapter 4	Prenatal Care

Overview

- Prenatal care involves nursing assessments and client education for expectant mothers. When providing prenatal care, nurses must take into account cultural considerations.

- Prenatal education encompasses a great deal of information provided to a client who is pregnant. Major areas of focus include assisting the client in self-care of the discomforts of pregnancy, promoting a safe outcome to pregnancy, and fostering positive feelings by the pregnant woman and her family regarding the childbearing experience.

- Prenatal care dramatically reduces infant and maternal morbidity and mortality rates by early detection and treatment of potential problems. A majority of birth defects occur between 2 and 8 weeks of gestation.

Nursing Assessments

- Nurses play an integral role in assessing a client's current knowledge, previous pregnancies, and birthing experiences.

- Nursing assessment in prenatal care includes obtaining information regarding:

  o Reproductive and obstetrical history (contraception use, gynecological diagnoses, and obstetrical difficulties).

  o Medical history, including the woman's immune status (rubella and hepatitis B).

  o Family history, such as genetic disorders.

  o Any recent or current illnesses or infections.

  o Current medications, including substance abuse and alcohol consumption. The nurse should display a nonjudgmental, matter-of-fact demeanor when interviewing a client regarding substance abuse and observe for signs and symptoms such as lack of grooming.

  o Psychosocial history (a client's emotional response to pregnancy, adolescent pregnancy, spouse, support system, history of depression, domestic violence issues).

  o Any hazardous environmental exposures; current work conditions.

  o Current exercise and diet habits.

- A nurse should ascertain what a client's goals are for the birthing process. The nurse should discuss various birthing methods, such as Lamaze, and pain control options (epidural, natural childbirth).

- Prenatal care begins with an initial assessment and then continues throughout pregnancy. In an uneventful pregnancy, prenatal visits are scheduled every month for 7 months, every 2 weeks during the eighth month, and every week during the last month.

  o At the initial prenatal visit:

    ▪ Determine estimated date of delivery based on the last menstrual period. A vaginal ultrasound may be done to establish the estimated date of delivery.

    ▪ Obtain medical and nursing history to include: past medical health, family history, social supports, and review of systems (to determine risk factors) and past obstetrical history.

    ▪ Perform a physical assessment to include a client's baseline weight, vital signs, and pelvic examination. Have the client empty her bladder prior to the exam.

    ▪ Obtain initial laboratory work to induce blood type, Rh factor, HIV status, hepatitis B, venereal disease research laboratory, rubella status, urinalysis, and Papanicolaou test. An indirect Coombs' test will determine if a client is sensitized to Rh-positive blood.

  o Ongoing prenatal visits include:

    ▪ Monitoring weight, blood pressure, and urine for glucose, protein, and leukocytes.

    ▪ Monitor a client for the presence of edema.

    ▪ Monitoring fetal development.

      ▫ FHR can be heard by Doppler at 10 to 12 weeks of gestation or heard with an ultrasound stethoscope at 16 to 20 weeks of gestation. Listen at the midline, right above the symphysis pubis, by holding the stethoscope firmly on the abdomen.

      ▫ Start measuring fundal height after 12 weeks of gestation. Between 18 and 30 weeks of gestation, the fundal height measured in centimeters should equal the week of gestation. Have the client empty her bladder and measure from the level of the symphysis pubis to the upper border of the fundus.

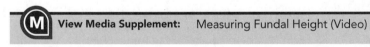

View Media Supplement: Measuring Fundal Height (Video)

      ▫ Begin assessing for fetal movement between 16 and 20 weeks of gestation.

    ▪ Providing education for self-care to include ways to manage common discomforts and concerns of pregnancy (nausea and vomiting, fatigue, backache, varicosities, heartburn, activity, sexuality).

ROUTINE LABORATORY TESTS IN PRENATAL CARE	
LABORATORY TEST	PURPOSE
Blood type, Rh-factor, and presence of irregular antibodies	Determines the risk for maternal-fetal blood incompatibility (erythroblastosis fetalis) or neonatal hyperbilirubinemia. For clients who are Rh-negative and not sensitized, the indirect Coombs' test will be repeated between 24 to 28 weeks of gestation.
CBC with differential, Hgb, and Hct	Detects infection and anemia.
Hgb electrophoresis	Identifies hemoglobinopathies (sickle cell anemia and thalassemia).
Urinalysis with microscopic examination of pH, specific gravity, color, sediment, protein, glucose, albumin, RBCs, WBCs, casts, acetone, and human chorionic gonadotropin	Identifies diabetes mellitus, gestational hypertension, renal disease, and infection.
One-hour glucose tolerance (Oral ingestion or IV administration of concentrated glucose with venous sample taken 1 hr later [fasting not necessary])	Identifies hyperglycemia; done at initial visit for at-risk clients, and at 24 to 28 weeks of gestation for all pregnant women (> 140 mg/dL requires follow up).
Three-hour glucose tolerance (Fasting overnight prior to oral ingestion or IV administration of concentrated glucose with a venous sample taken 1, 2, and 3 hr later)	Used in clients with elevated 1-hr glucose test as a screening tool for diabetes mellitus. A diagnosis of gestational diabetes requires two elevated blood-glucose readings.
Papanicolaou (PAP) test	Screens for cervical cancer, herpes simplex type 2, and/or human papillomavirus.
Vaginal/cervical culture	Detects streptococcus ß-hemolytic, Group B (routinely obtained at 35 to 37 weeks of gestation), bacterial vaginosis, or sexually transmitted infections (gonorrhea and Chlamydia).
Rubella titer	Determines immunity to rubella.
PPD (tuberculosis screening), chest screening after 20 weeks of gestation with positive purified protein derivative	Identifies exposure to tuberculosis.
Hepatitis B screen	Identifies carriers of hepatitis B.
Venereal disease research laboratory	Syphilis screening mandated by law.
HIV	Detects HIV infection (The Centers for Disease Control and Prevention and The American Congress of Obstetricians and Gynecologists recommends testing all clients who are pregnant unless the client refuses testing).

ROUTINE LABORATORY TESTS IN PRENATAL CARE	
LABORATORY TEST	PURPOSE
Toxoplasmosis, other infections, rubella, cytomegalovirus, and herpes virus (TORCH) screening when indicated	Screening for a group of infections capable of crossing the placenta and adversely affecting fetal development.
Maternal serum alpha-fetoprotein (MSAFP)	Screening occurs between 15 to 22 weeks of gestation. Used to rule out Down syndrome (low level) and neural tube defects (high level). The provider may decide to use a more reliable indicator and opt for the Quad screening instead of the MSAFP at 16 to 18 weeks of gestation. This includes AFP, inhibin-A, a combination analysis of human chorionic gonadotropin, and estriol.

- o Perform or assist with Leopold maneuvers to palpate presentation and position of the fetus.

- o Assist the primary care provider with the pelvic examination. This examination is performed to determine the status of a client's reproductive organs and birth canal. Pelvic measurements determine whether the pelvis will allow for the passage of the fetus at delivery.

  - ■ The nurse should encourage the client to empty her bladder and take deep breaths during the examination to decrease discomfort.

- o Assess for costovertebral angle tenderness, which is indicative of renal infection.

  - ■ Administer $Rh_o(D)$ immune globulin (RhoGAM) IM around 28 weeks of gestation for clients who are Rh-negative.

Client Education

- Components of prenatal education include health promotion, preparation for pregnancy and birth, common discomforts of pregnancy, and danger signs to report.

- Health Promotion

  - o Preconception and prenatal education should stress healthy behaviors that promote the health of the pregnant woman and her fetus.

    - ■ A client should be instructed to avoid all over-the-counter medications, supplements, and prescriptive medications unless the obstetrician who is supervising her care has knowledge of this practice.

    - ■ Alcohol (birth defects) and tobacco (low birth weight) are contraindicated during pregnancy.

    - ■ Substance abuse of any kind is to be avoided during pregnancy and during lactation.

- ○ The nurse should educate a client about the following:
  - Encourage the client to receive a flu vaccine during the fall months.
  - Encourage smoking cessation.
  - Treat current infections.
  - Obtain genetic testing and provide counseling.
  - Ascertain maternal exposure to hazardous materials.
- ○ Exercise during pregnancy yields positive benefits and should consist of 30 min of moderate exercise (walking or swimming) daily if not medically or obstetrically contraindicated.
  - Avoid the use of hot tubs or saunas.
  - Consume at least 2 to 3 L of water each day from food and beverage sources.
- Preparation for Pregnancy and Birth
  - ○ Nurses should provide anticipatory teaching to the pregnant client and her family about:
    - Physical and emotional changes during pregnancy and interventions that can be implemented to provide relief.
    - Danger signs and symptoms to report to the primary care provider.
    - Various birthing options available to enhance the birthing process.
  - ○ Maternal adaptation to pregnancy and the attainment of the maternal role – whereby the idea of pregnancy is accepted and assimilated into the client's way of life – includes hormonal and psychological aspects.
    - Emotional lability is experienced by many women with unpredictable mood changes and increased irritability, tearfulness, and anger alternating with feelings of joy and cheerfulness. This all may result from profound hormonal changes.
    - A feeling of ambivalence about the pregnancy, which is a normal response, may occur early in the pregnancy resolving before the third trimester. It consists of conflicting feelings (joy, pleasure, sorrow, hostility) about the pregnancy. These feelings can occur simultaneously whether the pregnancy was planned or not.
  - ○ The nurse should anticipate prenatal education topics that should be reviewed with a client based on her current knowledge and previous pregnancy and birth experiences. The client's readiness to learn is enhanced when the nurse provides teaching during the appropriate trimester based on learning needs. Using a variety of educational methods, such as pamphlets and videos, and having the client verbalize and demonstrate learned topics will ensure that learning has taken place.
    - First Trimester
      - □ Physical and psychosocial changes
      - □ Common discomforts of pregnancy and measures to provide relief

- Lifestyle: exercise/stress/nutrition, sex, dental care, over-the-counter and prescription medications, tobacco, alcohol, substance abuse (discuss strategies to decrease or discontinue use), and STDs (encourage safe sexual practices)
- Possible complications and signs to report
- Fetal growth and development
- Prenatal exercise
- Expected laboratory testing

- **Second Trimester**
  - Benefits of breastfeeding.
  - Common discomforts and relief measures
  - Lifestyle: sex and pregnancy, rest and relaxation, posture, body mechanics, clothing, seat-belt safety, and travel
  - Fetal movement
  - Complications (preterm labor, gestational hypertension, gestational diabetes mellitus, premature rupture of membranes)
  - Childbirth preparation

- **Third Trimester**
  - Childbirth preparations
    - Childbirth classes or birth plan.
    - Breathing and relaxation techniques (deep cleansing breaths at one-half the usual respiratory rate during contractions can promote relaxation of the abdominal muscles, which lessens the discomfort of uterine contractions)
    - Discussion regarding pain management during labor and birth (natural childbirth, epidural)
    - Signs and symptoms of preterm labor and labor
    - Labor process
    - Infant care
    - Postpartum care
  - Fetal movement/kick counts to ascertain fetal well-being. A client should be instructed to count and record fetal movements or kicks daily.
    - It is recommended that mothers count fetal activity 2 or 3 times a day for 60 min each time. Fetal movements of less than 3 in/hr or movements that cease entirely for 12 hr indicate a need for further evaluation.
  - Diagnostic testing for fetal well-being (nonstress test, biophysical profile, ultrasound, and contraction stress test).

- Common Discomforts of Pregnancy

  - Nausea and vomiting may occur during the first trimester. The client should eat crackers or dry toast $1/_2$ to 1 hr before rising in the morning to relieve discomfort. Instruct the client to avoid having an empty stomach and ingesting spicy, greasy, or gas-forming foods. Encourage the client to drink fluids between meals.

  - Breast tenderness may occur during the first trimester. The client should wear a bra that provides adequate support.

  - Urinary frequency may occur during the first and third trimesters. The client should empty her bladder frequently, decrease fluid intake before bedtime, and use perineal pads. The client should be taught how to perform Kegel exercises (alternate tightening and relaxation of pubococcygeal muscles) to reduce stress incontinence (leakage of urine with coughing and sneezing).

  - Urinary tract infections (UTI) are common during pregnancy because of renal changes and the vaginal flora becoming more alkaline.

    - UTI risks can be decreased by encouraging the client to wipe the perineal area from front to back after voiding; avoiding bubble baths; wearing cotton underpants; avoiding tight-fitting pants; and consuming plenty of water (8 glasses per day).

    - The client should urinate before and after intercourse to flush bacteria from the urethra that can be introduced during intercourse.

    - Advise the client to urinate as soon as the urge occurs because retaining urine provides an environment for bacterial multiplication.

    - Advise the client to notify her primary care provider if her urine is malodorous or contains blood or pus.

  - Fatigue may occur during the first and third trimesters. The client should be encouraged to engage in frequent rest periods.

  - Heartburn may occur during the second and third trimesters due to the stomach being displaced by the enlarging uterus and a slowing of the gastrointestinal tract motility and digestion brought about by increased progesterone levels. The client should eat small frequent meals, not allow the stomach to get too empty or too full, sit up for 30 min after meals, and check with her primary care provider prior to using any over-the-counter antacids.

  - Constipation may occur during the second and third trimesters. The client should be encouraged to drink plenty of fluids, eat a diet high in fiber, and exercise regularly.

  - Hemorrhoids may occur during the second and third trimesters. A warm sitz bath, witch hazel pads, and topical ointments applied to the area will help relieve discomfort.

  - Backaches are common during the second and third trimesters. The client should be encouraged to exercise regularly, perform pelvic tilt exercises (alternately arching and straightening the back), use proper body mechanics using the legs to lift rather than the back, and use the side-lying position.

○ Shortness of breath and dyspnea may occur because the diaphragm is elevated about 4 cm by the enlarged uterus. This limits diaphragm expansion on inspiration. The client should maintain good posture, sleep with extra pillows, and contact her primary care provider if symptoms worsen.

○ Leg cramps during the third trimester may occur due to the compression of lower extremity nerves and blood vessels by the enlarging uterus. This can result in poor peripheral circulation as well as an imbalance in the calcium/phosphorus ratio. Homans' sign should be checked and if it is negative, the client should extend the affected leg, keeping the knee straight and dorsiflexing the foot (toes toward head). Massaging and applying heat over the affected muscle or a foot massage while the leg is extended can help relieve cramping. The client should notify her primary care provider if frequent cramping occurs.

○ Varicose veins and lower extremity edema can occur during the second and third trimesters. The client should rest with her legs elevated, avoid constricting clothing, wear support hose, avoid sitting or standing in one position for extended periods of time, and should not sit with her legs crossed at the knees. She should sleep in the left-lateral position and exercise moderately with frequent walking to stimulate venous return.

○ Gingivitis, nasal stuffiness, and epistaxis (nosebleed) can occur as a result of elevated estrogen levels causing an increased vascularity and proliferation of connective tissue. The client should gently brush her teeth, observe good dental hygiene, use a humidifier, and use normal saline nose drops or spray.

○ Braxton Hicks contractions, which occur from the first trimester onward, may increase in intensity and frequency during the third trimester. Inform the client that a change of position and walking should cause contractions to subside. If contractions increase in intensity and frequency (true contractions) with regularity, the client should notify her primary care provider.

○ Supine hypotension occurs when a woman lies on her back and the weight of the gravid uterus compresses her ascending vena cava. This reduces blood supply to the fetus. The client may experience feelings of lightheadedness and faintness. Teach the client to lie in a side-lying or semi-sitting position with her knees slightly flexed.

● Danger Signs During Pregnancy

○ The following indicate potential dangerous situations that should be reported to the primary care provider immediately if experienced by a client.

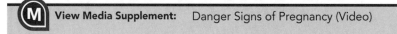

View Media Supplement: Danger Signs of Pregnancy (Video)

■ Gush of fluid from the vagina (rupture of amniotic fluid) prior to 37 weeks of gestation

■ Vaginal bleeding (placental problems such as abruption or previa)

■ Abdominal pain (premature labor, abruptio placenta, or ectopic pregnancy)

■ Changes in fetal activity (decreased fetal movement may indicate fetal distress)

- Persistent vomiting (hyperemesis gravidarum)

- Severe headaches (pregnancy-induced hypertension)

- Elevated temperature (infection)

- Dysuria (urinary tract infection)

- Blurred vision (pregnancy-induced hypertension)

- Edema of face and hands (pregnancy-induced hypertension)

- Epigastric pain (pregnancy-induced hypertension)

- Concurrent occurrence of flushed dry skin, fruity breath, rapid breathing, increased thirst and urination, and headache (hyperglycemia)

- Concurrent occurrence of clammy pale skin, weakness, tremors, irritability, and lightheadedness (hypoglycemia)

○ During the client's second trimester, the nurse should begin to present and review various options of birthing methods, assist the client in making an informed decision regarding her birth plan, and encourage her to schedule childbirth preparation classes. Exploration may continue into the third trimester.

○ Signs of preterm labor should be reviewed with the client at each pregnant visit.

○ Birth plans can be verbal or written agreements that describe what the pregnant woman wishes to occur during labor and delivery.

○ Common birthing methods prepare a pregnant woman for the labor and delivery process and may decrease her anxiety. The couple will also receive education about maternal relaxation techniques and partner support during the birthing process.

- Dick-Read method – refers to "childbirth without fear." Uses controlled breathing and conscious and progressive relaxation of different muscle groups throughout the entire body. This method instructs a woman to relax completely between contractions and keep all muscles except the uterus relaxed during contractions.

- Lamaze – the mission of Lamaze International is to promote a healthy, natural, and safe approach to pregnancy, childbirth, and early parenting by advocating and working with health care providers, parents, and professional childbirth educators.

- Leboyer – is a method of childbirth that is based on the idea of "birth without violence." Environmental variables are stressed to ease the transition of the fetus from the uterus to the external environment (dim lights, soft voices, warm birthing room). Water births are based on this method.

- Bradley – stresses the partner's involvement as the birthing coach. This method emphasizes increasing self-awareness and teaching the woman to deal with the stress of labor by tuning into her own body. The mother is encouraged to trust her body and use natural breathing, relaxation, nutrition, exercise, and education throughout her pregnancy.

CHAPTER 4: PRENATAL CARE

 Application Exercises

1. A nurse is teaching a group of women who are pregnant about measures to relieve backache during pregnancy. The nurse should teach the women which of the following? (Select all that apply.)

_____ Avoid any lifting.

_____ Perform Kegel exercises twice a day.

_____ Perform the pelvic rock exercise every day.

_____ Use good body mechanics.

_____ Avoid constrictive clothing.

2. A nurse is teaching a group of clients who are pregnant about behaviors to avoid during pregnancy. The nurse determines that a client needs further instruction when the client states,

A. "I can have a drink of wine with dinner."

B. "Smoking is a major cause of low birth weight in babies."

C. "Signs of infection should be reported to my primary care provider."

D. "I should not take over-the-counter medications without checking with my primary care provider first."

3. A client who is at 8 weeks of gestation tells the nurse that she isn't sure she is happy about being pregnant. The nurse should respond to the client by stating,

A. "I will inform the primary care provider that you are having these feelings."

B. "It is normal to have feelings during the first few months of pregnancy."

C. "You should be happy that you are going to bring new life into the world."

D. "I am going to make an appointment with the counselor for you to discuss these thoughts."

4. A client who is pregnant should promptly report which of the following symptoms to the primary care provider?

A. Vaginal bleeding

B. Swelling of the ankles

C. Heartburn after eating

D. Faintness when lying on her back

5. A client who is at 7 weeks of gestation is experiencing nausea and vomiting in the morning. The nurse in the prenatal clinic provides teaching that should include which of the following?

A. Eat crackers or plain toast before getting out of bed.

B. Wake during the night to eat to prevent an empty stomach.

C. Skip breakfast and eat lunch after nausea has subsided.

D. Eat a large supper to prevent an empty stomach in the morning.

CHAPTER 4: PRENATAL CARE

 Application Exercises Answer Key

1. A nurse is teaching a group of women who are pregnant about measures to relieve backache during pregnancy. The nurse should teach the women which of the following? (Select all that apply.)

_____ Avoid any lifting.

_____ Perform Kegel exercises twice a day.

__X__ **Perform the pelvic rock exercise every day.**

__X__ **Use good body mechanics.**

_____ Avoid constrictive clothing.

The pelvic rock or tilt exercises stretch out the muscles of the lower back and help relieve lower back pain. Good body mechanics will help prevent injury to the back that can occur from using incorrect muscles. Lifting can be done, but use the knees to lift rather than the back. Kegel exercises are done to strengthen the perineal muscles. Avoiding constrictive clothing will help prevent vaginitis, heat rash, or varicoses.

 NCLEX® Connection: Health Promotion and Maintenance, Ante/Intra/Postpartum and Newborn Care

2. A nurse is teaching a group of clients who are pregnant about behaviors to avoid during pregnancy. The nurse determines that a client needs further instruction when the client states,

A. "I can have a drink of wine with dinner."

B. "Smoking is a major cause of low birth weight in babies."

C. "Signs of infection should be reported to my primary care provider."

D. "I should not take over-the-counter medications without checking with my primary care provider first."

No alcohol should be consumed during pregnancy. All medications should be approved with the primary care provider. Signs of infection or any concerns should be reported to the primary care provider. Smoking is a major cause of low birth weight infants.

 NCLEX® Connection: Health Promotion and Maintenance, Ante/Intra/Postpartum and Newborn Care

3. A client who is at 8 weeks of gestation tells the nurse that she isn't sure she is happy about being pregnant. The nurse should respond to the client by stating,

    A. "I will inform the primary care provider that you are having these feelings."

    B. "It is normal to have feelings during the first few months of pregnancy."

    C. "You should be happy that you are going to bring new life into the world."

    D. "I am going to make an appointment with the counselor for you to discuss these thoughts."

Ambivalence during the first trimester is a normal response. The client usually overcomes ambivalence before the second trimester. The other responses are nontherapeutic statements.

 NCLEX® Connection: Health Promotion and Maintenance, Developmental Stages and Transitions

4. A client who is pregnant should promptly report which of the following symptoms to the primary care provider?

    A. Vaginal bleeding

    B. Swelling of the ankles

    C. Heartburn after eating

    D. Faintness when lying on back

Vaginal bleeding during pregnancy is always a dangerous sign and the client should notify her primary care provider. Swelling of the ankles is a normal occurrence that can be relieved by the client elevating her lower extremities and not sitting or standing for prolonged periods of time. Heartburn frequently occurs because of the slowed gastrointestinal motility and compression of the stomach by the enlarging uterus. Supine hypotension, which can be experienced by the client as a faintness felt when lying on the back, occurs because of the gravid uterus compressing the ascending vena cava. This compression can be detrimental to the fetus. Supine hypotension is easily rectified by instructing the client to lie on her side or in a semi-sitting position.

 NCLEX® Connection: Health Promotion and Maintenance, Ante/Intra/Postpartum and Newborn Care

5. A client who is at 7 weeks of gestation is experiencing nausea and vomiting in the morning. The nurse in the prenatal clinic provides teaching that should include which of the following?

    A. Eat crackers or plain toast before getting out of bed.

    B. Wake during the night to eat to prevent an empty stomach.

    C. Skip breakfast and eat lunch after nausea has subsided.

    D. Eat a large supper to prevent an empty stomach in the morning.

Nausea and vomiting may occur during the first trimester. The client should eat crackers or dry toast ½ to 1 hr before rising in the morning to relieve discomfort. Instruct the client to avoid an empty stomach, spicy, greasy, or gas-forming foods. Encourage the client to drink fluids between meals.

NCLEX® Connection: Health Promotion and Maintenance, Ante/Intra/Postpartum and Newborn Care

UNIT 1	ANTEPARTUM NURSING CARE
Section	Low-Risk, Uncomplicated Pregnancy: Changes During Pregnancy
Chapter 5	Nutrition During Pregnancy

Overview

- Adequate nutritional intake by a client during pregnancy is essential to promoting fetal and maternal health.

- Recommended weight gain during pregnancy is usually 11.2 to 15.9 kg (25 to 35 lb). The general rule is that clients should gain 1 to 2 kg (3 to 4 lb) during the first trimester and after that, a weight gain of approximately 0.4 kg (1 lb) per week for the last two trimesters.

- It is important for the nurse to evaluate the pregnant client's nutritional choices, possible risk factors, and diet history, and the nurse should also review specific nutritional guidelines for at-risk clients. Assistance should be given to a client to develop a postpartum nutritional plan.

Nursing Assessment and Interventions

- Obtain both subjective and objective dietary information from the client.

  o Journal

  o Daily food sheets

  o Questionnaires

  o Client's weight on first prenatal visit and follow-up visit

  o Laboratory reports such as Hgb and iron levels

- Encourage the client to record caloric intake.

  o Have client first record everything eaten. The nurse, dietician, or client can identify the caloric value of each item. Often, this count gives a better objective finding of the nutritional status of the client's intake.

PLAN OF CARE FOR A PREGNANT CLIENT		
EXPECTED OUTCOMES	INTERVENTIONS	EVALUATION OF THE PLAN
• The client will consume the recommended dietary allowances/ nutrients during her pregnancy.	• The nurse will assess the client's dietary journal on the next prenatal visit. • The nurse will provide educational materials regarding nutritional benefits to the mother and her newborn. • The nurse will provide encouragement and answer questions that the client has regarding her dietary plans. • The nurse will weigh the client and monitor for signs of inadequate weight gain. • The nurse will make a referral if needed.	• Is there adequate weight gain? • Is the client compliant with the nursing plan of care?

- Instruct the client to adhere and maintain the following during pregnancy.

  o An increase of 340 calories/day is recommended during the second trimester. An increase of 452 calories/day is recommended during the third trimester.

  o If the client is breastfeeding during the postpartum period, an additional intake of 330 calories/day is recommended during the first 6 months, and an additional intake of 400 calories/day is recommended during the second 6 months.

  o Increasing protein intake is essential to basic growth. Also, increasing the intake of foods high in folic acid is crucial for neurological development and the prevention of neural tube defects. Foods high in folic acid include leafy vegetables, dried peas and beans, seeds, and orange juice. Breads, cereals, and other grains are fortified with folic acid. Increased intake of folic acid should be encouraged for clients who wish to become pregnant and clients of childbearing age. It is recommended that 600 mcg of folic acid should be taken during pregnancy. Current recommendations for clients who are lactating include consuming 500 mcg of folic acid.

  o Iron supplements are often added to the prenatal plan to facilitate an increase of the maternal RBC mass. Iron is best absorbed between meals and when given with a good source of vitamin C. Milk and caffeine interfere with the absorption of iron supplements. Good food sources of iron include beef liver, red meats, fish, poultry, dried peas and beans, and fortified cereals and breads. A stool softener may need to be added to decrease constipation experienced with iron supplements.

- o Calcium, which is important to a developing fetus, is involved in bone and teeth formation.

  - Good sources of calcium include milk, calcium-fortified soy milk, fortified orange juice, nuts, legumes, and dark green leafy vegetables. Daily recommendation is 1,000 mg/day for pregnant and nonpregnant women over the age of 19, and 1,300 mg/day for those under 19 years of age.

- o 2 to 3 L of fluids is recommended daily. Fluids that are preferable include water, fruit juice, or milk.

- o Caffeine intake should be limited to 300 mg/day. The equivalent of 500 to 750 mL/day of coffee may increase the risk of a spontaneous abortion or fetal intrauterine growth restriction.

- o It is recommended that women abstain from alcohol consumption during pregnancy.

Risk Factors to Ensuring Adequate Nutrition During Pregnancy

- Age, culture, education, and socioeconomic issues may affect adequate nutrition during pregnancy. Also, certain conditions specific to each client may inhibit adequate caloric intake.

  - o Adolescents may have poor nutritional habits (a diet low in vitamins and protein, not taking prescribed iron supplements).

  - o Vegetarians may have low protein, calcium, iron, zinc, and vitamin B_{12}.

  - o Nausea and vomiting during pregnancy

  - o Anemia

  - o Eating disorders such as anorexia nervosa or bulimia

  - o Pregnant clients diagnosed with the appetite disorder pica (craving to eat nonfood substances such as dirt or red clay). This disorder may diminish the amount of nutritional foods taken in.

  - o Excessive weight gain can lead to macrosomia and labor complications.

  - o Inability to gain weight may result in low birth weight of the newborn.

  - o Financially unable to purchase/access food. Therefore, the nurse should advise the client of "Women Infants and Children" programs that are federally available for pregnant women and their children (up to 5 years old).

Dietary Complications During Pregnancy

- Nausea and constipation are common during pregnancy.

  - o For nausea, tell the client to eat dry crackers or toast. Have her avoid alcohol, caffeine, fats, and spices. Also avoid drinking fluids with meals, and DO NOT take a medication to control nausea without first checking with the primary care provider.

  - o For constipation, increase fluid consumption and include extra fiber in the diet. Fruits, vegetables, and whole grains all contain fiber.

- Maternal phenylketonuria (PKU) – this is a maternal genetic disease in which high levels of phenylalanine pose danger to the fetus.

  o It is important for the female client to resume the PKU diet for at least 3 months prior to pregnancy and continue the diet throughout pregnancy.

  o The diet should include foods that are low in phenylalanine. Foods high in protein, such as fish, poultry, meat, eggs, nuts, and dairy products, must be avoided due to high phenylalanine levels.

- The client's blood phenylalanine levels should be monitored during pregnancy.

- These interventions will prevent fetal complications such as mental retardation and behavioral problems.

Creating a Postpartum Nutritional Plan

- A lactating woman's nutritional plan should include instructions to:

  o Increase caloric intake.

  o Increase oral fluids.

  o Increase protein intake.

  o Avoid alcohol and caffeine.

  o Avoid food substances that do not agree with the newborn (foods that may cause increased gas).

  o Adhere to a recommended, well-balanced diet.

  o Take calcium supplements if she consumes an inadequate amount of dietary calcium.

- A nutritional plan for a woman who is not breastfeeding should include:

  o Resuming a previous diet plan.

  o Adhering to a recommended well-balanced diet.

Desired Client Outcomes

  o A client should gain the recommended amount of weight throughout her pregnancy.

  o A client should consume adequate dietary intake during pregnancy and lactation based on current recommendations.

CHAPTER 5: NUTRITION DURING PREGNANCY

Ⓐ Application Exercises

1. A nurse working in a prenatal clinic is providing education to a client who is pregnant. The client states that she does not like milk. What is a good source of calcium that the nurse can recommend to the client?

    A. Dark green, leafy vegetables

    B. Deep red or orange vegetables

    C. Citrus fruits and juices

    D. Meat, poultry, and fish

2. Which of the following clients should the nurse be concerned about regarding weight gain? A client who has gained

    A. 1.8 kg (4 lb) and is in her first trimester.

    B. 3.6 kg (8 lb) and is in her first trimester.

    C. 6.8 kg (15 lb) and is in her second trimester.

    D. 11.3 kg (25) lb and is in her third trimester.

3. A prenatal nurse recommends folic acid supplements to a client who is of childbearing age. Which of the following defects can occur in the fetus or neonate as a result of folic acid deficiency?

    A. Iron deficiency anemia

    B. Poor bone formation

    C. Macrosomic fetus

    D. Neural tube defects

4. A client who is pregnant is diagnosed with iron deficiency anemia and has been prescribed iron supplements. The nurse should advise the client to take the iron supplements with which of the following?

    A. Ice water

    B. Low-fat or whole milk

    C. Tea or coffee

    D. Orange juice

CHAPTER 5: NUTRITION DURING PREGNANCY

 Application Exercises Answer Key

1. A nurse working in a prenatal clinic is providing education to a client who is pregnant. The client states that she does not like milk. What is a good source of calcium that the nurse can recommend to the client?

   A. Dark green, leafy vegetables

   B. Deep red or orange vegetables

   C. Citrus fruits and juices

   D. Meat, poultry, and fish

   Calcium is very important to a developing fetus. It is involved in bone and teeth formation. Good sources of calcium include calcium-fortified orange juice, nuts, legumes, and low oxalate, dark green, leafy vegetables. The other food choices are not good sources of calcium.

   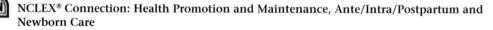 NCLEX® Connection: Health Promotion and Maintenance, Ante/Intra/Postpartum and Newborn Care

2. Which of the following clients should the nurse be concerned about regarding weight gain? A client who has gained

   A. 1.8 kg (4 lb) and is in her first trimester.

   B. 3.6 kg (8 lb) and is in her first trimester.

   C. 6.8 kg (15 lb) and is in her second trimester.

   D. 11.3 kg (25) lb and is in her third trimester.

   A client who has gained 3.6 kg (8 lb) in her first trimester has gained too much weight. Recommended weight gain during pregnancy is usually 11.2 to 15.9 kg (25 to 35 lb). The general rule is that clients should gain 1 to 2 kg (3 to 4 lb) during the first trimester and after that a weight gain of approximately 0.4 kg (1 lb) per week for the last two trimesters.

   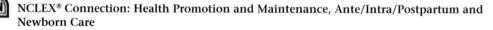 NCLEX® Connection: Health Promotion and Maintenance, Ante/Intra/Postpartum and Newborn Care

3. A prenatal nurse recommends folic acid supplements to a client who is of childbearing age. Which of the following defects can occur in the fetus or neonate as a result of folic acid deficiency?

    A. Iron deficiency anemia

    B. Poor bone formation

    C. Macrosomic fetus

D. Neural tube defects

Folic acid supplements are recommended to prevent neural tube defects in the fetus. It is recommended that all women of childbearing age take this supplement. Excellent food sources of folic acid are fresh green, leafy vegetables, liver, peanuts, cereals, and whole-grain breads. Iron deficiency anemia can occur as a result of a lack of iron-rich sources of food such as meat, chicken, and fish. Calcium deficiency can result in poor teeth and bone formation. Maternal obesity can lead to a macrosomic fetus.

 NCLEX® Connection: Health Promotion and Maintenance, Ante/Intra/Postpartum and Newborn Care

4. A client who is pregnant is diagnosed with iron deficiency anemia and has been prescribed iron supplements. The nurse should advise the client to take the iron supplements with which of the following?

    A. Ice water

    B. Low-fat or whole milk

    C. Tea or coffee

D. Orange juice

Orange juice contains vitamin C, which aids in the absorption of iron. Milk and caffeine interfere with iron absorption. Also, caffeine intake from tea and coffee should be limited to 300 mg/day because caffeine increases the risk of a spontaneous abortion or fetal intrauterine growth restriction. Water will not help the absorption of iron, but drinking plenty of water should be encouraged to prevent constipation, which is a side effect of iron supplements.

 NCLEX® Connection: Health Promotion and Maintenance, Ante/Intra/Postpartum and Newborn Care

UNIT 1	ANTEPARTUM NURSING CARE
Section	Low-Risk, Uncomplicated Pregnancy: Changes During Pregnancy
Chapter 6	Assessment of Fetal Well-Being

Overview

- This chapter covers the assessments that are used to determine the well-being of a fetus during pregnancy.

- The diagnostic procedures listed include ultrasound (abdominal, transvaginal, Doppler), biophysical profile, nonstress test, contraction stress test (nipple, oxytocin [Pitocin]), amniocentesis, percutaneous umbilical cord blood sampling, chorionic villus sampling, quad marker screening, and maternal serum alpha-fetoprotein.

DIAGNOSTIC PROCEDURE AND NURSING MANAGEMENT: ULTRASOUND (ABDOMINAL, TRANSVAGINAL, DOPPLER)

Overview

- Ultrasound – a procedure lasting approximately 20 min that consists of high-frequency sound waves used to visualize internal organs and tissues by producing a real time three-dimensional pictorial image of the developing fetus and maternal structures (FHR, pelvic anatomy). An ultrasound allows for an early diagnosis of complications, permitting earlier interventions, and thereby decreasing the neonate's and mother's morbidity and mortality. Currently, there are three types of ultrasounds: external abdominal, transvaginal, and Doppler.

  o External abdominal ultrasound – a noninvasive, painless, and safe procedure. An abdominal ultrasound is more useful after the first trimester when the gravid uterus is larger. The ultrasound transducer is moved over a client's abdomen to obtain an image.

  o Internal transvaginal ultrasound – an invasive procedure in which a probe is inserted vaginally and allows for a more accurate evaluation. An advantage of this procedure is that it does not require a full bladder.

    ▪ It is especially useful in clients who are obese and those in the first trimester to detect an ectopic pregnancy, identify abnormalities, and help to establish gestational age.

    ▪ A transvaginal ultrasound may also be used in the third trimester in conjunction with abdominal scanning to evaluate for preterm labor.

- o Doppler ultrasound blood flow analysis – an external ultrasound method of noninvasively studying the maternal-fetal blood flow by measuring the velocity at which RBCs are traveling in the uterine and fetal vessels using a handheld ultrasound device that reflects sound waves from a moving target. It is especially useful in fetal intrauterine growth restriction (IUGR), identifying poor placental perfusion, and as an adjunct in pregnancies at risk because of hypertension, diabetes mellitus, multiple fetuses, or preterm labor.

- Indications for the use of an Ultrasound During Pregnancy

  - o Potential diagnoses for:

    - Confirming pregnancy.
    - Confirming gestational age by biparietal diameter (side-to-side) measurement.
    - Identifying multifetal pregnancy.
    - Site of fetal implantation (uterine or ectopic).
    - Assessing fetal growth and development.
    - Assessing maternal structure.
    - Confirming fetal viability or death.
    - Ruling out or verifying fetal abnormalities.
    - Locating the site of placental attachment.
    - Determining amniotic fluid volume.
    - Fetal movement observation (fetal heartbeat, breathing, and activity).
    - Placental grading (evaluating placental maturation).
    - Adjunct for other procedures (e.g., amniocentesis, biophysical profile).

  - o Client presentation

    - Vaginal bleeding evaluation
    - Questionable fundal height measurement in relationship to gestational weeks
    - Reports decreased fetal movements
    - Preterm labor
    - Questionable rupture of membranes

- Nursing Actions for an Ultrasound

  - o Preparation of a client

    - Explain the procedure to the client and that it presents no known risk to her or her fetus.
    - Advise the client to drink 1 to 2 quarts of fluid prior to the ultrasound to fill the bladder to lift and stabilize the uterus, displace the bowels away, and act as an echolucent to better reflect sound waves and to get a better image of the fetus.

- Assist the client into a supine position with a wedge placed under her right hip to displace the uterus (prevent supine hypotension).
    - Ongoing care
        - Apply an ultrasonic/transducer gel to the client's abdomen before the transducer is moved over the skin to obtain a better fetal image, assuring that the gel is at room temperature or warmer to prevent uterine cramping.
        - Allow the client to empty her bladder at the termination of the procedure.
- Nursing Actions for a Transvaginal Ultrasound
    - Preparation of a client
        - Assist the client into a lithotomy position. The vaginal probe is covered with a protective device, lubricated with a water-soluble gel, and the client or examiner may insert the probe.
    - Ongoing care
        - During the procedure, the position of the probe or tilt of the table may be changed to facilitate the complete view of the pelvis.
        - Inform the client that some pressure may be felt as the probe is moved.
    - Interventions
        - Fetal and maternal structures may be pointed out to the client as the ultrasound procedure is performed.

DIAGNOSTIC PROCEDURE AND NURSING MANAGEMENT: BIOPHYSICAL PROFILE

Overview

- Biophysical profile (BPP) – uses a real-time ultrasound to visualize physical and physiological characteristics of the fetus and observes for fetal biophysical responses to stimuli.

- BPP assesses the fetal well-being by measuring the following five variables with a score of 2 for each normal finding, and 0 for each abnormal finding for each variable.

    - Reactive FHR (reactive nonstress test) = 2; nonreactive = 0.

    - Fetal breathing movements (at least 1 episode of 30 sec in 30 min) = 2; absent or less than 30 sec duration = 0.

    - Gross body movements (at least 3 body or limb extensions with return to flexion in 30 min) = 2; less than 3 episodes = 0.

    - Fetal tone (at least 1 episode of extension with return to flexion) = 2; slow extension and flexion, lack of flexion, or absent of movement = 0.

    - Amniotic fluid volume (at least 1 pocket of fluid that measures at least 1 cm in 2 perpendicular planes) = 2; pockets absent or less than 1 cm = 0.

- Interpretation of Findings

    o Total score of 8 to 10 is being normal

    o 6 is equivocal

    o < 4 is abnormal

- Potential Diagnoses

    o Nonreactive stress test

    o Suspected oligohydramnios or polyhydramnios

    o Suspected fetal hypoxemia and/or hypoxia

- Client Presentation

    o Premature rupture of membranes

    o Maternal infection

    o Decreased fetal movement

    o Intrauterine growth restriction

- Nursing Actions

    o Preparation of a client

        ▪ Follow the same nursing management techniques as those used for an ultrasound.

DIAGNOSTIC PROCEDURE AND NURSING MANAGEMENT: NONSTRESS TEST (NST)

Overview

- Nonstress test (NST) – most widely used technique for antepartum evaluation of fetal well-being performed during the third trimester. It is a noninvasive procedure that monitors response of the FHR to fetal movement. A Doppler transducer, used to monitor the FHR, and a tocotransducer, used to monitor uterine contractions, is attached externally to a client's abdomen to obtain paper tracing strips. The client pushes a button attached to the monitor whenever she feels a fetal movement, which is then noted on the paper tracing. This allows a nurse to assess the FHR in relationship to the fetal movement.

- Indications for the use of a Nonstress Test During Pregnancy

    o Potential diagnoses for:

        ▪ Assessing for an intact fetal CNS during the third trimester.

        ▪ Ruling out the risk for fetal death in clients who have diabetes mellitus. Used twice a week or, until after 28 weeks of gestation.

- o Client presentation

  - Decreased fetal movement

  - Intrauterine growth restriction

  - Postmaturity

  - Gestational diabetes mellitus

  - Pregnancy-induced hypertension

  - Maternal chronic hypertension

  - History of previous fetal demise

  - Advanced maternal age

  - Sickle cell disease

- Interpretation of Findings

  - o The NST is interpreted as reactive if the FHR is a normal baseline rate with moderate variability, accelerates to 15 beats/min for at least 15 seconds and occurs two or more time during a 20-min period.

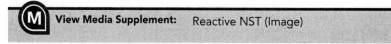

View Media Supplement: Reactive NST (Image)

  - o Nonreactive NST indicates that the fetal heart rate does not accelerate adequately with fetal movement. It does not meet the above criteria after 40 minutes. If this is so, a further assessment such as a contraction stress test (CST) or biophysical profile (BPP) is indicated.

  - o Nursing Actions

  - o Preparation of a client

    - Seat the client in a reclining chair or place in a semi-Fowler's or left-lateral position.

    - Apply conduction gel to the client's abdomen.

    - Apply two belts to the client's abdomen and attach the FHR and uterine contraction monitors.

  - o Ongoing care

    - Instruct the client to press the button on the handheld event marker each time she feels the fetus move.

    - If there are no fetal movements (fetus sleeping), vibroacoustic stimulation (sound source, usually laryngeal stimulator) may be activated for 3 seconds on the maternal abdomen over the fetal head to awaken a sleeping fetus.

    - If NST is still nonreactive, anticipate a CST and/or BPP.

- Miscellaneous

  o Disadvantages of a NST include a high rate of false nonreactive results with the fetal movement response blunted by sleep cycles of the fetus, fetal immaturity, maternal medications, and chronic smoking.

DIAGNOSTIC PROCEDURE AND NURSING MANAGEMENT: CONTRACTION STRESS TEST (CST)

Overview

- Nipple stimulated CST consists of a woman lightly brushing her palm across her nipple for 2 or 3 min, which causes the pituitary gland to release endogenous oxytocin, and then stopping the nipple stimulation when a contraction begins. The same process is repeated after a 5 min rest period.

  o Stimulates contractions (which decrease placental blood flow) and analyze the FHR in conjunction with the contractions to determine how the fetus will tolerate the stress of labor. A pattern of at least three contractions within a 10-min time period with duration of 40 to 60 seconds each must be obtained to use for assessment data.

  o Hyperstimulation of the uterus (uterine contraction longer than 90 seconds or more frequent than every 2 min) should be avoided by stimulating the nipple intermittently with rest periods in between and avoiding bimanual stimulation of both nipples unless stimulation of one nipple is unsuccessful.

- Oxytocin (Pitocin) administration CST is used if nipple stimulation fails and consists of the IV administration of oxytocin to induce uterine contractions.

  o Contractions started with oxytocin may be difficult to stop and can lead to preterm labor

- Indications for the use of a contraction stress test during pregnancy

  o Potential diagnoses

    ■ High-risk pregnancies (gestational diabetes mellitus, postterm pregnancy).

    ■ Nonreactive stress test.

  o Client presentation

    ■ Decreased fetal movement

    ■ Intrauterine growth restriction

    ■ Postmaturity

    ■ Gestational diabetes mellitus

    ■ Pregnancy-induced hypertension

    ■ Maternal chronic hypertension

- - History of previous fetal demise
  - Advanced maternal age
  - Sickle-cell disease
- Interpretation of Findings
  - A negative CST (normal finding) is indicated if within a 10-min period, with three uterine contractions, there are no late decelerations of the FHR.
  - A positive CST (abnormal finding) is indicated with persistent and consistent late decelerations on more than half of the contractions. This is suggestive of uteroplacental insufficiency. Variable deceleration may indicate cord compression, and early decelerations may indicate fetal head compression. Based on these findings, the primary care provider may determine to induce labor or perform a cesarean birth.

 View Media Supplement: Positive CST (Image)

- Nursing Actions
  - Preparation of a client
    - Obtain a baseline of the FHR, fetal movement, and contractions for 10 to 20 min and document.
    - Explain the procedure to the client and obtain an informed consent form from her.
    - Complete an assessment without artificial stimulation if contractions are occurring spontaneously.
  - Ongoing care
    - Initiate nipple stimulation if there are no contractions. Instruct the client to roll a nipple between her thumb and fingers or brush her palm across her nipple. The client should stop when a uterine contraction begins.
    - Monitor and provide adequate rest periods for the client to avoid hyperstimulation of the uterus.
  - Interventions
    - Initiate IV oxytocin administration if nipple stimulation fails to elicit a sufficient uterine contraction pattern. If hyperstimulation of the uterus and/or preterm labor occurs:
      - Monitor for contractions lasting longer than 90 seconds and/or occurring more frequently than every 2 min.
      - Provide administration of tocolytics as prescribed.
      - Maintain bed rest during the procedure.
      - Observe the client for 30 min afterward to see that contractions have ceased and preterm labor does not begin.

- Complications

  o Potential for preterm labor

DIAGNOSTIC PROCEDURE AND NURSING MANAGEMENT: AMNIOCENTESIS

Overview

- Amniocentesis – the aspiration of amniotic fluid for analysis by insertion of a needle transabdominally into a client's uterus and amniotic sac under direct ultrasound guidance locating the placenta and determining the position of the fetus. It may be performed after 14 weeks of gestation.

- Indications for the use of an Amniocentesis During Pregnancy

  o Potential diagnoses

    - Maternal age greater than 35 years

    - Previous birth with a chromosomal anomaly

    - A parent who is a carrier of a chromosomal anomaly

    - A family history of neural tube defects

    - Prenatal diagnosis of a genetic disorder or congenital anomaly of the fetus

    - Alpha fetoprotein level for fetal abnormalities

    - Lung maturity assessment

    - Fetal hemolytic disease diagnosis

    - Meconium in the amniotic fluid

- Interpretation of Findings

  o Alpha-fetoprotein (AFP) can be measured from the amniotic fluid between 16 and 18 weeks of gestation and may be used to assess for neural tube defects in the fetus or chromosomal disorders. May be evaluated to follow up a high level of AFP in maternal serum.

    - High levels of AFP are associated with neural tube defects such as anencephaly (incomplete development of fetal skull and brain), spina bifida (open spine), or omphalocele (abdominal wall defect). High AFP levels may also be present with normal multifetal pregnancies.

    - Low levels of AFP are associated with chromosomal disorders (Down syndrome) or gestational trophoblastic disease (hydatidiform mole).

  o Tests for fetal lung maturity may be performed if gestation is less than 37 weeks, in the event of a rupture of membranes, for preterm labor, or for a complication indicating a cesarean birth. Amniotic fluid is tested to determine if the fetal lungs are mature enough to adapt to extrauterine life or if the fetus will likely have respiratory distress. Determination is made whether the fetus should be removed immediately or if the fetus requires more time in utero with the administration of glucocorticoids to promote fetal lung maturity.

- Fetal Lung Tests
  - Lecithin/sphingomyelin (L/S) ratio – a 2:1 indicating fetal lung maturity (2.5:1 or 3:1 for a client who has diabetes mellitus).
  - Presence of phosphatidylglycerol (PG) – absence of PG is associated with respiratory distress

- Preprocedure for an Amniocentesis
  - Nursing actions
    - Explain the procedure to the client and obtain an informed consent form from her.
  - Client education
    - Instruct the client to empty her bladder prior to the procedure to reduce its size and reduce the risk of inadvertent puncture.

- Intraprocedure
  - Nursing actions
    - Assist the client into a supine position and place a wedge or rolled towel under her right hip to displace the uterus off the vena cava and place a drape over the client exposing only her abdomen.
    - Prepare the client for an ultrasound to locate the placenta.
    - Obtain the client's baseline vital signs and FHR and document prior to the procedure.
    - Cleanse the client's abdomen with an antiseptic solution prior to the administration of a local anesthetic given by the primary care provider.
    - Take maternal blood pressure and obtain the FHR for baseline levels.
  - Client education
    - Advise the client that she will feel slight pressure as the needle is inserted for aspiration. However, she should continue breathing because holding her breath will lower the diaphragm against the uterus and shift the intrauterine contents.

- Postprocedure
  - Nursing actions
    - Monitor the client's vital signs, FHR, and uterine contractions throughout and 30 min following the procedure.
    - Have the client rest for 30 min.
    - Administer $Rh_o(D)$ immune globulin (RhoGAM) to the client if she is Rh-negative (standard practice after an amniocentesis for all women who are Rh-negative to protect against Rh isoimmunization).

- ○ Client education
  - Advise the client to report to her primary care provider if she experiences fever, chills, leakage of fluid, or bleeding from the insertion site, decreased fetal movement, vaginal bleeding, or uterine contractions after the procedure.
  - Encourage the client to drink plenty of liquids and rest for the next 24 hr postprocedure.
- ○ Complications
  - Amniotic fluid emboli
  - Maternal or fetal hemorrhage
  - Fetomaternal hemorrhage with Rh isoimmunization
  - Maternal or fetal infection
  - Inadvertent fetal damage or anomalies involving limbs
  - Fetal death
  - Inadvertent maternal intestinal or bladder damage
  - Miscarriage or preterm labor
  - Premature rupture of membranes
  - Leakage of amniotic fluid
- ○ Nursing actions
  - Monitor the client's vital signs, temperature, respiratory status, FHR, uterine contractions, and vaginal discharge for amniotic fluid or bleeding.
- ○ Client education
  - Provide medication administration as prescribed, client education, and support.

DIAGNOSTIC PROCEDURE AND NURSING MANAGEMENT: ADDITIONAL PRENATAL TESTING FOR HIGH-RISK PREGNANCY

Overview

- Percutaneous umbilical blood sampling (PUBS) – the most common method used for sampling a fetal blood transfusion. This procedure obtains fetal blood sampling from the umbilical cord by passing a fine-gauge fiber optic scope (fetoscope) into the amniotic sac using the amniocentesis technique. The needle is advanced into the umbilical cord under ultrasound guidance and blood is aspirated from the umbilical vein. Blood studies from the cordocentesis may consist of:
  - ○ Kleihauer-Betke test that ensures blood obtained is from the fetus.
  - ○ CBC count with differential.
  - ○ Indirect Coombs' test for Rh antibodies.

- o Karyotyping (visualization of chromosomes).

- o Blood gases.

- Indications for the use of PUBS

  - o Potential Diagnoses

    - Diagnosing prenatal blood and chromosomal disorders

    - Karyotyping of malformed fetuses

    - Detecting of fetal infection

    - Determining the acid-base balance status of fetuses with IUGR

- Interpretation of Findings

  - o Evaluate for isoimmune fetal hemolytic anemia and assessing the need for a fetal blood transfusion.

- Client Education

  - o Provide medication administration as prescribed.

  - o Educate client and provide support.

- Complications

  - o Cord laceration

  - o Preterm labor

  - o Amnionitis

DIAGNOSTIC PROCEDURE AND NURSING MANAGEMENT: ADDITIONAL PRENATAL TESTING FOR HIGH-RISK PREGNANCY

Overview

- Chorionic villus sampling (CVS) – assessment of a portion of the developing placenta (chorionic villi) is aspirated through a thin sterile catheter or syringe through the abdomen or intravaginally through the cervix under ultrasound guidance and analyzed.

  - o CVS is a first-trimester alternative to amniocentesis with one of its advantages being an earlier diagnosis of any abnormalities. CVS can be performed at 10 to 12 weeks of gestation and rapid results with chromosome studies are available in 24 to 48 hr following aspiration.

- Indications for the use of CVS During Pregnancy

  - o Potential diagnoses

    - Women at risk for giving birth to a neonate who has a genetic chromosomal abnormality (cannot determine spina bifida or anencephaly)

- ○ Client education

    - ■ Provide ongoing education and support.

    - ■ Instruct the client to drink plenty of fluid to fill the bladder prior to the procedure to assist in positioning the uterus for catheter insertion.

- • Complications

    - ■ Spontaneous abortion (higher risk with CVS than with amniocentesis)

    - ■ Risk for fetal limb loss

    - ■ Miscarriage

    - ■ Chorioamnionitis and rupture of membranes

- • Miscellaneous

    - ○ The advantage of an earlier diagnosis should be weighed against the increased risk of fetal anomalies and death.

DIAGNOSTIC PROCEDURE AND NURSING MANAGEMENT: QUAD MARKER AND ALPHA-FETOPROTEIN (MSAFP) SCREENING

Overview

- • Description of Procedure

    - ○ Quad Marker screening – a blood test done between 15 to 20 weeks of gestation that will ascertain information about the likelihood of fetal birth defects. It does not diagnose the actual defect. It may be performed instead of the maternal serum alpha-fetoprotein yielding more reliable findings. The test screens for the presence of hCG, AFP, estriol and Inhibin-A.

        - ■ Human chorionic gonadotropin (hCG) – a hormone produced by the placenta

        - ■ Alpha-fetoprotein (AFP) – a protein produced by the fetus

        - ■ Estriol – a protein produced by the fetus and placenta

        - ■ Inhibin-A – a protein produced by the ovaries and placenta

- • Indications

    - ○ Client presentation

        - ■ 15 to 20 weeks gestation

        - ■ Women at risk for giving birth to a neonate who has a genetic chromosomal abnormality

- • Interpretation of Findings

    - ○ Low levels of AFP may indicate a risk for Down syndrome

    - ○ High levels of AFP may indicate a risk for neural tube defects

- o Higher levels than normal of hCG and Inhibin-A indicates a risk for Down syndrome

- o Lower levels than normal of estriol may indicate a risk for Down syndrome

- Description of Procedure

  - o Maternal serum AFP is a screening tool used to detect neural tube defects. Clients with abnormal findings should be referred for a quad marker screening, genetic counseling, ultrasound, and an amniocentesis.

- Indications

  - o Potential diagnoses

    - All pregnant clients between 16 to 18 weeks of gestation

- Interpretation of Findings

  - o High levels may indicate a neural tube defect or open abdominal defect.

  - o Lower levels may indicate Down syndrome

- Nursing Actions

  - o Preparation of a client

    - Discuss testing with the client.

    - Draw blood sample.

  - o Client education

    - Offer support and education as needed.

CHAPTER 6: ASSESSMENT OF FETAL WELL-BEING

(A) Application Exercises

1. A nurse is evaluating a client's biophysical profile (BPP). Which of the following are variables should be included in this test? (Select all that apply.)

_____ Fetal weight

_____ Fetal breathing movement

_____ Fetal tone

_____ Reactive FHR

_____ Amniotic fluid volume

2. A nurse is caring for a client who is in preterm labor and is scheduled to undergo an amniocentesis. She is also scheduled for a fetal lung maturity test to determine if her fetus can adapt to extrauterine life or will develop respiratory distress. Which of the following is a test for fetal lung maturity?

A. Alpha-fetoprotein (AFP)

B. Lecithin/sphingomyelin (L/S) ratio

C. Kleihauer-Betke test

D. Indirect Coombs' test

3. A client who is undergoing a nonstress test asks a nurse to explain why she is using an acoustic vibration device. The nurse states that the device is used to

A. stimulate uterine contractions.

B. relax uterine contractions.

C. sooth the fetus to sleep.

D. awaken the sleeping fetus.

4. A nurse determines that a client who is pregnant needs further instructions about an amniocentesis when the client states,

A. "I must report cramping or signs of infection to the physician."

B. "I should drink lots of fluids for the next 24 hr following the procedure."

C. "I need to have a full bladder for the procedure to be done."

D. "The amniotic fluid can be used to detect genetic abnormalities."

5. Which of the following findings from a client who is pregnant should indicate to a nurse that the client should undergo a contraction stress test (CST)? (Select all that apply.)

_____ Decreased fetal movement

_____ Intrauterine growth restriction (IUGR)

_____ Postmaturity

_____ Advanced maternal age

_____ Urinary tract infection

CHAPTER 6: ASSESSMENT OF FETAL WELL-BEING

(A) Application Exercises Answer Key

1. A nurse is evaluating a client's biophysical profile (BPP). Which of the following are variables should be included in this test? (Select all that apply.)

_____	Fetal weight
__X__	**Fetal breathing movement**
__X__	**Fetal tone**
__X__	**Reactive FHR**
__X__	**Amniotic fluid volume**

BPP uses a real-time ultrasound to visualize physical and physiological characteristics of the fetus and observes for fetal biophysical responses to stimuli. BPP assesses the fetal well-being by measuring the following five variables with a score of 2 for each normal finding, and 0 for each abnormal finding for each variable. Fetal breathing, tone, reactive FHR, amniotic fluid volume, and gross body movements are variables to assess fetal well-being. Fetal weight is not included in a BPP.

(N) **NCLEX® Connection: Reduction of Risk Potential, Diagnostic Tests**

2. A nurse is caring for a client who is in preterm labor and is scheduled to undergo an amniocentesis. She is also scheduled for a fetal lung maturity test to determine if her fetus can adapt to extrauterine life or will develop respiratory distress. Which of the following is a test for fetal lung maturity?

A. Alpha fetoprotein (AFP)

B. Lecithin/sphingomyelin (L/S) ratio

C. Kleihauer-Betke test

D. Indirect Coombs' test

An L/S ratio of 2:1 indicates fetal lung maturity (2.5:1 or 3:1 for a client who has diabetes mellitus). AFP can be measured from the maternal serum between 16 and 18 weeks of gestation and may be used to assess for neural tube defects in the fetus or chromosomal disorders. A Kleihauer-Betke test is used to ensure blood is obtained from the fetus during a percutaneous umbilical blood sampling. An indirect Coombs' test is used to detect Rh antibodies in the mother's blood.

(N) **NCLEX® Connection: Reduction of Risk Potential, Diagnostic Tests**

3. A client who is undergoing a nonstress test asks a nurse to explain why she is using an acoustic vibration device. The nurse states that the device is used to

    A. stimulate uterine contractions.

    B. relax uterine contractions.

    C. sooth the fetus to sleep.

    D. awaken the sleeping fetus.

    If there is no fetal movement (fetus sleeping), vibroacoustic stimulation (sound source, usually a laryngeal stimulator) is activated for 3 seconds on the maternal abdomen over the fetal head to awaken a sleeping fetus. Vibroacoustic stimulation has no effect on uterine contractions.

 NCLEX® Connection: Reduction of Risk Potential, Diagnostic Tests

4. A nurse determines that a client who is pregnant needs further instructions about an amniocentesis when the client states,

    A. "I must report cramping or signs of infection to the physician."

    B. "I should drink lots of fluids for the next 24 hr following the procedure."

    C. "I need to have a full bladder for the procedure to be done."

    D. "The amniotic fluid can be used to detect genetic abnormalities."

    A full bladder may be necessary for an abdominal ultrasound and chorionic villus sampling. An amniocentesis requires an empty bladder to prevent an inadvertent puncture from occurring. The client should report any signs of infection to the primary care provider and should drink plenty of fluids and rest for 24 hr following the procedure. The amniocentesis is used to detect genetic abnormalities.

 NCLEX® Connection: Reduction of Risk Potential, Diagnostic Tests

5. Which of the following findings from a client who is pregnant should indicate to a nurse that the client should undergo a contraction stress test (CST)? (Select all that apply).

    _**X**_   **Decreased fetal movement**

    _**X**_   **Intrauterine growth restriction (IUGR)**

    _**X**_   **Postmaturity**

    _**X**_   **Advanced maternal age**

    _____   Urinary tract infection

    Decreased fetal movement, IUGR, postmaturity, and advanced maternal age are all findings that require interventions. Assessing fetal well-being by performing a CST would be indicated. A urinary tract infection would not require a CST.

 NCLEX® Connection: Reduction of Risk Potential, Diagnostic Tests

UNIT 1	ANTEPARTUM NURSING CARE
Section	Complications of Pregnancy
Chapter 7	Bleeding During Pregnancy

Overview

- Vaginal bleeding during pregnancy is always abnormal and must be carefully investigated to determine the cause. It can impair both the outcome of the pregnancy and the mother's life.

- The primary causes of bleeding are summarized in the following table according to common causes during each trimester of pregnancy.

SUMMARY OF CAUSES OF BLEEDING DURING PREGNANCY		
TIME	COMPLICATION	SIGNS AND SYMPTOMS
First trimester	Spontaneous abortion	Vaginal bleeding, uterine cramping, and partial or complete expulsion of products of conception
	Ectopic pregnancy	Abrupt unilateral lower-quadrant abdominal pain with or without vaginal bleeding
Second trimester	Gestational trophoblastic disease	Uterine size increasing abnormally fast, abnormally high levels of hCG, nausea and increased emesis, no fetus present on ultrasound, and scant or profuse dark brown or red vaginal bleeding
Third trimester	Placenta previa	Painless vaginal bleeding
	Abruptio placenta	Vaginal bleeding, sharp abdominal pain, and tender rigid uterus
	Vasa previa	Fetal vessel cross over the cervix abrupt bright red vaginal bleeding following rupture of membranes

- Other Causes of Bleeding

  - Incompetent cervix

    - Painless bleeding with cervical dilation leading to fetal expulsion o   Preterm labor

        ■ Pink-stained vaginal discharge, uterine contractions becoming regular, cervical dilation and effacement

SPONTANEOUS ABORTION

Overview

- Spontaneous abortion is when a pregnancy is terminated before 20 weeks of gestation (the point of fetal viability) or a fetal weight less than 500 g.

- Types of abortion are clinically classified according to symptoms and whether the products of conception are partially or completely retained or expulsed. Types of abortions include threatened, inevitable, incomplete, complete, and missed.

Risk Factors

- Chromosomal abnormalities (account for 50%)

- Maternal illness, such as insulin-dependent diabetes mellitus

- Advancing maternal age

- Premature cervical dilation

- Chronic maternal infections

- Maternal malnutrition

- Trauma or injury

- Anomalies in the fetus or placenta

- Substance abuse

Assessment

- Subjective and Objective Data

    o   Backache

    o   Rupture of membranes

    o   Dilation of the cervix

    o   Fever

    o   Abdominal tenderness

    o   Signs and symptoms of hemorrhage such as hypotension and tachycardia

SPONTANEOUS ABORTION (MISCARRIAGE) ASSESSMENT				
TYPE	CRAMPS	BLEEDING	TISSUE PASSED	CERVICAL OPENING
Threatened	With or without slight cramps	Spotting to moderate	None	Closed
Inevitable	Moderate	Mild to severe	None	Dilated with membranes or tissues bulging at cervix
Incomplete	Severe	Continuous and severe	Partial fetal tissue or placenta	Dilated with tissue in cervical canal or passage of tissue
Complete	Mild	Minimal	Complete expulsion of uterine contents	Closed with no tissue in cervical canal
Missed	None	Brownish discharge	None, prolonged retention of tissue	Closed
Septic	Malodorous	Malodorous discharge	Varies	Usually dilated
Recurrent	Varies	Varies	Yes	Usually dilated

- ○ Laboratory tests
    - ▪ Hgb and Hct, if considerable blood loss
    - ▪ Clotting factors monitored for disseminated intravascular coagulopathy (DIC) – a complication with retained products of conception
    - ▪ WBC for suspected infection
    - ▪ Serum human chorionic gonadotropin (hCG) levels to confirm pregnancy
- ○ Diagnostic procedures
    - ▪ An ultrasound is used to determine the presence of a viable or dead fetus, or partial or complete products of conception within the uterine cavity.
    - ▪ An examination of the cervix to observe if it is opened or closed.
    - ▪ Dilation and curettage (D&C) is done to dilate and scrape the uterine walls to remove uterine contents for inevitable and incomplete abortions.
    - ▪ Dilation and evacuation (D&E) is done to dilate and evacuate uterine contents after 16 weeks of gestation.

- Prostaglandin is administered into the amniotic sac or by a vaginal suppository to augment or induce labor to expulse the products of conception for a late term, incomplete, inevitable, or missed abortion.

Collaborative Care

- Nursing Care

  ○ Observe bleeding amount and color (counting pads).

  ○ Perform a pregnancy test.

  ○ Use the lay term "miscarriage" with clients, because abortion will likely sound insensitive.

  ○ Place the client on bed rest with the administration of sedation for threatened, inevitable, and incomplete abortions.

  ○ Avoid a vaginal exam.

  ○ Assist with an ultrasound.

  ○ Administer analgesics and blood products as prescribed.

  ○ Determine how much tissue has passed and saving all passed tissue for examination.

  ○ Assist with termination of pregnancy (D&C, D&E) as indicated based on duration of pregnancy.

  ○ Provide client education and emotional support.

- Medications

  ○ $Rh_O(D)$ immune globulin (RhoGAM)

- Therapeutic Intent

  ○ $Rh_O(D)$ immune globulin (RhoGAM) suppresses the immune response of clients who are Rh-negative to Rh-positive RBCs from the fetus.

- Nursing Considerations

  ○ $Rh_O(D)$ immune globulin (RhoGAM), as indicated, to clients who are Rh-negative.

  ○ Administer prostaglandins or IV oxytocin (Pitocin) as prescribed to expulse products of conception in late, incomplete, inevitable, or missed abortions.

  ○ Administer broad-spectrum antibiotics as prescribed for treatment of septic abortion.

- Health Promotion and Disease Prevention

  ○ Discharge instructions

    - Instruct the client to notify the primary care provider of heavy, bright red vaginal bleeding.

    - Take prescribed antibiotics.

    - Tell the client that a small amount of discharge is normal for 1 to 2 weeks.

- Refrain from sexual intercourse or placing anything into the vagina for 2 weeks.
- Provide contacts for bereavement support groups.
- Instruct the client to avoid pregnancy for 2 months.

- Client Outcomes

  o The client will experience no psychological or physiological signs or symptoms of complications.

ECTOPIC PREGNANCY

Overview

- Ectopic pregnancy is the abnormal implantation of a fertilized ovum outside of the uterine cavity. The implantation is usually in the fallopian tube, which can result in a tubal rupture causing a fatal hemorrhage.
- Ectopic pregnancy is the second most frequent cause of bleeding in early pregnancy.

Risk Factors

- Risk factors for an ectopic pregnancy include any factor that compromises tubal patency (pelvic inflammatory disease, contraceptive intrauterine device [IUD])

Assessment

- Subjective Data

  o One or two missed menses

  o Unilateral stabbing pain and tenderness in the lower-abdominal quadrant

  o Scant, dark red, or brown vaginal spotting if tube ruptures (bleeding may be into intraperitoneal area)

  o Referred shoulder pain from blood irritation of the diaphragm or phrenic nerve (common symptom)

  o Frequent nausea and vomiting after tube rupture

- Objective Data

  o Signs of hemorrhage and shock (hypotension, tachycardia, pallor)

- Laboratory Tests

  o Hormone levels of progesterone and hCG elevated

  o WBC count elevated to 15,000/mm^3

- Diagnostic Procedures

  o Transvaginal ultrasound showing an empty uterus

  o Rapid surgical treatment

- Linear salpingostomy is done to salvage the fallopian tube if not ruptured.

- Laparoscopic salpingostomy (removal of the tube) is performed when the tube has ruptured.

Collaborative Care

- Nursing Care

  ○ Replace fluids that are lost and maintain electrolyte balance.

  ○ Provide client education and psychological support.

  ○ Prepare the client for surgery and postoperative nursing care.

- Medication

  ○ Methotrexate (MTX)

- Classification and Therapeutic Intent

  ○ Methotrexate is used to inhibit cell division and enlargement of the embryo. It also prevents rupture of the fallopian tube to preserve it.

- Nursing Considerations

  ○ Obtain serum hCG levels, liver and renal function studies, CBC, and type and Rh.

- Health Promotion and Disease Prevention

  ○ Client education

    - Instruct the client who is prescribed methotrexate to avoid alcohol consumption and vitamins containing folic acid to prevent a toxic response to the medication.

    - Advise the client to protect herself from sun exposure (photosensitivity).

  ○ Client outcomes

    - The client will experience no psychological or physiological signs or symptoms of complications.

GESTATIONAL TROPHOBLASTIC DISEASE (HYDATIDIFORM MOLE, CHORIOCARCINOMA, AND MOLAR PREGNANCY)

Overview

- Gestational trophoblastic disease is the proliferation and degeneration of trophoblastic villi in the placenta that becomes swollen, fluid-filled, and takes on the appearance of grape-like clusters. The embryo fails to develop beyond a primitive state and these structures are associated with choriocarcinoma, which is a rapidly metastasizing malignancy. Two types of molar growths are identified by chromosomal analysis.

- In the complete mole, all genetic material is paternally derived.

  ○ The ovum has no genetic material or the material is inactive.

  ○ The complete mole contains no fetus, placenta, amniotic membranes, or fluid.

  ○ There is no placenta to receive maternal blood; therefore, hemorrhage into the uterine cavity occurs and vaginal bleeding results.

  ○ Approximately 20% of complete moles progress toward a choriocarcinoma.

- In the partial mole, genetic material is derived both maternally and paternally.

  ○ A normal ovum is fertilized by two sperm or one sperm in which meiosis or chromosome reduction and division did not occur.

  ○ A partial mole often contains abnormal embryonic or fetal parts, an amniotic sac, and fetal blood, but congenital anomalies are present.

  ○ Approximately 6% of partial moles progress toward a choriocarcinoma.

Risk Factors

- Low protein intake

- Under 18 years of age

- Older than 35 years of age

Assessment

- Subjective Data

  ○ Vaginal bleeding at approximately 16 weeks of gestation

  ○ Excessive vomiting (hyperemesis gravidarum) due to elevated hCG levels

- Objective Data

  ○ Physical assessment findings

    ■ Rapid uterine growth larger than expected for the duration of the pregnancy due to the overproliferation of trophoblastic cells

    ■ Bleeding is often dark brown resembling prune juice, or bright red that is either scant or profuse and continues for a few days or intermittently for a few weeks

    ■ Bleeding accompanied by discharge from the clear fluid-filled vesicles

    ■ Symptoms of pregnancy-induced hypertension (PIH), including hypertension, edema, and proteinuria, that occur prior to 20 weeks of gestation (PIH usually does not occur until after 20 weeks of gestation)

- Laboratory tests

  - Urinalysis for proteinuria

    - Serial hCG immunoassays for pregnancy are strongly positive (1 to 2 million IU compared with a normal pregnancy level of 400,000 IU), and secondary hCG is produced by the overgrowing trophoblastic cells.

  - Analysis of serum hCG every 1 to 2 weeks until levels are normal, every 2 to 4 weeks for 6 months, and every 2 months for 1 year. These analyses should be performed in this manner because levels that plateau or increase suggest a malignant transformation.

- Diagnostic procedures

  - An ultrasound will reveal a dense growth with characteristic vesicles, but no fetus in utero.

  - Suction curettage is done to aspirate and evacuate the mole.

  - Following mole evacuation, the client should undergo a baseline pelvic exam and ultrasound scan of the abdomen in addition to frequent follow-up pelvic exams.

Collaborative Care

- Nursing Care

  - Measure fundal height.

  - Assess vaginal bleeding and discharge.

  - Assess gastrointestinal status and appetite.

  - Assess the client's extremities and face for edema.

  - Administer chemotherapy for choriocarcinoma in the event of an abnormal rising hCG titer, an enlarging uterus, and findings of malignant cells.

- Medications

  - Administer $Rh_o(D)$ immune globulin (RhoGAM) to the client who is Rh-negative.

- Health Promotion and Disease Prevention

  - Discharge instructions

    - Advise the client to bring any clots or tissue passed to the provider for evaluation.

  - Client education

    - Provide client education about the disease and emotional support regarding the loss of an anticipated pregnancy.

    - Instruct the client to use reliable contraception for 12 months because a pregnancy would make it impossible to monitor the decline in hCG levels, which is a significant component of follow-up care.

    - Instruct the client about the critical importance of follow up because of the increased risk of choriocarcinoma.

- Client outcomes

  - The client will experience no psychological or physiological signs or symptoms of complications.

PLACENTA PREVIA

 Overview

- Placenta previa occurs when the placenta abnormally implants in the lower segment of the uterus near or over the cervical os instead of attaching to the fundus. The abnormal implantation results in bleeding during the third trimester of pregnancy as the cervix begins to dilate and efface.

> **View Media Supplement:** Placenta Previa (Image)

- Placenta previa is classified into three types dependent on the degree to which the cervical os is covered by the placenta.

  - Complete or total – when the cervical os is completely covered by the placental attachment

  - Incomplete or partial – when the cervical os is only partially covered by the placental attachment

  - Marginal or low-lying – when the placenta is attached in the lower uterine segment but does not reach the cervical os

Risk Factors

- Risk factors for placenta previa

  - Previous placenta previa

  - Uterine scarring (previous cesarean birth, curettage, endometritis)

  - Maternal age greater than 35 years

  - Multifetal gestation

  - Multiple gestations or closely spaced pregnancies

Assessment

- Subjective Data

  - Painless, bright red vaginal bleeding that increases as the cervix dilates

- Objective Data

  - Physical assessment findings

    - A soft, relaxed, nontender uterus with normal tone

    - A fundal height that is greater than usually expected for gestational age

- A fetus in a breech, oblique, or transverse position
- A palpable placenta
- Vital signs that are usual and within normal limits
- A decreasing urinary output
- Laboratory tests
  - Hgb and Hct for blood loss assessment
  - CBC
  - ABO blood typing and Rh-factor
  - Coagulation profile
  - Kleihauer-Betke test (used to detect fetal blood in maternal circulation)
- Diagnostic Procedures
  - Transabdominal or transvaginal ultrasound for placement of the placenta
  - Fetal monitoring for fetal well-being assessment

Collaborative Care

- Nursing Care
  - Assess the client for bleeding, leakage, or contractions.
  - Assess fundal height.
  - Perform Leopold maneuvers (fetal position and presentation).
  - Refrain from performing vaginal exams (may exacerbate bleeding).
  - Administer IV fluids to the client as prescribed.
  - Have oxygen equipment available in case of fetal distress.
- Medications
  - Corticosteroids such as betamethasone (Celestone) are prescribed for fetal lung maturation if delivery of the fetus is anticipated (cesarean birth).
- Health Promotion and Disease Prevention
  - Discharge instructions
    - Bed rest
    - Nothing inserted vaginally
    - Blood replacement as prescribed

○ Client education

- The client's pregnancy will be maintained without any maternal or fetal compromise.

ABRUPTIO PLACENTA

 Overview

- Abruptio placenta is the premature separation of the placenta from the uterus, which can be a partial or complete detachment. This separation occurs after 20 weeks of gestation, which is usually in the third trimester. It has significant maternal and fetal morbidity and mortality and is a leading cause of maternal death.

View Media Supplement: Abruptio Placenta (Image)

- Coagulation defect, such as disseminated intravascular coagulopathy, is often associated with moderate to severe abruption.

Risk Factors

- Maternal hypertension
- Blunt external abdominal trauma (motor-vehicle crash, maternal battering)
- Cocaine abuse resulting in vasoconstriction
- Previous incidents of abruptio placenta
- Cigarette smoking
- Premature rupture of membranes
- Multifetal pregnancy

Assessment

- Subjective Data
  ○ Sudden onset of intense localized uterine pain with bright red vaginal bleeding
- Objective Data
  ○ Physical assessment findings
    - Vaginal bleeding that is bright red or dark
    - A board-like abdomen that is tender
    - A firm, rigid uterus with contractions (uterine hypertonicity)
    - Fetal distress
    - Signs of hypovolemic shock

- ○ Laboratory tests
  - Hgb and Hct decreased
  - Coagulation factors decreased
  - Clotting defects (disseminated intravascular coagulation)
  - Cross and type match for possible blood transfusions
  - Kleihauer-Betke test (used to detect fetal blood in maternal circulation)
- ○ Diagnostic procedures
  - Ultrasound for fetal well-being and placental assessment
  - Biophysical profile to ascertain fetal well-being

Collaborative Care

- Nursing Care
  - ○ Palpate the uterus for tenderness and tone.
  - ○ Assess FHR pattern.
  - ○ Administer IV fluids as prescribed.
  - ○ Administer oxygen 8 to 10 L via face mask.
- Medications
  - ○ Administer blood products and fluid volume replacements to maintain the client's urine output at 30 mL/hr or more and Hct at 30% or greater.
  - ○ Administer corticosteroids to promote fetal lung maturity.
  - ○ Client education
    - Provide emotional support for the client and family.
  - ○ Client outcomes
    - Birth of viable neonate

VASA PREVIA

Overview

- A vasa previa is the presence of fetal blood vessels crossing the amniotic membranes over the cervical os. There is a high newborn mortality rate associated with this condition. The risk is associated with fetal hemorrhage, as the client's cervix dilates or membranes rupture.
- Diagnosing this condition during the antepartum period is associated with improved outcomes. However, this condition is rarely diagnosed prior to the onset of labor.

Assessment

- Objective Data

    o Physical assessment findings

        ▪ Painless heavy bleeding upon rupture of membranes

        ▪ Fetal bradycardia

    o Laboratory tests

        ▪ Hgb and Hct decreased

        ▪ Cross and type match for possible blood transfusions

    o Diagnostic procedures

        ▪ Confirmation by sonography

Collaborative Care

- Nursing Care

    o Assess bleeding rate, amount, and color.

    o Administer IV fluids as prescribed.

    o Administer oxygen 8 to 10 L via face mask.

    o Prepare for an emergency cesarean birth.

- Medications

        ▪ Administer blood products and fluid volume replacements to maintain the client's urine output at 30 mL/hr or more and Hct at 30% or greater.

    o Health promotion and disease prevention

        ▪ Client Education

            □ Provide emotional support for the client and family.

    o Client outcomes

        ▪ Birth of viable neonate

CHAPTER 7: BLEEDING DURING PREGNANCY

 Application Exercises

1. A woman arrives in the emergency department with abrupt, sharp right-sided lower-quadrant abdominal pain, and bright red vaginal spotting. She has missed one menstrual cycle. She tells the nurse that she cannot be pregnant because she has been using an intrauterine device. The nurse should suspect which of the following?

    A. Missed abortion

    B. Ectopic pregnancy

    C. Severe preeclampsia

    D. Hydatidiform mole

2. A nurse at an antepartum clinic is caring for a client who is at 4 months of gestation. The client reports continued nausea and vomiting and scant, prune-colored discharge. She has experienced no weight loss and has a fundal height larger than expected for the duration of pregnancy. Which of the following complications should the nurse suspect?

    A. Hyperemesis gravidarum

    B. Threatened abortion

    C. Hydatidiform mole

    D. Preterm labor

3. A nurse is providing care for a client who is diagnosed with a marginal abruptio placenta. The nurse is aware that which of the following findings are risk factors for developing the condition? (Select all that apply.)

    _____ Maternal hypertension

    _____ Blunt abdominal trauma

    _____ Cocaine abuse

    _____ Maternal age

    _____ Cigarette smoking

4. A nurse is providing care for a client who is at 32 weeks of gestation and is diagnosed with a placenta previa. The nurse notes that the client is actively bleeding. Which of the following types of medications should the nurse anticipate the primary care provider will prescribe?

    A. Betamethasone (Celestone)

    B. Indomethacin (Indocin)

    C. Terbutaline (Brethine)

    D. Methylergonovine (Methergine)

5. A client presents to labor and delivery with stabbing abdominal pain, rigid abdomen and heavy, bright red bleeding. The nurse is aware that these findings are associated with which of the following?

    A. Placenta previa

    B. Vasa previa

    C. Abruptio placenta

    D. Threatened abortion

CHAPTER 7: BLEEDING DURING PREGNANCY

Ⓐ Application Exercises Answer Key

1. A woman arrives in the emergency department with abrupt, sharp right-sided lower-quadrant abdominal pain, and bright red vaginal spotting. She has missed one menstrual cycle. She tells the nurse that she cannot be pregnant because she has been using an intrauterine device. The nurse should suspect which of the following?

    A. Missed abortion

    B. Ectopic pregnancy

    C. Severe preeclampsia

    D. Hydatidiform mole

Signs and symptoms of an ectopic pregnancy include unilateral lower-quadrant abdominal pain with or without bleeding. A missed abortion occurs when products of conception are retained and there is a brownish discharge. Severe preeclampsia does not have vaginal bleeding unless initiated by worsening complications and presents with an epigastric, right upper quadrant pain. Hydatidiform mole causes dark brown bleeding in the second trimester and is not generally accompanied by abdominal pain.

Ⓝ **NCLEX® Connection: Physiological Adaptation, Alterations in Body Systems**

2. A nurse at an antepartum clinic is caring for a client who is at 4 months of gestation. The client reports continued nausea and vomiting and scant, prune-colored discharge. She has experienced no weight loss and has a fundal height larger than expected for the duration of pregnancy. Which of the following complications should the nurse suspect?

    A. Hyperemesis gravidarum

    B. Threatened abortion

    C. Hydatidiform mole

    D. Preterm labor

Hydatidiform mole (gestational trophoblastic disease) exhibits a uterine size that increases abnormally fast. The trophoblastic tissue causes abnormally high levels of hCG that result in excessive nausea and emesis. There is no fetus present on the ultrasound. There may be scant or profuse dark brown or red vaginal bleeding that first occurs in the second trimester, usually around the 16th week of gestation. Hyperemesis gravidarum is accompanied by weight loss and dehydration. Threatened abortion occurs in the first trimester and is indicated by spotting to moderate bleeding, but the uterus is not abnormally enlarged. Preterm labor presents prior to 37 weeks of gestation and is accompanied by pink-stained vaginal discharge and uterine contractions that become more regular.

 NCLEX® Connection: Physiological Adaptation, Alterations in Body Systems

3. A nurse is providing care for a client who is diagnosed with a marginal abruptio placenta. The nurse is aware that which of the following findings are risk factors for developing the condition? (Select all that apply.)

   X   **Maternal hypertension**

   X   **Blunt abdominal trauma**

   X   **Cocaine abuse**

         Maternal age

   X   **Cigarette smoking**

Maternal hypertension, blunt abdominal trauma, cocaine abuse, and cigarette smoking are risk factors for abruption placenta. Maternal age is not an associated risk for this condition. However, it is a risk factor for placenta previa.

 NCLEX® Connection: Physiological Adaptation, Alterations in Body Systems

4. A nurse is providing care for a client who is at 32 weeks of gestation and is diagnosed with placenta previa. The nurse notes that the client is actively bleeding. Which of the following medications should the nurse anticipate that the primary care provider will prescribe?

   A. Betamethasone (Celestone)

   B. Indomethacin (Indocin)

   C. Terbutaline (Brethine)

   D. Methylergonovine (Methergine)

Corticosteroids (Betamethasone) will be prescribed for fetal lung maturation if delivery of the fetus is anticipated (cesarean birth). Indocin and terbutaline are used to treat preterm labor. Methergine is used to treat postpartum hemorrhage.

 NCLEX® Connection: Pharmacological and Parenteral Therapies, Expected Actions/ Outcomes

5. A client presents to labor and delivery with stabbing abdominal pain, rigid abdomen and heavy, bright red bleeding. The nurse is aware that these findings are associated with which of the following?

   A. Placenta previa

   B. Vasa previa

   C. Abruptio placenta

   D. Threatened abortion

Abruptio placenta is the sudden onset of intense localized uterine pain with bright red vaginal bleeding. An abdomen that is both rigid and tender is also a common assessment finding. Placenta previa and vasa previa are conditions with painless vaginal bleeding. A threatened abortion may have slight abdominal cramping with spotting to moderate vaginal bleeding.

 NCLEX® Connection: Physiological Adaptation, Alterations in Body Systems

UNIT 1	ANTEPARTUM NURSING CARE
Section	Complications of Pregnancy
Chapter 8	Infections

Overview

- Maternal infections during pregnancy require prompt identification and treatment by a primary care provider. This section will explore HIV, TORCH infections, streptococcus ß-hemolytic, Group B, chlamydia, gonorrhea, and *Candida albicans*. Risk factors, assessment findings, collaborative care, and desired outcomes will be discussed.

HIV/AIDS

Overview

- HIV is a retrovirus that attacks and causes destruction of T lymphocytes. It causes immunosuppression in a client. HIV is transmitted from the mother to a neonate perinatally through the placenta and postnatally through the breast milk.

- Routine laboratory testing in the early prenatal period includes testing for HIV. Early identification and treatment significantly decreases the incidence of perinatal transmission.

- Testing is also recommended in the third trimester clients who are at an increased risk.

- Procedures, such as amniocentesis and an episiotomy, should be avoided due to the risk of maternal blood exposure.

- Use of internal fetal monitors, vacuum extraction, and forceps during labor should be avoided because of the risk of fetal bleeding.

- Administering injections and blood testing should not take place until the first bath is given to the neonate.

Risk Factors

- Risk Factors

  - IV drug use

  - Multiple sexual partners

  - Bisexuality

  - Maternal history of multiple STDs

  - Blood transfusion (rare occurrence)

Assessment

- Subjective Data

  o Fatigue

- Objective Data

  o Physical assessment findings

    ▪ Diarrhea

    ▪ Weight loss

    ▪ Anemia

  o Laboratory tests

    ▪ Obtain informed maternal consent prior to testing. Testing begins with an antibody screening test such as enzyme immunoassay. Confirmation of positive results is confirmed by Western blot testing.

    ▪ Screen the client for STDs such as, gonorrhea, Chlamydia, syphilis, and hepatitis B.

    ▪ Obtain frequent viral load levels and CD4 cell counts throughout the pregnancy.

Collaborative Care

- Nursing Care

  o Provide counseling prior to and after testing.

  o Refer the client for a mental health consultation, legal assistance, and financial resources.

  o Use standard precautions.

  o Administer antiviral combination therapy as prescribed.

  o Obtain prescribed laboratory testing.

- Medications

  o Retrovir (Zidovudine)

    ▪ Antiretroviral agent

    ▪ Nucleoside reverse transcriptase inhibitor

  o Nursing considerations

    ▪ Administer retrovir at 14 weeks of gestation, throughout the pregnancy, and before the onset of labor or cesarean birth.

    ▪ Administer retrovir to a neonate following delivery and for 6 weeks following.

- Health Promotion and Disease Prevention

  o Discharge instructions

    ▪ Instruct the client not to breastfeed.

    ▪ Discuss HIV and safe sexual relations with the client.

- Client Outcomes

  o The client will remain free from injury during pregnancy.

TORCH INFECTIONS

Overview

- TORCH is an acronym for a group of infections that can negatively affect a woman who is pregnant. These infections can cross the placenta and have teratogenic affects on the fetus. TORCH does not include all the major infections that present risks to the mother and fetus.

Risk Factors

- Toxoplasmosis is caused by consumption of raw or undercooked meat or handling cat feces. The symptoms are similar to influenza or lymphadenopathy.

- Rubella (German measles) is contracted through children who have rashes or neonates who are born to mothers who had rubella during pregnancy.

- Cytomegalovirus (member of herpes virus family) is transmitted by droplet infection from person to person, a virus found in semen, cervical and vaginal secretions, breast milk, placental tissue, urine, feces, and blood. Latent virus may be reactivated and cause disease to the fetus in utero or during passage through the birth canal.

- The herpes simplex virus (HSV) is spread by direct contact with oral or genital lesions. Transmission to the fetus is greatest during vaginal birth if the woman has active lesions.

Assessment

- Subjective Data

  o Toxoplasmosis symptoms similar to influenza or lymphadenopathy

  o Malaise, muscle aches, (flu-like symptoms)

  o Rubella joint and muscle pain

  o Cytomegalovirus has asymptomatic or mononucleosis-like symptoms

- Objective Data

  o Physical assessment findings

    ▪ Signs of rubella include rash, mild lymphedema, fever, and fetal consequences, which include miscarriage, congenital anomalies, and death.

    ▪ Herpes simplex virus initially presents with lesions.

- Signs of toxoplasmosis include fever and tender lymph nodes.
  - ○ Laboratory tests
    - For herpes simplex, obtain cultures from women who have HSV or are at or near term.
  - ○ Diagnostic procedures
    - A TORCH screen is an immunologic survey that is used to identify the existence of these infections in the mother (to identify fetal risks) or in her newborn (detection of antibodies against infections).
    - Prenatal screenings

Collaborative Care

- Nursing Care
  - ○ Monitor fetal well-being.
  - ○ Educate the client on prevention practices including good hand hygiene and cooking meat properly.
- Medications
  - ○ Administer antibiotics as prescribed.
  - ○ For toxoplasmosis treatment includes sulfonamides or a combination of pyrimethamine and sulfadiazine (potentially harmful to the fetus, but parasitic treatment essential).
- Health Promotion and Disease Prevention
  - ○ Client education
    - For rubella, vaccination of women who are pregnant is contraindicated because rubella infection may develop. These women should avoid crowds of young children. Women with low titers prior to pregnancy should receive immunizations.
    - Because no treatment for cytomegalovirus exists, tell client to prevent exposure by frequent hand hygiene before eating, and avoiding crowds of young children.
    - Emphasize to the client the importance of compliance with prescribed treatment.
    - Provide client with emotional support.
  - ○ Client outcomes
    - The client will remain free from infection.

STREPTOCOCCUS ß-HEMOLYTIC, GROUP B

Overview

- Streptococcus ß-hemolytic, Group B (GBS) is a bacterial infection that can be passed to a neonate during labor and delivery.

Risk Factors

- Risk Factors

  o History of positive culture with previous pregnancy

  o Risk factors for neonatal GBS

    ▪ Positive culture with pregnancy

    ▪ Prolonged rupture of membranes

    ▪ Preterm delivery

Assessment

- Objective Data

  o Physical assessment findings

    ▪ Positive GBS may have maternal and fetal effects including premature rupture of membranes, preterm labor and delivery, chorioamnionitis, infections of the urinary tract, and maternal sepsis.

  o Laboratory tests

    ▪ Vaginal and rectal cultures are performed at 35 to 37 weeks of gestation.

Collaborative Care

- Nursing Care

  o Administer prophylaxis antibiotics during labor.

- Medications

  o Penicillin G or ampicillin (Principen) may be prescribed to treat positive GBS.

    ▪ Administer penicillin 5 million units initially IV bolus, followed by 2.5 million units intermittent IV bolus every 4 hr. The client may be prescribed ampicillin 2 grams IV initially, followed by 1 g every 4 hr.

    ▪ Bactericidal antibiotic is used to destroy the GBS.

- Health Promotion and Disease Prevention

  o Client education

    ▪ Instruct the client to notify the labor and delivery nurse of GBS status.

- Client Outcomes

  o The newborn's blood culture is negative for GBS with no clinical signs of sepsis.

CHLAMYDIA

Overview

- Chlamydia is a bacterial infection caused by *Chlamydia trachomatis*. It is the most common STD. The infection is often difficult to diagnose because it is typically asymptomatic. According to current guidelines from the Centers for Disease Control and Prevention, all women and adolescents ages 20 to 25 who are sexually active should be screened for STDs.

Risk Factors

- Risk Factors
  - Multiple sexual partners
  - Unprotected sexual practices

Assessment

- Subjective Data
  - Vaginal spotting
  - Vulvar itching
- Objective Data
  - Physical assessment findings
    - White, watery vaginal discharge
  - Laboratory tests
    - Endocervical culture

Collaborative Care

- Nursing Care
  - Instruct the client to take the entire prescription as prescribed.
  - Identify and treat all sexual partners.
  - Clients who are pregnant should be retested 3 weeks after completing the prescribed regimen.
- Medications
  - Azithromycin (Zithromax), amoxicillin (Amoxil), and erythromycin (Ery-Tab) are prescribed during pregnancy.
    - Broad-spectrum antibiotic
    - Bactericidal action

- Nursing Care
  - □ Administer erythromycin (Romycin) to all neonates following delivery. This is the medication of choice for ophthalmia neonatorum. This antibiotic is both bacteriostatic and bactericidal, thus it provides prophylaxis against *Neisseria gonorrhoeae* and *Chlamydia trachomatis*.
- Client Education
  - □ Instruct the client to take all prescription as prescribed.
  - □ Educate the client about the possibility of decreasing effectiveness of oral contraceptives.
- Client Outcomes
  - The client will remain free from infection.

GONORRHEA

 Overview

- *Neisseria gonorrhoeae* is the causative agent of gonorrhea. Gonorrhea is a bacterial infection that is primarily spread by genital to genital contact. However, it can also be spread by anal to genital contact or oral to genital contact. It can also be transmitted to a neonate during delivery. Women are frequently asymptomatic.

Risk Factors

- Risk Factors
  - Multiple sexual partners
  - Unprotected sexual practices

Assessment

- Subjective Data (Male)
  - Urethral discharge
  - Painful urination
  - Frequency
- Subjective Data (Female)
  - Lower abdominal pain
  - Dysmenorrhea
- Objective Data – Male/Female
  - Physical assessment findings
    - Urethral discharge
    - Yellowish-green vaginal discharge

- ■ Reddened vulva and vaginal walls
- ■ If gonorrhea is left untreated, it can cause pelvic inflammatory disease, heart disease, and arthritis.
  - ○ Laboratory tests
    - ■ Urethral and vaginal cultures
    - ■ Urine culture

Collaborative Care

- Nursing Care
  - ○ Provide client education regarding disease transmission.
  - ○ Instruct the client to take the entire prescription as prescribed.
  - ○ Identify and treat all sexual partners.
- Medications
  - ○ Ceftriaxone (Rocephin) IM and azithromycin (Zithromax) PO for chlamydia
    - ■ One dose prescription
    - ■ Broad-spectrum antibiotic
    - ■ Bactericidal action
  - ○ Client education
    - ■ Instruct the client to take entire prescription as prescribed.
    - ■ Instruct the client to repeat the culture to assess for medication effectiveness.
    - ■ Educate the client regarding safe-sex practices.
- Client Outcomes
  - ○ The client will remain free from infection.

CANDIDA ALBICANS

Overview

- A fungal infection caused by *Candida albicans*.

Risk Factors

- Risk Factors
  - ○ Diabetes mellitus
  - ○ Oral contraceptives
  - ○ Recent antibiotic treatment

Assessment

- Subjective Data

    o Vulvar itching

- Objective Data

    o Physical assessment findings

        ■ Thick, creamy white vaginal discharge

        ■ Vulvar redness

        ■ White patches on vaginal walls

        ■ Gray-white patches on the tongue and gums (neonate)

    o Laboratory tests

        ■ Wet prep

    o Diagnostic procedures

        ■ Potassium hydroxide (KOH) prep

        ■ Presence of hyphae and pseudohyphae indicates positive findings

Collaborative Care

- Nursing Care

    o Medications

        ■ Fluconazole (Diflucan)

            □ Antifungal agent

            □ Fungicidal action

            □ Over-the-counter treatments, such as clotrimazole (Monistat), is available to treat candidiasis. However, it is important for the provider to diagnosis candidiasis initially.

- Health Promotion and Disease Prevention

    o Client education

        ■ Instruct the client to avoid tight-fitting clothing.

        ■ Instruct client to wear cotton-lined underpants.

        ■ Instruct client to limit wearing damp clothing.

        ■ Instruct client to void before and after intercourse and avoid douching.

        ■ Instruct client to increase dietary intake of yogurt with active cultures.

- Client outcomes

    o The client will remain free from infection.

CHAPTER 8: INFECTIONS

 Application Exercises

1. A nurse on the obstetrical unit is admitting client who is in labor. The client has a positive HIV status. The nurse is aware that which of the following is contraindicated for this client?

_____ Episiotomy

_____ Vacuum extraction

_____ Forceps

_____ Cesarean birth

_____ Internal fetal monitor

2. A nurse in an antepartum clinic is providing care for a client. Which of the following clinical findings are suggestive of TORCH? (Select all that apply.)

_____ Joint pain

_____ Malaise

_____ Rash

_____ Urinary frequency

_____ Tender lymph nodes

3. A nurse is caring for a client who is diagnosed with gonorrhea. Which of the following medications should the nurse anticipate the provider will prescribe?

A. Ceftriaxone (Rocephin)

B. Fluconazole (Diflucan)

C. Metronidazole (Flagyl)

D. Zidovudine (Retrovir)

4. A nurse is caring for a client who is in labor. The nurse is aware that which of the following conditions has medications that can be prescribed as prophylactic treatment during labor or immediately following delivery? (Select all that apply.)

_____ Gonorrhea

_____ Chlamydia

_____ HIV

_____ Streptococcus ß-hemolytic, Group B

_____ TORCH

CHAPTER 8: INFECTIONS

 Application Exercises Answer Key

1. A nurse on the obstetrical unit is admitting client who is in labor. The client has a positive HIV status. The nurse is aware that which of the following is contraindicated for this client?

X	**Episiotomy**
X	**Vacuum extraction**
X	**Forceps**
_____	Cesarean birth
X	**Internal fetal monitor**

An episiotomy is contraindicated for clients who are HIV positive due to the risk of maternal blood exposure. Additionally, the use of internal fetal monitors, vacuum extraction, and forceps during labor should be avoided because of the risk of fetal bleeding. A cesarean birth is not a contraindication for this client.

 NCLEX® Connection: Physiological Adaptation, Alterations in Body Systems

2. A nurse in an antepartum clinic is providing care for a client. Which of the following clinical findings are suggestive of TORCH? (Select all that apply.)

X	**Joint pain**
X	**Malaise**
X	**Rash**
_____	Urinary frequency
X	**Tender lymph nodes**

Symptoms of TORCH are flu-like in presentation. They may include reports of joint pain, malaise, rash, and tender lymph nodes. Urinary frequency is not a symptom associated with TORCH.

 NCLEX® Connection: Physiological Adaptation, Alterations in Body Systems

3. A nurse is caring for a client who is diagnosed with gonorrhea. Which of the following medications should the nurse anticipate the provider will prescribe?

A. Ceftriaxone (Rocephin)

B. Fluconazole (Diflucan)

C. Metronidazole (Flagyl)

D. Zidovudine (Retrovir)

Ceftriaxone IM or doxycycline (Vibramycin) orally for 7 days is prescribed for the treatment of gonorrhea. Fluconazole is used to treat candidiasis. Metronidazole is used in the treatment of bacterial vaginosis and trichomoniasis. Zidovudine is used to treat HIV/AIDS.

NCLEX® Connection: Physiological Adaptation, Alterations in Body Systems

4. A nurse is caring for a client who is in labor. The nurse is aware that which of the following conditions has medications that can be prescribed as prophylactic treatment during labor or immediately following delivery? (Select all that apply.)

__X__	**Gonorrhea**
__X__	**Chlamydia**
__X__	**HIV**
__X__	**Streptococcus ß-hemolytic, Group B**
_____	TORCH

Erythromycin (Romycin) is the medication of choice for ophthalmia neonatorum. This antibiotic is both bacteriostatic and bactericidal, thus it provides prophylaxis against *Neisseria gonorrhoeae* and *Chlamydia trachomatis*. It is administered to the neonate immediately following delivery. Retrovir (Zidovudine) is prescribed to the client in labor who is HIV positive. It is also administered to the neonate following delivery and for 6 weeks thereafter. Penicillin G or ampicillin (Principen) may be prescribed to treat positive GBS.

Ⓝ NCLEX® Connection: Physiological Adaptation, Alterations in Body Systems

UNIT 1	ANTEPARTUM NURSING CARE
Section	Complications of Pregnancy
Chapter 9	Medical Conditions

Overview

- Unexpected medical conditions may occur during pregnancy. Awareness, early detection, and interventions are crucial components to ensure fetal well-being and maternal health.

- Unexpected medical conditions include incompetent cervix, hyperemesis gravidarum, anemia, gestational diabetes mellitus, gestational hypertension/pregnancy-induced hypertension, and heart disease.

INCOMPETENT CERVIX

Overview

- Incompetent cervix is the painless dilation of the cervix in the absence of uterine contractions. The cervix is incapable of supporting the weight and pressure of the growing fetus and results in expulsion of the products of conception during the second trimester of pregnancy. This usually occurs around 20 weeks of gestation.

Risk Factors

- History of cervical trauma (previous lacerations, excessive dilations, and curettage for biopsy)

- In utero, exposure to diethylstilbestrol (ingested by the client's mother during pregnancy)

- Congenital structural defects

- Increased maternal age

Assessment

- Subjective Data

  o Increase in pelvic pressure

- Objective Data

  o Physical assessment findings

    ▪ Pink-stained vaginal discharge or bleeding

    ▪ Possible gush of fluid (rupture of membranes)

- Uterine contractions with the expulsion of the fetus

- Postoperative (cerclage) monitoring for uterine contractions, rupture of membranes, and signs of infection

  o Diagnostic and therapeutic procedures

- An ultrasound showing a short cervix (less than 20 mm in length) indicates a reduced cervical competence.

- Prophylactic cervical cerclage is the surgical reinforcement of the cervix with a heavy ligature that is placed submucosally around the cervix to strengthen it and prevent premature cervical dilation. The cerclage is removed at 37 weeks of gestation.

Collaborative Care

- Nursing Care

  o Evaluate the client's support systems and availability of assistance if activity restrictions and/or bed rest are prescribed.

  o Assess vaginal discharge.

  o Monitor client reports of pressure and contractions.

  o Check the client's vital signs and temperature.

- Medications

  o Administer tocolytics prophylactically to inhibit uterine contractions.

- Health Promotion and Disease Prevention

  o Discharge instructions

- Place the client on activity restriction/bed rest.

- Encourage hydration to promote a relaxed uterus (dehydration stimulates uterine contractions).

- Advise the client to refrain from intercourse, prolonged standing for more than 90 min, and heavy lifting.

  o Client education

- Provide client education about signs and symptoms to report to the primary care provider for preterm labor, rupture of membranes, infection, strong contractions less than 5 min apart, severe perineal pressure, and an urge to push.

- Instruct the client about using the home uterine activity monitor to monitor for uterine contractions.

- Arrange for the client to follow up with a home-health agency for close observation and supervision.

- Remove the cerclage around 37 weeks of gestation.

○   Client outcomes

- The client will remain free of injury during pregnancy.
- The client will maintain the pregnancy until term.

HYPEREMESIS GRAVIDARUM

Overview

- Hyperemesis gravidarum is excessive nausea and vomiting (related to elevated hCG levels) that is prolonged past 12 weeks of gestation and results in a 5% weight loss from prepregnancy weight, electrolyte imbalance, acetonuria, and ketosis.

- Hyperemesis gravidarum may be accompanied with liver dysfunction.

- There is a risk to the fetus for intrauterine growth restriction (IUGR) or preterm birth if the condition persists.

Risk Factors

- Maternal age younger than 20 years

- Obesity

- First pregnancy

- Multifetal gestation

- Gestational trophoblastic disease

- Women with a history of psychiatric disorders

- Transient hyperthyroidism

- Vitamin B deficiencies

- High stress levels

Assessment

- Objective Data

  ○   Physical assessment findings

  - Excessive vomiting for prolonged periods
  - Dehydration with possible electrolyte imbalance
  - Weight loss
  - Increased pulse rate
  - Decreased blood pressure
  - Poor skin turgor

o Laboratory tests

- Urinalysis for ketones and acetones (breakdown of protein and fat) is the most important initial laboratory test

- Elevated specific gravity

- Chemistry profile revealing electrolyte imbalances such as:

  □ Sodium, potassium, and chloride reduced from low intake.

  □ Acidosis resulting from excessive vomiting.

  □ Elevated liver enzymes

- Thyroid test indicating hyperthyroidism

- Hct concentration is elevated because inability to retain fluid results in hemoconcentration.

Collaborative Care

- Nursing Care

  o Monitor the client's I&O.

  o Assess the client's skin turgor and mucus membranes.

  o Monitor the client's vital signs.

  o Monitor the client's weight.

  o Have the client remain NPO for 24 to 48 hr.

  o Give the client IV fluids of lactated Ringer's solution for hydration.

- Medications

  o Give pyridoxine (Vitamin B_6) and other vitamin supplements as tolerated.

  o Use antiemetic medications cautiously for uncontrollable nausea and vomiting (promethazine [Phenergan], metoclopramide [Reglan]).

  o Use corticosteroids to treat refractory hyperemesis gravidarum.

- Health Promotion and Disease Prevention

  o Discharge instructions

    - Advance the client to clear liquids after 24 hr if no vomiting.

    - Advance the client's diet, as tolerated, with frequent, small meals. Start with dry toast, crackers, or cereal, then move to a soft diet, and finally to a normal diet as tolerated.

    - In severe cases, or if vomiting returns, enteral nutrition per feeding tube or total parental nutrition (TPN) may be considered.

     o   Client outcomes

         ■   The client will maintain fluid and electrolyte balance, stabilize weight, and retain meals.

ANEMIA

 Overview

- Iron-deficiency anemia occurs during pregnancy due to inadequacy in maternal iron stores and consuming insufficient amounts of dietary iron.

Risk Factors

- Risk Factors

     o   Less than 2 years between pregnancies

     o   Heavy menses

     o   Diet low in iron

Assessment

- Subjective Data

     o   Fatigue

     o   Irritability

     o   Headache

     o   Shortness of breath with exertion

     o   Palpitations

     o   Craving unusual food (pica)

- Objective Data

     o   Physical assessment findings

         ■   Pallor

         ■   Brittle nails

         ■   Shortness of breath

     o   Laboratory tests

         ■   Hgb < 12 mg/dL

         ■   Hct < 33%

Collaborative Care

- Nursing Care

     o   Prophylactic treatment of prenatal supplements with 60 mg of iron is suggested.

- o Increase dietary intake of foods rich in iron (legumes, fruit, green, leafy vegetables, and meat).

  - o Educate the client about ways to minimize gastrointestinal side effects.

- Medications

  - o Ferrous sulfate iron supplements

    - Used to increase Hgb and Hct levels

  - o Nursing considerations and client education

    - Instruct the client to take the supplement on an empty stomach.

    - Encourage the intake of vitamin C to increase absorption.

    - Suggest that the client increase roughage in diet to assist with discomforts of constipation.

  - o Iron dextran (Imferon)

    - Used in the treatment of iron-deficiency anemia when oral iron supplements cannot be tolerated by the client who is pregnant

  - o Client Outcomes

    - The client's Hgb and Hct levels will increase during the pregnancy.

GESTATIONAL DIABETES MELLITUS

Overview

- Gestational diabetes mellitus is an impaired tolerance to glucose with the first onset or recognition during pregnancy. The ideal blood glucose level during pregnancy should fall between 70 and 110 mg/dL.

- Symptoms of diabetes mellitus may disappear a few weeks following delivery. However, approximately 50% of women will develop diabetes mellitus within 5 years.

- Gestational diabetes mellitus causes increased risks to the fetus including:

  - o Spontaneous abortion, which is related to poor glycemic control.

  - o Infections (urinary and vaginal), which are related to increased glucose in the urine and decreased resistance because of altered carbohydrate metabolism.

  - o Hydramnios, which can cause overdistention of the uterus, premature rupture of membranes, preterm labor, and hemorrhage.

  - o Ketoacidosis from diabetogenic effect of pregnancy (increased insulin resistance), untreated hyperglycemia, or inappropriate insulin dosing.

  - o Hypoglycemia, which is caused by overdosing in insulin, skipped or late meals, or increased exercise.

  - o Hyperglycemia, which can cause excessive fetal growth (macrosomia).

Risk Factors

- Obesity

- Maternal age older than 25 years

- Family history of diabetes mellitus

- Previous delivery of an infant that was large or stillborn

Assessment

- Subjective Data

  o Hypoglycemia (nervousness, headache, weakness, irritability, hunger, blurred vision, tingling of mouth or extremities)

  o Hyperglycemia (thirst, nausea, abdominal pain, frequent urination, flushed dry skin, fruity breath)

- Objective Data

  o Physical assessment findings

    ▪ Hypoglycemia

    ▪ Shaking

    ▪ Clammy pale skin

    ▪ Shallow respirations

    ▪ Rapid pulse

    ▪ Hyperglycemia

    ▪ Vomiting

    ▪ Excess weight gain during pregnancy

  o Laboratory tests

    ▪ Routine urinalysis with glycosuria

    ▪ A Glucola screening test/1 hr glucose tolerance test (50 g oral glucose load, followed by plasma glucose analysis 1 hr later performed at 24 to 28 weeks of gestation – fasting not necessary; a positive blood glucose screening is 140 mg/dL or greater; additional testing with a 3-hr glucose tolerance test is indicated)

    ▪ A 3-hr glucose tolerance test (following overnight fasting, avoidance of caffeine, and abstinence from smoking for 12 hr prior to testing; a fasting glucose is obtained, a 100 g glucose load is given, and serum glucose levels are determined at 1, 2, and 3 hr following glucose ingestion)

    ▪ Ketones tested to assess the severity of ketoacidosis

  o Diagnostic procedures

    ▪ Biophysical profile to ascertain fetal well-being

- Amniocentesis with alpha-fetoprotein
- Nonstress test to assess fetal well-being

Collaborative Care

- Nursing Care

  o Monitor the client's blood glucose.

  o Monitor the fetus.

  o Instruct the client to perform daily kick counts.

- Medications

  o Administer insulin as prescribed.

    - Most oral hypoglycemic agents are contraindicated for gestational diabetes mellitus, but there is limited use of glyburide (DiaBeta) at this time. The provider will need to make the determination if these medications may be used.

- Health Promotion and Disease Prevention

  o Client education

    - Educate the client about diet and exercise.

    - Instruct the client about self-administration of insulin.

  o Desired client outcomes

    - The client will effectively manage and control blood glucose level throughout her pregnancy to ensure maternal/fetal well-being.

GESTATIONAL HYPERTENSION/PREGNANCY-INDUCED HYPERTENSION

Overview

- Hypertensive disease in pregnancy is divided into clinical subsets of the disease based on end-organ effects and progresses along a continuum from mild gestational hypertension, mild and severe preeclampsia, eclampsia, and hemolysis, elevated liver enzymes, and low platelets (HELLP) syndrome.

- Vasospasm contributing to poor tissue perfusion is the underlying mechanism for the signs and symptoms of pregnancy hypertensive disorders.

- Gestational hypertension (GH), which begins after the 20th week of pregnancy, describes hypertensive disorders of pregnancy whereby the woman has an elevated blood pressure at 140/90 mm Hg or greater, or a systolic increase of 30 mm Hg or a diastolic increase of 15 mm Hg from the prepregnancy baseline. There is no proteinuria or edema. The client's blood pressure returns to baseline by 12 weeks postpartum.

- Mild preeclampsia is GH with the addition of proteinuria of 1 to 2+ and a weight gain of more than 2 kg (4.4 lb) per week in the second and third trimesters. Mild edema will also begin to appear in the upper extremities or face.

- Severe preeclampsia consists of blood pressure that is 160/100 mm Hg or greater, proteinuria 3 to 4+, oliguria, elevated serum creatinine greater than 1.2 mg/dL, cerebral or visual disturbances (headache and blurred vision), hyperreflexia with possible ankle clonus, pulmonary or cardiac involvement, extensive peripheral edema, hepatic dysfunction, epigastric and right upper-quadrant pain, and thrombocytopenia.

- Eclampsia is severe preeclampsia symptoms along with the onset of seizure activity or coma. Eclampsia is usually preceded by headache, severe epigastric pain, hyperreflexia, and hemoconcentrations, which are warning signs of probable convulsions.

- HELLP syndrome is a variant of GH in which hematologic conditions coexist with severe preeclampsia involving hepatic dysfunction. HELLP syndrome is diagnosed by laboratory tests, not clinically.

  o H – hemolysis resulting in anemia and jaundice

  o EL – elevated liver enzymes resulting in elevated alanine aminotransferase (ALT) or aspartate transaminase (AST), epigastric pain, and nausea and vomiting

  o LP – low platelets (< 100,000/mm^3), resulting in thrombocytopenia, abnormal bleeding and clotting time, bleeding gums, petechiae, and possibly DIC

- Gestational hypertensive disease and chronic hypertension may occur simultaneously

- Gestational hypertensive diseases are associated with placental abruption, acute renal failure, hepatic rupture, preterm birth, and fetal and maternal death

Risk Factors

- No single profile identifies risks for gestational hypertensive disorders, but some high risks include:

  o Maternal age younger than 20 or older than 40.

  o First pregnancy.

  o Morbid obesity.

  o Multifetal gestation.

  o Chronic renal disease.

  o Chronic hypertension.

  o Familiar history of preeclampsia.

  o Diabetes mellitus.

  o Rh incompatibility.

  o Molar pregnancy.

  o Previous history of GH.

Assessment

- Subjective Data
  - Severe continuous headache
  - Nausea
  - Blurring of vision
  - Flashes of lights or dots before the eyes
- Objective Data
  - Physical assessment findings
    - Hypertension
    - Proteinuria
    - Periorbital, facial, hand, and abdominal edema
    - Pitting edema of lower extremities
    - Vomiting
    - Oliguria
    - Hyperreflexia
    - Scotoma
    - Epigastric pain
    - Right-upper quadrant pain
    - Dyspnea
    - Diminished breath sounds
    - Seizures
    - Jaundice
    - Signs of progression of hypertensive disease with indications of worsening liver involvement, renal failure, worsening hypertension, cerebral involvement, and developing coagulopathies
    - Rapid weight gain (2 kg [4.4 lb]) per week in the second and third trimesters
- Abnormal Laboratory Findings
  - Elevated liver enzymes (LDH, AST)
  - Increased creatinine
  - Increased plasma uric acid
  - Thrombocytopenia
  - Decreased Hgb
  - Hyperbilirubinemia

- Laboratory Tests

  o Liver enzymes

  o Serum creatinine, BUN, uric acid, and magnesium increase as renal function decreases

  o CBC

  o Clotting studies

  o Chemistry profile

- Diagnostic Procedures

  o Dipstick testing of urine for proteinuria

  o Twenty-four hour urine collection for protein and creatinine clearance

  o Nonstress test, contraction stress test, biophysical profile, and serial ultrasounds to assess fetal status

  o Doppler blood flow analysis to assess fetal well-being

Collaborative Care

- Nursing Care

  o Assess the client's level of consciousness.

  o Obtain pulse oximetry.

  o Monitor the client's urine output and obtain a clean-catch urine sample to assess for proteinuria.

  o Obtain daily weights.

  o Monitor vital signs.

  o Discuss lateral positioning.

  o Perform NST and daily kick counts as prescribed.

  o Instruct the client to monitor I&O.

- Medications

  o Magnesium sulfate

    ■ Anticonvulsant

    ■ Administer IV magnesium sulfate, which is the medication of choice for prophylaxis or treatment. It will lower blood pressure and depress the CNS.

  o Nursing considerations

    ■ Use an infusion control device to maintain a regular flow rate.

    ■ Inform the client that she may initially feel flushed, hot, and sedated with the magnesium sulfate bolus.

- Monitor the client's blood pressure, pulse, respiratory rate, deep-tendon reflexes, level of consciousness, urinary output (indwelling urinary catheter for accuracy), presence of headache, visual disturbances, epigastric pain, uterine contractions, and FHR and activity.

- Place the client on fluid restriction of 100 to 125 mL/hr, and maintain a urinary output of 30 mL/hr or greater.

- Monitor the client for signs of magnesium sulfate toxicity.

  □ Absence of patellar deep tendon reflexes

  □ Urine output less than 30 mL/hr

  □ Respirations less than 12/min

  □ Decreased level of consciousness

  □ Cardiac dysrhythmias

  ○ If magnesium toxicity is suspected:

- Immediately discontinue infusion.

- Administer antidote calcium gluconate.

- Prepare for actions to prevent respiratory or cardiac arrest.

- Health Promotion and Disease Prevention

  ○ Discharge instructions

- Maintain the client on bed rest and encourage her to lie in a side-lying position.

- Promote diversional activities.

- Have the client avoid foods that are high in sodium.

- Have the client avoid alcohol and limit caffeine.

- Instruct the client to increase her fluid intake to 8 glasses/day.

- Maintain a dark quiet environment to avoid stimuli that may precipitate a seizure.

- Maintain a patent airway in the event of a seizure.

- Administer antihypertensive medications as prescribed.

  ○ Client outcomes

- The client will maintain blood pressure within acceptable parameters.

- The client and fetus will remain free of injury.

HEART DISEASE

Overview

- Cardiovascular disease in pregnancy warrants early identification and monitoring to decrease incidence of maternal or fetal complications. Congenital cardiac anomaly and valvular disorders are the most commonly seen cardiovascular diseases in a client who is pregnant.

NEW YORK HEART ASSOCIATION'S CLASSIFICATION OF HEART DISEASE	
• Class I	• Client exhibits no symptoms with activity.
• Class II	• Client has symptoms with ordinary exertion.
• Class III	• Client displays symptoms with minimal exertion.
• Class IV	• Client has symptoms at rest.

- The above classification system will guide the primary care provider in the management of cardiovascular disease during the antepartum, intrapartum, and postpartum periods and assist with predicting client outcomes.

- The provider will evaluate the client's classification at 3 and 7 months gestation to determine appropriate treatment and interventions.

- Clients meeting classification I and II should experience a normal pregnancy and delivery. Total bed rest is indicated for clients in classification III. Clients within classification IV are not good candidates for pregnancy and all risk factors should be discussed with the client.

Risk Factors

- Preterm labor

- Miscarriage

- Intrauterine growth restriction

Assessment

- Subjective Data

  ○ Dizziness

  ○ Shortness of breath

  ○ Weakness

  ○ Fatigue

- o Chest pain on exertion

- o Anxiety

- Objective Data

  - o Physical assessment findings

    - Arrhythmias

    - Irregular heart rate

    - Tachycardia

    - Heart murmur

    - Distended jugular veins

    - Cyanosis of nails or lips

    - Pallor

    - Generalized edema

    - Diaphoresis

    - Increased respirations

    - Cough

    - Hemoptysis

    - Intrauterine growth restriction

    - Decreased amniotic fluid

    - FHR with decreased variability

  - o Laboratory tests

    - Hgb

    - Hct

    - WBC

    - Chemistry profile

    - Sedimentation rate

    - Maternal ABGs

    - Clotting studies

  - o Diagnostic procedures

    - Echocardiogram

    - Holter monitoring

    - Chest x-ray

    - Ultrasound

    - Pulse oximetry

- NST
- Biophysical profile

- Complications

  ○ Clients with cardiac disease may experience complications including right-sided heart failure, hypertension, arrhythmias, pulmonary hypertension, heart failure, aneurysm, aortic dissection, and maternal/fetal death.

Collaborative Care

- Nursing Care

  ○ Instruct the client to adhere to bed rest.

  ○ Provide the client with education related to restricting dietary sodium and adhering to a cardiac diet.

  ○ Instruct the client to decrease physical activity.

  ○ Monitor the client's vital signs.

  ○ Monitor FHR and uterine contractions.

  ○ Administer influenza and pneumococcus vaccines.

  ○ Encourage the client to take prenatal vitamins and iron supplements.

  ○ Administer oxygen to the client as prescribed.

  ○ Monitor the client's daily weight and urinary output.

  ○ Perform diagnostic procedures and laboratory studies as indicated.

  ○ Instruct the client to perform daily kick counts to assess fetal well-being.

  ○ Perform NST as prescribed.

- Medications

  ○ Pharmacological management is determined by the client's cardiac diagnoses and clinical presentation.

    - Propranolol (Inderal)
      □ Beta blocker
      □ Used to treat tachyarrhythmias and to lower maternal blood pressure
    - Gentamicin (Garamycin)
      □ Aminoglycoside antibiotic
      □ Prophylaxis that is given to prevent endocarditis
    - Ampicillin (Polycillin)
      □ Antibiotic
      □ Prophylaxis that is given to prevent endocarditis

- ■ Heparin sodium
    - □ Anticoagulant
    - □ Used in treating clients with pulmonary embolus, deep vein thrombosis, prosthetic valves, cyanotic heart defects, and rheumatic heart disease
- ■ Nursing considerations
    - □ Educate the client regarding self-administrations of anticoagulants.
    - □ Provide nutritional education regarding avoiding foods that are high in vitamin K.
- ■ Digoxin (Lanoxin)
    - □ Cardiac glycoside
    - □ Used to increase cardiac output during pregnancy, and may be prescribed if fetal tachycardia is present
- ○ Health promotion and disease prevention
- ○ Client education
    - ■ Instruct the client to notify the nurse of signs or symptoms of infection.
    - ■ Reinforce education related to medication therapy.
    - ■ Instruct the client to perform daily kick counts.
- ○ Client outcomes
    - ■ The client will remain free of injury during pregnancy.
    - ■ The client will be free of infection.

CHAPTER 9: MEDICAL CONDITIONS

 Application Exercises

1. A nurse is caring for a 16-year-old client who is gravida 1 para 0. The client is admitted to the labor unit showing signs of early labor. She has a blood pressure of 168/102 mm Hg, 3+ protein in her urine, and her face and hands are swollen. Which of the following medications should the nurse anticipate the primary care provider will prescribe for this client?

    A. Calcium gluconate

    B. Oxytocin

    C. Magnesium sulfate

    D. Prostaglandin

2. A nurse is caring for a client at 14 weeks of gestation who is diagnosed with hyperemesis gravidarum. The nurse is aware that which of the following are risk factors for the client? (Select all that apply.)

    _____ Obesity

    _____ Multifetal pregnancy

    _____ Maternal age greater than 40

    _____ Vitamin B deficiencies

    _____ Oligohydramnios

3. A nurse is administering magnesium sulfate IV to a client who has severe preeclampsia for seizure prophylaxis. Which of the following indicates magnesium sulfate toxicity? (Select all that apply.)

    _____ Respirations less than 12/min

    _____ Urinary output less than 30 mL/hr

    _____ Hyperreflexic deep-tendon reflexes

    _____ Decreased level of consciousness

    _____ Flushing and sweating

4. Which of the following classifications of heart disease is the client symptomatic with marked limitations on physical activity?

    A. Class I

    B. Class II

    C. Class III

    D. Class IV

5. A nurse is caring for a client who is diagnosed with mitral valve prolapse. The client's ECG findings reveal tachyarrhythmias. Which of the following medications should the nurse anticipate the provider will prescribe?

    A. Propranolol (Inderal)

    B. Gentamicin (Garamycin)

    C. Digoxin (Lanoxin)

    D. Nifedipine (Procardia)

CHAPTER 9: MEDICAL CONDITIONS

 Application Exercises Answer Key

1. A nurse is caring for a 16-year-old client who is gravida 1 para 0. The client is admitted to the labor unit showing signs of early labor. She has a blood pressure of 168/102 mm Hg, 3+ protein in her urine, and her face and hands are swollen. Which of the following medications should the nurse anticipate the primary care provider will prescribe for this client?

    A. Calcium gluconate

    B. Oxytocin

    C. Magnesium sulfate

    D. Prostaglandin

    Magnesium sulfate is an anticonvulsant that would be prescribed for a client who is exhibiting signs and symptoms of severe preeclampsia as evidenced by this client's elevated blood pressure and 3+ proteinuria. Depending on her gestational age, the primary care provider may want to augment the client's labor and order an oxytocin (Pitocin) drip. Calcium gluconate is the antidote for magnesium sulfate and will be a standing order to be administered in the event of magnesium sulfate toxicity. Prostaglandin is administered by a vaginal suppository to augment or induce labor.

     NCLEX® Connection: Physiological Adaptation, Alterations in Body Systems

2. A nurse is caring for a client at 14 weeks of gestation who is diagnosed with hyperemesis gravidarum. The nurse is aware that which of the following are risk factors for the client? (Select all that apply.)

    __X__   **Obesity**

    __X__   **Multifetal pregnancy**

    _____   Maternal age greater than 40

    __X__   **Vitamin B deficiencies**

    _____   Oligohydramnios

    Risk factors for hyperemesis gravidarum include obesity, multifetal gestation, vitamin B deficiencies, and maternal age less than 20. Oligohydramnios is not a risk factor for clients who have hyperemesis gravidarum.

     NCLEX® Connection: Physiological Adaptation, Alterations in Body Systems

3. A nurse is administering magnesium sulfate IV to a client who has severe preeclampsia for seizure prophylaxis. Which of the following indicates magnesium sulfate toxicity? (Select all that apply.)

   X   **Respirations less than 12/min**

   X   **Urinary output less than 30 mL/hr**

         Hyperreflexic deep-tendon reflexes

   X   **Decreased level of consciousness**

         Flushing and sweating

Signs of magnesium sulfate toxicity include the absence of patellar deep-tendon reflexes, urine output less than 30 mL/hr, respirations less than 12/min, and a decreased level of consciousness. Flushing and sweating are side effects of magnesium sulfate but are not signs of toxicity.

 NCLEX® Connection: Physiological Adaptation, Alterations in Body Systems

4. Which of the following classifications of heart disease is the client symptomatic with marked limitations on physical activity?

A. Class I

B. Class II

C. Class III

D. Class IV

The classification system will guide the provider in the management of cardiovascular disease. Clients exhibiting symptoms with marked limitations on physical activity are in Class III. Clients exhibits no symptoms with activity in Class I. Class II clients have symptoms with ordinary exertion. Class IV clients have symptoms at rest.

 NCLEX® Connection: Physiological Adaptation, Alterations in Body Systems

5. A nurse is caring for a client who is diagnosed with mitral valve prolapse. The client's ECG findings reveal tachyarrhythmias. Which of the following medications should the nurse anticipate the primary care provider will prescribe?

A. Propranolol (Inderal)

B. Gentamicin (Garamycin)

C. Digoxin (Lanoxin)

D. Nifedipine (Procardia)

Propranolol is prescribed to treat arrhythmias. Gentamicin is an antibiotic prophylaxis prescribed to prevent endocarditis. Digoxin is used to increase cardiac output during pregnancy. Nifedipine is given late in pregnancy to control high blood pressure.

 NCLEX® Connection: Physiological Adaptation, Alterations in Body Systems

UNIT 1	ANTEPARTUM NURSING CARE
Section	Complications of Pregnancy
Chapter 10	Early Onset of Labor

◎ Overview

- Understanding the importance of identifying the onset of early labor in a client who is pregnant is crucial for maternal and fetal well-being.

- Preterm labor, premature rupture of membranes, and preterm premature rupture of membranes will be mentioned in this chapter.

PRETERM LABOR

◎ Overview

- Preterm labor is defined as uterine contractions and cervical changes that occur between 20 and 37 weeks of gestation.

- It is important for a nurse to have a thorough understanding of the risk factors, assessment findings, and nursing interventions to care for the client who has preterm labor.

Risk Factors

- Infections of the urinary tract, vagina, or chorioamnionitis (infection of the amniotic sac)

- Previous preterm birth

- Multifetal pregnancy

- Hydramnios (excessive amniotic fluid)

- Age below 17 or above 35

- Low socioeconomic status

- Smoking

- Substance abuse

- Domestic violence

- History of multiple miscarriages or abortions

- Diabetes mellitus or hypertension

- Lack of prenatal care

- Incompetent cervix

- Placenta previa or abruptio placentae

- Preterm premature rupture of membranes

- Short interval between pregnancies

- Uterine abnormalities

- Diethylstilbestrol (DES) exposure in utero

    o DES was an agent widely used from 1948 to 1971 to diminish miscarriages; however, it is no longer used. DES exposure is now known to cause increased incidents of vaginal clear cell carcinoma in women who were exposed to DES while in utero.

Assessment

- Subjective Data

    o Persistent low backache

    o Pressure in the pelvis and cramping

    o Gastrointestinal cramping, sometimes with diarrhea

    o Urinary frequency

    o Vaginal discharge

- Objective Data

    o Physical assessment findings

        ■ Increase, change, or blood in vaginal discharge

        ■ Change in cervical dilation

        ■ Regular uterine contractions with a frequency of every 10 min or greater, lasting 1 hr or longer

        ■ Premature rupture of membranes

    o Laboratory tests

        ■ Obtain a vaginal swab for fetal fibronectin testing.

        ■ Assist with the collection of cervical cultures.

        ■ Perform a CBC.

        ■ Perform a urinalysis.

- Diagnostic procedures
  - Test for fetal fibronectin, a protein in the amniotic fluid that appears between 24 and 34 weeks of gestation. This protein can be found in the vaginal secretions when the fetal membrane integrity is lost.
  - Measure endocervical length with an ultrasound to assess for a shortened cervix, which is suggested in certain studies to precede preterm labor.
  - Use home uterine activity monitoring (HUAM), which is a uterine contraction monitoring device that can be used by the client at home.
  - HUAM is not considered to be effective in preventing preterm labor.
  - Obtain cervical cultures to detect if there is a presence of infectious organisms. Culture and sensitivity results guide prescription of an appropriate antibiotic, if indicated.
  - Perform a biophysical profile and/or a nonstress test to provide information about the fetal well-being.

Collaborative Care

- Nursing Care
  - Management of a client who is in preterm labor includes focusing on stopping uterine contractions.
    - Activity restriction
      - Instruct the client to remain on modified bed rest with bathroom privileges.
      - Encourage the client to rest in the left lateral position to increase blood flow to the uterus and decrease uterine activity.
      - Tell the client to avoid sexual intercourse.
    - Ensuring hydration
      - Dehydration stimulates the pituitary gland to secrete an antidiuretic hormone and oxytocin. Preventing dehydration will prevent the release of oxytocin, which stimulates uterine contractions.
    - Identifying and treating any infection
      - Have the client report any vaginal discharge, noting color, consistency, and odor.
      - Monitor maternal vital signs and temperature.
    - Chorioamnionitis should be suspected with the occurrence of elevated maternal temperature and tachycardia.
    - Monitor FHR and contraction pattern.
      - Fetal tachycardia, a prolonged increase in the FHR greater than 160/min may indicate infection, which is frequently associated with preterm labor.

- Medications

    o Terbutaline (Brethine)

        ■ Classification and therapeutic intent

            □ Terbutaline is a beta-adrenergic agonist that relaxes uterine smooth muscle by stimulating beta-2 receptors in the smooth muscle fibers to inhibit uterine activity.

        ■ Nursing considerations

            □ Monitor the client closely. Tocolytic therapy should be discontinued immediately if the client exhibits signs and symptoms of pulmonary edema, which includes chest pain, shortness of breath, respiratory distress, audible wheezing and crackles, and/or a productive cough containing blood-tinged sputum.

        ■ Vital signs

            □ Monitor the client's pulmonary function.

            □ Monitor the client's daily weights.

            □ Restrict the client's oral and IV fluid to 1,500 to 2,400 mL/24 hr to reduce the risk of pulmonary edema.

            □ Record the client's respiratory effort.

            □ Withhold the client's medication and contact the primary care provider if the maternal heart rate is 120 to 140/min, or if the client reports chest pain or cardiac arrhythmias

            □ Observe the injection site for infection if administered subcutaneously.

        ■ Client education

            □ Educate the client and family about adverse effects to observe for and when to notify the primary care provider.

            □ Inform the client that oral medication is frequently prescribed to take while at home.

    o Magnesium sulfate

        ■ Classification and therapeutic intent

            □ Magnesium sulfate is a commonly used tocolytic that relaxes the smooth muscle of the uterus and thus inhibits uterine activity by suppressing contractions.

        ■ Nursing considerations

            □ Monitor the client closely. Tocolytic therapy should be discontinued immediately if the client exhibits signs and symptoms of pulmonary edema, which includes chest pain, shortness of breath, respiratory distress, audible wheezing and crackles, and/or a productive cough containing blood-tinged sputum.

            □ Monitor for side effects.

□ Monitor for magnesium sulfate toxicity and discontinue for any of the following adverse effects, which include loss of deep tendon reflexes, urinary output less than 30 mL/hr, respiratory depression less than 12/min, pulmonary edema, and/or chest pain.

□ Administer calcium gluconate as an antidote for magnesium sulfate toxicity.

□ Contraindications for tocolysis include, but is not limited to, active vaginal bleeding, dilation of the cervix greater than 6 cm, chorioamnionitis, greater than 34 weeks of gestation and acute fetal distress.

■ Client education

□ Notify the nurse of blurred vision, headache, nausea, vomiting, or difficulty breathing.

○ Indomethacin (Indocin)

■ Classification and therapeutic Intent

□ Indomethacin is a nonsteroidal anti-inflammatory drug (NSAID) that suppresses preterm labor by blocking the production of prostaglandins. This inhibition of prostaglandins suppresses uterine contractions.

■ Inhibit uterine activity by suppressing contractions.

■ Nursing considerations

□ Monitor the client closely. Tocolytic therapy should be discontinued immediately if the client exhibits signs and symptoms of pulmonary edema, which includes chest pain, shortness of breath, respiratory distress, audible wheezing and crackles, and/or a productive cough containing blood-tinged sputum.

□ Indomethacin treatment should not exceed 48 hr.

□ Indomethacin should only be used if gestational age is less than 32 weeks of gestation.

□ Monitor the client for postpartum hemorrhage related to reduced platelet aggregation.

□ Administer indomethacin with food or rectally to decrease gastrointestinal distress.

□ Notify the nurse if the client reports blurred vision, headache, nausea, vomiting, or difficulty breathing.

□ Monitor the neonate at birth.

○ Betamethasone (Celestone)

■ Classification and therapeutic intent

□ Betamethasone is a glucocorticoid that is administered IM and requires a 24-hr period to be effective. The therapeutic action is to enhance fetal lung maturity and surfactant production.

- Nursing considerations
  - Administer the medication deep into the client's gluteal muscle 24 to 48 hr prior to birth of a preterm neonate.
  - Monitor the mother and neonate for pulmonary edema by assessing lung sounds.
  - Monitor for maternal and neonate hyperglycemia.
  - Monitor the neonate for heart rate changes.
- Client education
  - Educate the client regarding signs of pulmonary edema (chest pain, shortness of breath, and crackles).

- Health Promotion and Disease Prevention
  - Client outcomes
    - Client will maintain pregnancy until term.
    - Client's pregnancy will continue to promote fetal lung maturity.

PREMATURE RUPTURE OF MEMBRANES AND PRETERM PREMATURE RUPTURE OF MEMBRANES

Overview

- Premature rupture of membranes (PROM) is the spontaneous rupture of the amniotic membranes 1 hr or more prior to the onset of true labor. For most women, PROM signifies the onset of true labor if gestational duration is at term.

- Preterm premature rupture of membranes (PPROM) is the premature spontaneous rupture of membranes after 20 weeks of gestation and prior to 37 weeks of gestation.

Risk Factors

- Infection is the major risk of PROM and PPROM for both the client and the fetus. Once the amniotic membranes have ruptured, microorganisms can ascend from the vagina into the amniotic sac. PPROM is often preceded by infection.

- Chorioamnionitis is the infection of the amniotic membranes.
  - There is an increased risk of infection if there is a lag period over the 24-hr period from when the membranes rupture to delivery.

Assessment

- Subjective data
  - The client reports a gush or leakage of clear fluid from the vagina.

- ○ Objective data
  - ■ Physical assessment findings
    - □ Maternal temperature
    - □ Increased maternal or FHR
    - □ Foul-smelling fluid or vaginal discharge
    - □ Abdominal tenderness
  - ■ Assess the client for a prolapsed umbilical cord.
    - □ Abrupt FHR variable or prolonged deceleration
    - □ Visible or palpable cord at the introitus
- ○ Laboratory tests
  - ■ A positive Nitrazine paper test (blue, pH 6.5 to 7.5) or positive ferning test is conducted on amniotic fluid to verify rupture of membranes.

Collaborative Care

- Nursing Care
  - ○ Prepare for birth if indicated.
  - ○ Nursing management for PROM and PPROM is dependent on gestational duration, if there is evidence of infection, or an indication of fetal or maternal compromise.
  - ○ Provide reassurance to reduce maternal anxiety.
  - ○ Assess cervical dilation, effacement, and station.
  - ○ Assess vital signs every 2 hr.
  - ○ Notify the primary care provider of a temperature greater than 38° C (100° F).
  - ○ Assess FHR and uterine contractions.
  - ○ Advise the client to adhere to bed rest with bathroom privileges.
  - ○ Avoid vaginal exams.
  - ○ Encourage hydration.
  - ○ Obtain vaginal cultures for streptococcus ß-hemolytic, Group B, Chlamydia, and *Neisseria gonorrhoeae*
  - ○ Collect a CBC.
  - ○ Instruct the client to perform daily fetal kick counts.
  - ○ Notify the nurse of uterine contractions.

- Medications
  - Ampicillin (Omnipen)
    - Classification and therapeutic intent
      - Ampicillin is an antibiotic that is used to treat infection.
  - Nursing care
    - Obtain vaginal, urine, and blood cultures prior to administration of antibiotic.
  - Betamethasone (Celestone)
    - Classification and therapeutic intent
      - Betamethasone is a glucocorticoid that is administered IM in 2 injections, 24 hr apart and requires a 24-hr period to be effective. The therapeutic action is to enhance fetal lung maturity and surfactant production.
  - Nursing considerations
    - Administer the medication deep into the client's gluteal muscle 24 and 48 hr prior to birth of a preterm neonate.
    - Monitor the mother and neonate for pulmonary edema by assessing lung sounds.
    - Monitor for maternal and neonate hyperglycemia.
    - Monitor the neonate for heart rate changes.
  - Client education
    - Educate the client regarding signs of pulmonary edema (chest pain, shortness of breath, and crackles).
- Health Promotion and Disease Prevention
  - Discharge instructions
    - Expect that the client will be discharged home if dilation is less than 3 cm, no signs of infection, no contractions, and no malpresentation.
    - Advise the client to adhere to bed rest with bathroom privileges.
    - Encourage hydration.
  - Client education for PROM and PPROM
    - The client should conduct a self-assessment for uterine contractions.
    - The client should record daily kick counts for fetal movement.
    - The client should monitor for foul-smelling vaginal discharge.
      - Refrain from inserting anything into the vagina.
    - The client should abstain from intercourse.
    - The client should avoid tub baths.

- The client should wipe her perineal area from front to back after voiding and fecal elimination.

- The client should take her temperature every 4 hr when awake and report a temperature that is greater than 38° C (100° F).

- Desired Client Outcomes

  ○ The client will have no presence of fetal or maternal compromise.

CHAPTER 10: EARLY ONSET OF LABOR

 Application Exercises

1. A nurse is caring for a client who is prescribed terbutaline (Brethine) 0.25 mg subcutaneously. Which of the following is an adverse effect of this medication?

    A. Increased maternal heart rate

    B. Urinary frequency

    C. Low blood-glucose level

    D. Hyporeflexia

2. A nurse on a labor and delivery unit is providing care for a client who is at 32 weeks of gestation and is diagnosed with preterm labor. Which of the following medications should the nurse anticipate the primary care provider will prescribe to hasten fetal lung maturity?

    A. Terbutaline (Brethine)

    B. Indomethacin (Indocin)

    C. Nifedipine (Procardia)

    D. Betamethasone (Celestone)

3 Match the following terms with their appropriate phrases.

_____	Uterine contractions and cervical changes that occur between 20 and 37 weeks of gestation	A. Preterm premature rupture of membranes
_____	Spontaneous rupture of the amniotic membranes 1 hr or more prior to the onset of true labor	B. Chorioamnionitis
_____	Spontaneous rupture of membranes after 20 weeks of gestation and prior to 37 weeks of gestation	C. Preterm labor
_____	Infection of the amniotic membranes	D. Premature rupture of membranes

4. A nurse is caring for a client who is prescribed magnesium sulfate. The nurse recognizes that which of the following is a contraindication for use of this medication. (Select all that apply.)

    _____ Acute fetal distress

    _____ Preterm labor

    _____ Vaginal bleeding

    _____ Cervical dilation greater than 6 cm

    _____ Severe pregnancy-induced hypertension

CHAPTER 10: EARLY ONSET OF LABOR

 Application Exercises Answer Key

1. A nurse is caring for a client who is prescribed terbutaline (Brethine) 0.25 mg subcutaneously. Which of the following is an adverse effect of this medication?

   A. Increased maternal heart rate

   B. Urinary frequency

   C. Low blood-glucose level

   D. Hyporeflexia

   Maternal tachycardia is a normal adverse effect that will decrease over time. Urinary frequency and hyporeflexia are not adverse effects of terbutaline. Hyperglycemia, not hypoglycemia, is an adverse effect of the medication.

 NCLEX® Connection: Physiological Adaptation, Alterations in Body Systems

2. A nurse on a labor and delivery unit is providing care for a client who is at 32 weeks of gestation and is diagnosed with preterm labor. Which of the following medications should the nurse anticipate the primary care provider will prescribe to hasten fetal lung maturity?

   A. Terbutaline (Brethine)

   B. Indomethacin (Indocin)

   C. Nifedipine (Procardia)

   D. Betamethasone (Celestone)

   Betamethasone is a glucocorticoid that is given to clients in preterm labor to hasten surfactant production. Terbutaline, indomethacin and nifedipine are used for the treatment of preterm labor to maintain the pregnancy. However, these medications have no effect on fetal-lung maturity.

 NCLEX® Connection: Physiological Adaptation, Alterations in Body Systems

3. Match the following terms with their appropriate phrases.

__C__	Uterine contractions and cervical changes that occur between 20 and 37 weeks of gestation	A. Preterm premature rupture of membranes
__D__	Spontaneous rupture of the amniotic membranes 1 hr or more prior to the onset of true labor	B. Chorioamnionitis
__A__	Spontaneous rupture of membranes after 20 weeks of gestation and prior to 37 weeks of gestation	C. Preterm labor
__B__	Infection of the amniotic membranes	D. Premature rupture of membranes

 NCLEX® Connection: Physiological Adaptation, Alterations in Body Systems

4. A nurse is caring for a client who is prescribed magnesium sulfate. The nurse recognizes that which of the following is a contraindication for use of this medication. (Select all that apply.)

   X   **Acute fetal distress**

          Preterm labor

   X   **Vaginal bleeding**

   X   **Cervical dilation greater than 6 cm**

          Severe pregnancy-induced hypertension

Acute fetal distress and vaginal bleeding are complications that are contraindicated by the use of magnesium sulfate to stop labor. These clinical presentations would require immediate delivery of the fetus. Magnesium sulfate is also contraindicated for cervical dilation greater than 6 cm. Preterm labor and severe pregnancy-induced hypertension are indications for the use of magnesium sulfate.

Ⓝ NCLEX® Connection: Reduction of Risk Potential, Potential for Complications of Diagnostic Tests/Treatments/Procedures

UNIT 2: INTRAPARTUM NURSING CARE

- Labor and Delivery

- Complications of Labor and Delivery

NCLEX® CONNECTIONS

When reviewing the chapters in this unit, keep in mind the relevant sections of the NCLEX® outline, in particular:

CLIENT NEEDS: HEALTH PROMOTION AND MAINTENANCE

Relevant topics/tasks include:
- Ante/Intra/Postpartum and Newborn Care
  - Provide intrapartum care and education.

CLIENT NEEDS: PHYSIOLOGICAL ADAPTATION

Relevant topics/tasks include:
- Alterations in Body Systems
  - Provide care for the client experiencing complications of pregnancy/labor and/or delivery.

CLIENT NEEDS: PHARMACOLOGICAL AND PARENTERAL THERAPIES

Relevant topics/tasks include:
- Adverse Effects/Contraindications/Side Effects/Interactions
  - Identify contraindications to the administration of a medication to the client.
- Dosage Calculation
  - Use clinical decision making/critical thinking when calculating dosages.
- Medication Administration
  - Educate the client about medications.

CLIENT NEEDS: REDUCTION OF RISK POTENTIAL

Relevant topics/tasks include:
- Potential for Complications of Diagnostic Tests/Treatments/Procedures
  - Evaluate responses to procedures and treatments.
- Therapeutic Procedures
  - Assess the client's response to recovery from local, regional, or general anesthesia.

UNIT 2	INTRAPARTUM NURSING CARE
Section	Labor and Delivery
Chapter 11	**Labor and Delivery Processes**

Overview

- An intrapartum nurse should care for three clients during each labor and delivery:

  ○ Fetus.

  ○ Mother.

  ○ Family unit.

- Physiologic changes preceding labor (premonitory signs) include:

  ○ Backache – a constant low, dull backache, caused by pelvic muscle relaxation

  ○ Weight loss – a 0.5 to 1 kg (1 to 3 lb) weight loss

  ○ Lightening – fetal head descends into true pelvis about 14 days before labor; feeling that the fetus has "dropped;" easier breathing, but more pressure on bladder, resulting in urinary frequency; more pronounced in clients who are primigravida

  ○ Contractions – begin with irregular uterine contractions (Braxton Hicks) that eventually progress in strength and regularity

  ○ Bloody show – brownish or blood-tinged mucus discharge caused by expulsion of the cervical mucus plug resulting from the onset of cervical dilation and effacement

  ○ Energy burst – sometimes called "nesting" response

  ○ Gastrointestinal changes – less common, include nausea, vomiting, and indigestion

  ○ Rupture of membranes – spontaneous rupture of membranes can initiate labor or can occur anytime during labor, most commonly during the transition phase.

    ▪ Labor usually occurs within 24 hr of the rupture of membranes.

    ▪ Prolonged rupture of membranes greater than 24 hr before delivery of fetus may lead to an infection.

    ▪ Immediately following the rupture of membranes, a nurse should assess the FHR for abrupt decelerations, which are indicative of fetal distress to rule out umbilical cord prolapse.

  ○ Assessment of amniotic fluid – completed once the membranes rupture

    ▪ Color should be pale to straw yellow

- Odor should not be foul

- Clarity should appear watery and clear

- Volume is between 500 to 1,200 mL

- Nitrazine paper should be used by a nurse to test fluid to confirm that it is amniotic.

  □ Nitrazine tests the pH of the amniotic fluid. Deep blue (6.5 to 7.5) indicates fluid that is alkaline. If the fluid remains yellow, this indicates slight acidity because the fluid is urine.

- An intrapartum nurse should collect assessment data on maternal and fetal well-being during labor, the progress of labor, and psychosocial and cultural factors that affect labor.

- There are five factors (the five "Ps") that affect and define the labor and birth process: passenger, passageway, powers, position, and psychologic response.

  ○ Passenger – consists of the fetus and the placenta. The size of the fetal head, fetal presentation, lie, position, and attitude affect the ability of the fetus to navigate the birth canal. The placenta can be considered a passenger because it must also pass through the canal.

    - Lie – the relationship of the maternal longitudinal axis (spine) to the fetal longitudinal axis (spine).

      □ Transverse – fetal long axis is horizontal and forms a right angle to maternal axis and will not accommodate vaginal birth. The shoulder is the presenting part and may require delivery by cesarean birth if the fetus does not rotate spontaneously.

      □ Parallel or longitudinal – fetal long axis is parallel to maternal long axis, either a cephalic or breech presentation. Breech presentation may require a cesarean birth.

    - Attitude – relationship of fetal body parts to one another.

      □ Fetal flexion – chin flexed to chest, extremities flexed into torso.

      □ Fetal extension – chin extended away from chest, extremities extended.

    - Presentation – the part of the fetus that is entering the pelvic inlet first. It can be the back of the head (occiput), chin (mentum), shoulder (scapula), or breech (sacrum or feet).

    - Fetopelvic or fetal position – the relationship of the presenting part of the fetus (sacrum, mentum, or occiput) preferably the occiput, in reference to its directional position as it relates to one of the four maternal pelvic quadrants. It is labeled with three letters.

      □ The first letter references either the right (R) or left (L) side of the maternal pelvis.

      □ The second letter references the presenting part of the fetus, either occiput (O), sacrum (S), mentum (M), or scapula (Sc).

      □ The third letter references either the anterior (A), posterior (P), or transverse (T) part of the maternal pelvis.

    ■ Station – measurement of fetal descent in centimeters with station 0 being at the level of an imaginary line at the level of the ischial spines, minus stations superior to the ischial spines, and plus stations inferior to the ischial spines.

   ○ Passageway – the birth canal that is composed of the bony pelvis, cervix, pelvic floor, vagina, and introitus (vaginal opening). The size and shape of the bony pelvis must be adequate to allow the fetus to pass through it. The cervix must dilate and efface in response to contractions and fetal descent.

   ○ Powers – uterine contractions cause effacement and dilation of the cervix and descent of the fetus. Involuntary urge to push and voluntary bearing down in the second stage of labor helps in the expulsion of the fetus.

   ○ Position – of the woman who is in labor. The client should engage in frequent position changes during labor to increase comfort, relieve fatigue, and promote circulation. Position during the second stage is determined by maternal preference, primary care provider preference, and the condition of the mother and the fetus.

    ■ Gravity can aid in the fetal descent in upright, sitting, kneeling, and squatting positions.

   ○ Psychological response – maternal stress, tension, and anxiety can produce physiological changes that impair the progress of labor.

Nursing Interventions

- Preprocedure for Labor and Birth Process

   ○ Nursing actions

    ■ Leopold maneuvers – abdominal palpation of the number of fetuses, the fetal presenting part, lie, attitude, descent, and the probable location where fetal heart tones may be best auscultated on the woman's abdomen.

    ■ External electronic monitoring (tocotransducer) – separate transducer applied to the maternal abdomen over the fundus that measures uterine activity.

       □ Displays uterine contraction patterns

       □ Easily applied by the nurse, but must be repositioned with maternal movement to assure proper placement

    ■ External fetal monitoring (EFM) transducer applied to the abdomen of the client to assess FHR patterns during labor and birth.

    ■ Leopold maneuvers assist in identifying the best location for fetal heart tones.

   ○ Laboratory analysis

    ■ Urinalysis – clean-catch urine samples obtained to ascertain maternal:

       □ Hydration status via specific gravity.

       □ Nutritional status via ketones.

       □ Proteinuria, which is indicative of pregnancy-induced hypertension.

- ☐ Urinary tract infection via bacterial count.

- ☐ Beta-strep culture to check for streptococcus ß-hemolytic, Group B.

- ■ Blood tests

  - ☐ Hct level

  - ☐ ABO typing and Rh-factor if not previously done

- ○ Client education

  - ■ Provide the client/client's support network with ongoing education regarding the labor and delivery process and procedures.

- • Intraprocedure for Labor and Birth Process

  - ○ Nursing actions

    - ■ Assess maternal vital signs per agency protocol.

      - ☐ Check maternal temperature every 1 to 2 hr if membranes are ruptured.

    - ■ Assess FHR to determine fetal well-being. This may be performed by use of EFM or spiral electrode that is applied to the fetal scalp.

      - ☐ Prior to electrode placement, cervical dilation and rupture of membranes must occur.

    - ■ Assess uterine labor contraction characteristics by palpation (placing a hand over the fundus to assess contraction intensity, frequency, and duration) or by the use of the external or internal monitoring.

    - ■ Insert a solid, sterile, water-filled intrauterine pressure catheter inside the uterus to measure intrauterine pressure.

      - ☐ Displays uterine contraction patterns on monitor.

      - ☐ Requires the membranes to be ruptured and the cervix to be sufficiently dilated.

      - ☐ Frequency – established from the beginning of one contraction to the beginning of the next.

 View Media Supplement: Contraction Pattern (Image)

      - ☐ Duration – the time between the beginning of a contraction to the end of that same contraction.

      - ☐ Intensity – strength of the contraction at its peak described as mild, moderate, or strong.

      - ☐ Resting tone of uterine contractions – tone of the uterine muscle in between contractions.

        - ▸ A prolonged contraction duration or too frequent contractions without sufficient time for uterine relaxation in between can reduce blood flow to the placenta. This can result in fetal hypoxia and decreased FHR.

- Vaginal examination – performed digitally by the primary care provider or qualified nurse to assess for:

  □ Cervical dilation (stretching of cervical os adequate to allow fetal passage) and effacement (cervical thinning and shortening).

  □ Descent of the fetus through the birth canal as measured by fetal station in centimeters.

  □ Fetal position, presenting part, and lie.

  □ Membranes that are intact or ruptured.

CHARACTERISTICS OF TRUE VS. FALSE LABOR (BRAXTON HICKS CONTRACTIONS) TRUE LABOR LEADS TO CERVICAL DILATION AND EFFACEMENT	
TRUE LABOR	**FALSE LABOR**

• Contractions
  o May begin irregularly, but become regular in frequency
  o Stronger, last longer, and are more frequent
  o Felt in lower back, radiating to abdomen
  o Walking can increase contraction intensity
  o Continue despite comfort measures
	• Contractions
	  o Painless, irregular frequency, and intermittent
	  o Decrease in frequency, duration, and intensity with walking or position changes
	  o Felt in lower back or abdomen above umbilicus
	  o Often stop with sleep or comfort measures such as oral hydration or emptying of the bladder

• Cervix (assessed by vaginal exam)
  o Progressive change in dilation and effacement
  o Moves to anterior position
  o Bloody show
	• Cervix (assessed by vaginal exam)
	  o No significant change in dilation or effacement
	  o Often remains in posterior position
	  o No significant bloody show

• Fetus
  o Presenting part engages in pelvis
	• Fetus
	  o Presenting part is not engaged in pelvis

- Mechanism of labor – the adaptations the fetus makes as it progresses through the birth canal during the birthing process.

  □ Engagement – occurs when the presenting part, usually biparietal (largest) diameter of the fetal head passes the pelvic inlet at the level of the ischial spines. Referred to as station 0.

  □ Descent – the progress of the presenting part (preferably the occiput) through the pelvis. Measured by station during a vaginal examination, as either negative (#) station (measured in centimeters if superior to station 0 and not yet engaged) or positive (#) (station measured in centimeters if inferior to station 0).

    □   Flexion – when the fetal head meets resistance of the cervix, pelvic wall, or pelvic floor. The head flexes bringing the chin close to the chest, presenting a smaller diameter to pass through the pelvis.

    □   Internal rotation – the fetal occiput ideally rotates to a lateral anterior position as it progresses from the ischial spines to the lower pelvis in a corkscrew motion to pass through the pelvis.

    □   Extension – the fetal occiput passes under the symphysis pubis and then the head is deflected anteriorly and is born by extension of the chin away from the fetal chest.

    □   Restitution and external rotation – after the head is born, it rotates to the position it occupied as it entered the pelvic inlet (restitution) in alignment with the fetal body and completes a quarter turn to face transverse as the anterior shoulder passes under the symphysis.

    □   Expulsion – after birth of the head and shoulders the trunk of the neonate is born by flexing it toward the symphysis pubis.

STAGES OF LABOR			
STAGE	BEGINS WITH	ENDS WITH	MATERNAL CHARACTERISTICS
First stage: 12 1/2 hr (average)	• Onset of labor	• Complete dilation	• Cervical dilation 1 cm/hr for clients who are primigravida, and 1.5 cm/hr for clients who are multigravida, on average

Latent Phase:
 • Duration Primigravida:
   o 6 hr (approximately)
 • Duration Multigravida:
   o 4 hr (approximately)
	• Cervix 0 cm
	 • Irregular, mild to moderate contractions
	 • Frequency 5 to 30 min
	 • Duration 30 to 45 seconds
		• Cervix 3 cm	• Some dilation and effacement
			 • Talkative and eager

STAGES OF LABOR			
STAGE	BEGINS WITH	ENDS WITH	MATERNAL CHARACTERISTICS

Active Phase:
• Duration Primigravida:
  ○ 3 hr (approximately)
• Duration Multigravida:
  ○ 2 hr (approximately)
	• Cervix 4 cm
	• More regular, moderate to strong contractions
	• Frequency 3 to 5 min
	• Duration 40 to 70 seconds
		• Cervix 7 cm dilated	• Rapid dilation and effacement
			• Some fetal descent
			• Feelings of helplessness
			• Anxiety and restlessness increase as contractions become stronger

Transition: • Duration: ○ Approximately 20 to 40 min	• Cervix 8 cm • Strong to very strong contractions • Frequency 2 to 3 min • Duration 45 to 90 seconds	• Complete dilation at 10 cm	• Tired, restless, and irritable • Feeling out of control, client often states, "cannot continue" • May have nausea and vomiting • Urge to push • Increased rectal pressure and feelings of needing to have a bowel movement • Increased bloody show • Most difficult part of labor

Second Stage:
• Duration Primigravida:
  ○ 30 min to 2 hr
• Duration Multigravida:
  ○ 5 to 30 min
	• Full dilation
	• Intense contractions every 1 to 2 min
		• Birth	• Pushing results in birth of fetus

STAGES OF LABOR			
STAGE	BEGINS WITH	ENDS WITH	MATERNAL CHARACTERISTICS
Third Stage: • Duration Primigravida and Multigravida: ○ 5 to 30 min	• Delivery of the neonate	• Delivery of placenta	• Placental separation and expulsion • Schultze presentation: shiny fetal surface of placenta emerges first • Duncan presentation: dull maternal surface of placenta emerges first
Fourth Stage: • Duration Primigravida and Multigravida: ○ 1 to 4 hr	• Delivery of placenta	• Maternal stabilization of vital signs	• Achievement of vital sign homeostasis • Lochia scant to moderate rubra

View Media Supplement:
- Stages of Labor (Video)
- Schultze and Dirty Duncan Placenta (Images)

- Postprocedure for Labor and Delivery Process

  ○ Nursing assessments during fourth stage

  ▪ Maternal vital signs

  ▪ Fundus

  ▪ Lochia

  ▪ Perineum

  ▪ Urinary output

  ▪ Maternal/newborn bonding activities

  ○ Nursing interventions during the fourth stage

  ▪ Assess maternal vital signs every 15 min for the first hour and then according to facility protocol.

  ▪ Assess fundus and lochia every 15 min for the first hour and then according to facility protocol.

  ▪ Massage the uterine fundus and/or administer oxytocics as prescribed to maintain uterine tone to prevent hemorrhage.

- ■ Assess the client's perineum and provide comfort measures as indicated.

- ■ Encourage voiding to prevent bladder distention.

- ■ Promote an opportunity for maternal/newborn bonding.

○ Client education

- ■ Instruct the client to notify the nurse of increased vaginal bleeding or passage of blood clots. Offer assistance with breastfeeding and provide reassurance.

CHAPTER 11: LABOR AND DELIVERY PROCESSES

(A) Application Exercises

1. A client reports that her contractions started about 2 hr ago, did not go away when she had two glasses of water and rested, and became stronger since she started walking. She tells the nurse that the contractions occur every 10 min and last about half a minute. She hasn't had any fluid leak from her vagina; however, she did think she saw some blood when she wiped after voiding. Based on these reports, the nurse should recognize that the client is experiencing

   A. Braxton Hicks contractions.

   B. rupture of membranes.

   C. fetal descent.

   D. true contractions.

2. A nurse applies an external fetal monitor and tocotransducer to monitor the FHR and contractions of a client who is in labor. The FHR is around 140/min. Contractions are every 8 min and 30 to 40 seconds in duration. The nurse performs a vaginal exam and finds the cervix is 2 cm dilated, 50% effaced, and the fetus is at a -2 station. Which of the following stages and phases of labor is this client experiencing?

   A. The first stage, latent phase

   B. The first stage, active phase

   C. The first stage, transition phase

   D. The second stage of labor

3. A client experiences a large gush of fluid from her vagina while walking in the hallway of the birthing unit. The nurse's first nursing action after establishing that the fluid is amniotic fluid should be to

   A. assess the amniotic fluid for meconium.

   B. monitor the FHR for distress.

   C. dry the client and make her comfortable.

   D. monitor the client's uterine contractions.

4. While conducting an admission history for a client who is at 39 weeks of gestation, the client tells the nurse that she has been leaking fluid from her vagina for 2 days. The nurse knows that this client is at risk for

   A. cord prolapse.

   B. infection.

   C. postpartum hemorrhage.

   D. hydramnios.

5. A nurse is caring for a client who is in active labor and becomes nauseous and vomits. The client is also very irritable and feels that she needs to have a bowel movement. She states, "I've had enough. I can't do this anymore. I want to go home right now." The nurse knows that these signs indicate the client is in the

    A. second stage of labor.

    B. fourth stage of labor.

    C. transition phase of labor.

    D. latent phase of labor.

CHAPTER 11: LABOR AND DELIVERY PROCESSES

 Application Exercises Answer Key

1. A client reports that her contractions started about 2 hr ago, did not go away when she had two glasses of water and rested, and became stronger since she started walking. She tells the nurse that the contractions occur every 10 min and last about half a minute. She hasn't had any fluid leak from her vagina; however, she did think she saw some blood when she wiped after voiding. Based on these reports, the nurse should recognize that the client is experiencing

    A. Braxton Hicks contractions.

    B. rupture of membranes.

    C. fetal descent.

    D. true contractions.

    True contractions do not go away with hydration or walking. Instead, they are regular in frequency, duration, and intensity, and become stronger with walking. Braxton Hicks contractions decrease with hydration and walking. Fetal descent is the downward movement of the fetus in the birth canal. Rupture of membranes is when the amniotic membranes rupture and allow the amniotic fluid to escape.

 NCLEX® Connection: Health Promotion and Maintenance, Ante/Intra/Postpartum and Newborn Care

2. A nurse applies an external fetal monitor and tocotransducer to monitor the FHR and contractions of a client who is in labor. The FHR is around 140/min. Contractions are every 8 min and 30 to 40 seconds in duration. The nurse performs a vaginal exam and finds the cervix is 2 cm dilated, 50% effaced, and the fetus is at a -2 station. Which of the following stages and phases of labor is this client experiencing?

    A. The first stage, latent phase

    B. The first stage, active phase

    C. The first stage, transition phase

    D. The second stage of labor

    In stage 1, latent phase, the cervix dilates from 0 to 3 cm and contraction duration ranges from 30 to 45 seconds. In stage 1, active phase, the cervix dilates from 4 to 7 cm, and contraction duration ranges from 40 to 70 seconds. In stage 1, transition phase, the cervix dilates from 8 to 10 cm, and contraction duration ranges from 45 to 90 seconds. The second stage of labor consists of the expulsion of the fetus.

NCLEX® Connection: Health Promotion and Maintenance, Ante/Intra/Postpartum and Newborn Care

3. A client experiences a large gush of fluid from her vagina while walking in the hallway of the birthing unit. The nurse's first nursing action after establishing that the fluid is amniotic fluid should be to

    A. assess the amniotic fluid for meconium.

    B. monitor FHR for distress.

    C. dry the client and make her comfortable.

    D. monitor the client's uterine contractions.

    The greatest risk to the client and fetus is umbilical cord prolapse leading to fetal distress. Therefore, the first action the nurse should take is to monitor the FHR for distress. The nurse should then assess the color of the amniotic fluid, dry the client, and monitor the uterine contraction pattern.

    Ⓝ NCLEX® Connection: Physiological Adaptation, Alterations in Body Systems

4. While conducting an admission history for a client who is at 39 weeks of gestation, the client tells the nurse that she has been leaking fluid from her vagina for 2 days. The nurse knows that this client is at risk for

    A. cord prolapse.

    B. infection.

    C. postpartum hemorrhage.

    D. hydramnios.

    Rupture of membranes exceeding 24 hr before delivery increases the risk that infectious organisms will enter the vagina and then eventually into the uterus. While cord prolapse is a risk with rupture of membranes, it occurs when the fluid rushes out, rather than trickling or leaking out. The client is not at any greater risk for postpartum hemorrhage than other clients who are pregnant. Hydramnios means excess amniotic fluid. The client is more likely to have oligohydramnios or insufficient amniotic fluid.

    Ⓝ NCLEX® Connection: Physiological Adaptation, Alterations in Body Systems

5. A nurse is caring for a client who is in active labor and becomes nauseous and vomits. The client is also very irritable and feels that she needs to have a bowel movement. She states, "I've had enough. I can't do this anymore. I want to go home right now." The nurse knows that these signs indicate the client is in the

>   A. second stage of labor.
>
>   B. fourth stage of labor.
>
>   **C. transition phase of labor.**
>
>   D. latent phase of labor.

The transition phase of labor is the phase where the client becomes irritable, feels rectal pressure that can feel similar to the need to have a bowel movement, and can become nauseous with emesis. The second stage of labor is when the fetus is expulsed. The fourth stage is the recovery period. The latent phase of stage 1 is the beginning of labor, and the client is more relaxed, talkative, and eager for labor to progress.

Ⓝ NCLEX® Connection: Health Promotion and Maintenance, Ante/Intra/Postpartum and Newborn Care

UNIT 2	INTRAPARTUM NURSING CARE
Section	Labor and Delivery
Chapter 12	Pain Management

◎ Overview

- Pain is a subjective and individual experience, and each clients response to the pain of labor is unique.

- Sources of pain during the stages of labor

  - First stage – labor pain is an internal visceral pain that may be felt as back and leg pain, which is caused by:

    - Dilation, effacement, and stretching of the cervix.

    - Distention of the lower segment of the uterus.

    - Contractions of the uterus with resultant uterine ischemia.

  - Second stage – labor pain that is somatic and occurs with fetal descent and expulsion. Pain is caused by:

    - Pressure and distention of the vagina and the perineum, described by the client as "burning, splitting, and tearing."

    - Pressure and pulling on the pelvic structures (ligaments, fallopian tubes, ovaries, bladder, and peritoneum).

    - Lacerations of soft tissues (cervix, vagina, and perineum).

  - Third stage – labor pain with the expelling of the placenta is similar to the pain experienced during the first stage. Pain is caused by:

    - Uterine contractions.

    - Pressure and pulling of pelvic structures.

  - Fourth stage – pain is caused by:

    - Distention and stretching of the vagina and perineum incurred during the second stage with a splitting, burning, and tearing sensation.

- Safety for the mother and fetus must be the first consideration of the nurse when planning pain management measures.

Pain Assessment

- Pain level cannot always be assessed by monitoring the outward expressions of a client's pain. Client pain assessment may require persistent questioning and astute observation by the nurse. Cultural beliefs and behaviors of women during labor and delivery can affect the client's pain management.

  - Anxiety

    - Anxiety and fear are associated with pain. As fear and anxiety increase, muscle tension increases, and thus the experience of pain increases. This can become an increasing cycle of pain. The fear, tension, and pain cycle is illustrated below.

      - Fear

      - Fatigue

      - Full bladder

      - Individual pain tolerance

      - Previous experiences with pain

      - Fetal malposition

      - Cephalopelvic disproportion

      - Childbirth preparation

      - Level of support during labor

- Assess the beliefs and expectations related to discomfort, pain relief, and birth plans regarding pain relief methods for a client who is in labor.

- Assess the client's level, quality, frequency, duration, intensity, and location of pain through verbal and nonverbal cues. Use an appropriate pain scale allowing the client to indicate on a scale from 0 to 10 the severity of her pain with 10 representing the most severe pain.

  - Signs and symptoms of pain

    - Behavioral manifestations such as crying, moaning, screaming, gesturing, writhing, avoidance or withdrawal, and inability to follow instructions

    - Increasing blood pressure, tachycardia, and hyperventilation

- A nurse is responsible for helping the client maintain the proper position during administration of pharmacological interventions. She is also responsible for assisting the client with positioning for comfort after pharmacological administration during labor and birth.

- A nurse should provide client safety after the administration of any pharmacological intervention by putting the bed in a low position, maintaining side rails in the up position, placing the call light within the client's reach, and advising the client and her partner to call for assistance if she needs to leave the bed or ambulate.

- Evaluate the client's response to pain relief methods used (verbal report that pain is relieved or being relieved, appears relaxed between contractions).

TIMING AND EFFECTIVENESS OF PAIN RELIEF MEASURES DURING LABOR				
First Stage (Latent Phase)	First Stage (Active Phase)	Transition	Second Stage	Third Stage
Nonpharmacological methods ⟶				
Sedatives			Spinal block ━━━⟶	
	Opioids			
	Epidural ━━━━━━━━━━⟶			
			Pudendal ━━━⟶	
			Local infiltration ━━⟶	

Nonpharmacological Pain Management

- Nonpharmacological pain measures seek to reduce anxiety, fear, and tension, which are major contributing factors of pain in labor.

  ○ Gate-control theory of pain is based on the concept that the sensory nerve pathways that pain sensations use to travel to the brain will only allow a limited number of sensations to travel at any given time. By sending alternate signals through these pathways, the pain signals can be blocked from ascending the neurological pathway and inhibit the brain's perception and sensation of pain.

  ○ The gate-control theory of pain assists in the understanding of how nonpharmacological pain techniques can work to relieve pain.

- Interventions for nonpharmacological pain management

  ○ Childbirth preparation education, sensory and cutaneous strategies, and frequent maternal position changes

    ▪ Childbirth preparation methods such as Lamaze, Bradley, Dick-Read methods and/or pattern breathing methods are used to promote relaxation and pain relief.

      □ Nursing implications for breathing techniques include assessing for signs of hyperventilation (caused by low blood levels of PCO_2 from blowing off too much CO_2) such as light-headedness and tingling of the fingers.

      □ If hyperventilation occurs, have the client breathe into a paper bag or her cupped hands.

    ▪ Sensory stimulation strategies (based on the gate-control theory) to promote relaxation and pain relief

      □ Aroma therapy

      □ Breathing techniques

      □ Imagery

      □ Music

      □ Use of focal points

- Cutaneous strategies (based on the gate-control theory) to promote relaxation and pain relief
  - Back rubs and massage
  - Effleurage
    - Light, gentle circular stroking of the client's abdomen with the fingertips in rhythm with breathing during contractions
  - Sacral counterpressure
    - Consistent pressure is applied by the support person using the heel of the hand or fist against the client's sacral area to counteract pain in the lower back
  - Heat or cold therapy
  - Hydrotherapy (whirlpool or shower) increases maternal endorphin levels
  - Intradermal water block
  - Hypnosis
  - Acupressure
  - Transcutaneous electrical nerve stimulation (TENS) unit
- Frequent maternal position changes to promote relaxation and pain relief
  - Semi-sitting
  - Squatting
  - Kneeling
  - Kneeling and rocking back and forth
  - Supine position only with the placement of a wedge under one of the client's hips to tilt the uterus and avoid supine hypotension syndrome
- Client education
  - Teach the client who is in labor techniques to relieve labor pain, such as patterned breathing and progressive relaxation exercises.

Pharmacological Pain Management

- Pharmacological methods of pain relief include analgesia and local/regional anesthetics. To avoid slowing the progress of labor, prior to administering analgesic pain relief, the nurse should verify that labor is well established by performing a vaginal exam and evaluating uterine contraction pattern.

- Pharmacological Management
  - Alleviates pain sensations or raises the threshold for pain perception
  - Analgesia includes opioid analgesics and epidural and spinal regional analgesia.

- Sedatives (barbiturates) such as secobarbital (Seconal), pentobarbital (Nembutal), and phenobarbital (Luminal) are not typically used during birth, but can be used during the early or latent phase of labor to relieve anxiety and induce sleep.

  □ Adverse effects of sedatives

    ‣ Neonate respiratory depression secondary to the medication crossing the placenta and affecting the fetus

    ‣ Unsteady ambulation of the client

    ‣ Inhibition of the mother's ability to cope with the pain of labor. Sedatives should not be given if the client is experiencing pain, because apprehension can increase and cause the client to become hyperactive and disoriented.

  □ Client education

    ‣ Explain to the client that the medication will cause drowsiness.

    ‣ Instruct the client to request assistance with ambulation.

  □ Nursing actions

    ‣ Dim the lights and provide a quiet atmosphere.

    ‣ Provide safety for the client by lowering the position of the bed and elevate the side rails.

    ‣ Assist the mother to cope with labor.

    ‣ Assess the neonate for respiratory depression.

- Opioid analgesics such as meperidine hydrochloride (Demerol), fentanyl (Sublimaze), butorphanol (Stadol), and nalbuphine (Nubain) act in the CNS to decrease the perception of pain without the loss of consciousness. The client may be given opioid analgesics IM or IV, but the IV route is recommended during labor because action is quicker.

  □ Butorphanol (Stadol) and nalbuphine (Nubain) provide pain relief without causing significant respiratory depression in the mother or fetus. Both IM and IV routes are used.

  □ Adverse effects of opioid analgesics

    ‣ Crosses the placental barrier; if given to the mother too close to the time of delivery, opioid analgesics can cause respiratory depression in the neonate.

    ‣ Reduces gastric emptying; increases the risk for nausea and emesis

    ‣ Increases the risk for aspiration of food or fluids in the stomach

    ‣ Sedation

    ‣ Tachycardia

    ‣ Hypotension

    ‣ Decreased FHR variability

    ‣ Allergic reaction

□ Client education

▸ Explain to the client that the medication will cause drowsiness.

▸ Instruct the client to request assistance with ambulation.

□ Nursing actions

▸ Prior to administering analgesic or anesthetic pain relief, the nurse should verify that labor is well established with a fetus that is engaged.

▸ Administer antiemetics as prescribed.

▸ Monitor maternal vital signs, uterine contraction pattern, and continuous FHR monitoring.

■ Phenothiazine medications such as promethazine (Phenergan) or hydroxyzine (Vistaril) can control nausea and anxiety. They do not relieve pain and are used as an adjunct with opioids.

□ Adverse effects include dry mouth and sedation.

□ Nursing actions

▸ To avoid slowing the progress of labor, prior to administering analgesic pain relief, the nurse should verify that labor is well established by performing a vaginal exam that reveals cervical dilation of at least 4 cm with a fetus that is engaged.

▸ Provide ice chips or mouth swabs.

▸ Provide safety measures for the client.

■ Epidural and spinal regional analgesia consists of using analgesics such as fentanyl (Sublimaze) and sufentanil (Sufenta), which are short-acting opioids that are administered as a motor block into the epidural or intrathecal space without anesthesia. These opioids produce regional analgesia providing rapid pain relief while still allowing the client to sense contractions and maintain the ability to bear down.

□ Adverse effects of epidural and spinal analgesia

▸ Decreased gastric emptying resulting in nausea and vomiting

▸ Inhibition of bowel and bladder elimination sensations

▸ Bradycardia or tachycardia

▸ Hypotension

▸ Respiratory depression

▸ Allergic reaction and pruritus

▸ Elevated temperature

- □ Client education
  - ▸ Provide the client with ongoing education related to expectations for procedure.
- □ Nursing actions
  - ▸ Institute safety precautions, such as putting side rails up on the client's bed. The client may experience dizziness and sedation, which increases maternal risk for injury.
  - ▸ Assess the client for nausea and emesis and administer antiemetics as prescribed.
  - ▸ Monitor maternal vital signs per hospital protocol.
  - ▸ Monitor for allergic reaction.
  - ▸ Continue FHR pattern monitoring.

- Pharmacological Anesthesia
  - ○ Pharmacological anesthesia eliminates pain perceptions by interrupting the nerve impulses to the brain.
  - ○ Anesthesia used in childbirth includes regional blocks and general anesthesia.
    - ■ Regional blocks are most commonly used and consist of pudendal block, epidural block, spinal block, and paracervical nerve block.
      - □ Pudendal block consists of a local anesthetic such as lidocaine (Xylocaine) or bupivacaine (Marcaine) being administered transvaginally into the space in front of the pudendal nerve. This type of block has no maternal or fetal systemic effects, but it does provide local anesthesia to the perineum, vulva, and rectal areas during delivery, episiotomy, and episiotomy repair. It is administered during the second stage of labor 10 to 20 min before delivery providing analgesia prior to spontaneous expulsion of the fetus or forceps-assisted or vacuum-assisted birth.
      - □ Adverse effects of pudendal block
        - ▸ Broad ligament hematoma
        - ▸ Compromise of maternal bearing down reflex
      - □ Nursing actions
        - ▸ Instruct the client about the method.
        - ▸ Coach the client about when to bear down.
        - ▸ Assess the perineal and vulvar area postpartum for hematoma.

- An epidural block consists of a local anesthetic bupivacaine (Marcaine) along with an analgesic morphine (Duramorph) or fentanyl (Sublimaze) injected into the epidural space at the level of the fourth or fifth vertebrae. This eliminates all sensation from the level of the umbilicus to the thighs, relieving the discomfort of uterine contractions, fetal descent, and pressure and stretching of the perineum. It is administered when the client is in active labor and dilated to at least 4 cm. Continuous infusion or intermittent injections may be administered through an indwelling epidural catheter. Patient-controlled epidural analgesia is a new technique for labor analgesia and is becoming a favored method of acute pain relief management for labor and birth.

  □ Adverse effects of an epidural block

    ▸ Maternal hypotension

    ▸ Fetal bradycardia

    ▸ Inability to feel the urge to void

    ▸ Loss of the bearing down reflex

  □ Nursing actions

    ▸ Administer a bolus of IV fluids to help offset maternal hypotension as prescribed.

    ▸ Help to position and steady the client into either a sitting or side-lying modified Sims' position with her back curved to widen the intervertebral space for insertion of the epidural catheter.

    ▸ Encourage the client to remain in the side-lying position after insertion of the epidural catheter to avoid supine hypotension syndrome with compression of the vena cava.

    ▸ Coach the client in pushing efforts and request an evaluation of epidural pain management by anesthesia if pushing efforts are ineffective.

    ▸ Monitor maternal blood pressure and pulse, observe for hypotension, respiratory depression, and oxygen saturations.

    ▸ Assess FHR patterns continuously.

    ▸ Maintain the IV line and have oxygen and suction ready.

    ▸ Assess for orthostatic hypotension. If present, be prepared to administer an IV vasopressor such as ephedrine, position the client laterally, increase IV fluids, and initiate oxygen.

    ▸ Provide client safety such as raising the side rails of the bed. Do not allow the client to ambulate unassisted until all motor control has returned.

- Assess the maternal bladder for distention at frequent intervals and catheterize if necessary to assist with voiding.

- Monitor for the return of sensation in the client's legs after delivery but prior to standing. Assist the client with standing and walking for the first time after a delivery that included epidural anesthesia.

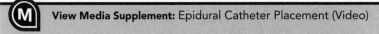
View Media Supplement: Epidural Catheter Placement (Video)

- Client education

  - Provide ongoing instructions related to the procedure and nursing actions.

- Spinal block consists of a local anesthetic that is injected into the subarachnoid space into the spinal fluid at the third, fourth, or fifth lumbar interspace. This can be done alone or in combination with an analgesic such as fentanyl (Sublimaze). The spinal block eliminates all sensations from the level of the nipples to the feet. It is commonly used for cesarean births. A low spinal block may be used for a vaginal birth, but is not used for labor. A spinal block is administered in the late second stage or before cesarean birth.

  - Adverse effects of a spinal block

    - Maternal hypotension

    - Fetal bradycardia

    - Loss of the bearing down reflex in the mother with a higher incidence of operative births

    - Potential headache from leakage of cerebrospinal fluid at the puncture site

    - Higher incidence of maternal bladder and uterine atony following birth

  - Nursing actions

    - Assess maternal vital signs every 10 min.

    - Manage maternal hypotension by administering an IV vasopressor, positioning the mother laterally, increasing IV fluids, and initiating oxygen.

    - Assess the client's uterine contractions.

    - Assess level of anesthesia.

    - Assess FHR patterns.

    - Provide client safety to prevent injury by raising the side rails of the bed, and assisting the client with repositioning and ambulating.

- ▸ Recognize signs of impending birth including sitting on one buttock, making grunting sounds, and bulging of the perineum.

- ▸ Encourage interventions to relieve a postpartum headache resulting from a cerebrospinal fluid leak. Interventions include placing the client in a supine position, promoting bed rest in a dark room, administering oral analgesics, caffeine, and fluids. An autologous blood patch is the most beneficial and reliable relief measure for cerebrospinal fluid leaks.

  □ Client education

  - ▸ Instruct the client about the method.

  - ▸ Instruct the client to bear down for expulsion of the fetus because during a vaginal birth, the mother will not feel her contractions.

- ■ General anesthesia is rarely used for vaginal or cesarean births when there are no complications present. It is only used in the event of a delivery complication or emergency when there is a contraindication to nerve block analgesia or anesthesia. General anesthesia produces unconsciousness.

  □ Nursing actions

  - ▸ Monitor maternal vital signs.

  - ▸ Monitor FHR patterns.

  - ▸ Ensure that the client has had nothing by mouth.

  - ▸ Ensure that the IV infusion is in place.

  - ▸ Premedicate the client with clear oral antacid to neutralize acidic stomach contents.

  - ▸ Administer a histamine H_2-receptor blocker such as ranitidine (Zantac) to decrease gastric acid production.

  - ▸ Administer metoclopramide (Reglan) to increase gastric emptying as prescribed.

  - ▸ Administer a short-acting barbiturate, such as thiopental sodium (Pentothal), to render the client unconscious as prescribed.

  - ▸ Administer succinylcholine chloride (Anectine), a muscle relaxant to facilitate passage of an endotracheal tube as prescribed.

  - ▸ Place a wedge under one of the client's hips to displace the uterus.

  - ▸ Assist with applying cricoid pressure before intubation.

  - ▸ Maintain an open airway and cardiopulmonary function.

  - ▸ Assess the client postpartum for maternal signs of decreased uterine tone, which can lead to hemorrhage and fetal narcosis, both of which can be produced by pharmacological agents used in general anesthesia.

  □ Client education for general anesthesia

  - ▸ Facilitate parent-newborn attachment as soon as possible.

CHAPTER 12: PAIN MANAGEMENT

 Application Exercises

1. A nurse is caring for a client who is at 40 weeks of gestation and experiencing contractions that are every 3 to 5 min, which are becoming stronger. A vaginal exam reveals that the client's cervix is 3 cm dilated, 80% effaced, and -1 station. The client states that she wants pain medication at this time. Which of the following interventions should the nurse suggest to the client at this time? (Select all that apply.)

_____ Patterned breathing techniques

_____ Insertion of indwelling urinary catheter

_____ Butorphanol (Stadol) 2 mg IV as prescribed

_____ Application of heat or cold

_____ Distraction or a focal point

2. A nurse is caring for a client who is in active labor. The client reports lower back pain. The nurse suspects that this pain is persistent occiput posterior presentation. Which of the following nonpharmacological nursing interventions should best alleviate this pain?

A. Abdominal effleurage

B. Sacral counterpressure

C. Hydrotherapy if not contraindicated

D. Back rub and massage

3. A nurse anesthetist is explaining an epidural procedure to a client who agrees that this is the best way to help suppress her pain. What is the role of the nurse before, during, and after administration of an epidural? (Select all that apply.)

_____ Administer a bolus of IV fluids prior to epidural insertion.

_____ Position the client in the lithotomy position for epidural catheter insertion.

_____ Have oxygen and suction ready in the event of respiratory depression.

_____ Palpate the client's bladder for distention and insert an indwelling urinary catheter if necessary.

_____ Encourage the client to ambulate to the bathroom every 1 to 2 hr to void.

4. A nurse is caring for a client who is primipara and in active labor. The client received meperidine (Demerol) 50 mg IV for pain 30 min prior to precipitous delivery. Which of the following medications should the nurse be prepared to administer?

A. Naloxone (Narcan) to the mother

B. Promethazine (Phenergan) to the mother

C. Naloxone (Narcan) to the neonate

D. Promethazine (Phenergan) to the neonate

5. A nurse is caring for a client who is in labor. Which of the following should the nurse assess for following placement of an epidural?

    A. Tachycardia in the fetus

    B. Hypotension in the mother

    C. Facial edema in the mother

    D. Irregular heartbeats in the fetus

6. A client in the labor and delivery unit is in the second stage of labor. Her labor has been progressing well without complications and she is expected to deliver vaginally in 20 min. The primary care provider is preparing to administer lidocaine (Xylocaine) for pain relief and perform an episiotomy. The nurse knows that this type of regional anesthetic block will likely be used with which of the following?

    A. Pudendal block

    B. Epidural block

    C. Spinal block

    D. Paracervical block

7. A nurse is caring for a client in labor. The client experiences hypotension and fetal bradycardia. Which of the following nursing actions should the nurse implement? (Select all that apply.)

    _____   Administer an ephedrine IV bolus.

    _____   Place the client in side-lying position.

    _____   Increase IV fluids.

    _____   Administer O_2 via face mask.

    _____   Administer naloxone (Narcan).

CHAPTER 12: PAIN MANAGEMENT

 Application Exercises Answer Key

1. A nurse is caring for a client who is at 40 weeks of gestation and experiencing contractions that are every 3 to 5 min, which are becoming stronger. A vaginal exam reveals that the client's cervix is 3 cm dilated, 80% effaced, and -1 station. The client states that she wants pain medication at this time. Which of the following interventions should the nurse suggest to the client at this time? (Select all that apply.)

   X   **Patterned breathing techniques**

          Insertion of indwelling urinary catheter

   X   **Butorphanol (Stadol) 2 mg IV as prescribed**

   X   **Application of heat or cold**

   X   **Distraction or a focal point**

Nonpharmacological comfort measures can be safely used at this time while the client is in the latent phase of labor. In addition, she may have the opioid analgesic. There is no indication for insertion of an indwelling urinary catheter.

 NCLEX® Connection: Basic Care and Comfort, Complementary and Alternative Therapies

2. A nurse is caring for a client who is in active labor. The client reports lower back pain. The nurse suspects that this pain is persistent occiput posterior presentation. Which of the following nonpharmacological nursing interventions should best alleviate this pain?

   A. Abdominal effleurage

   B. Sacral counterpressure

   C. Hydrotherapy if not contraindicated

   D. Back rub and massage

Sacral counterpressure is the application of steady pressure to the lower back to counteract the pressure exerted on the spinal nerves by the fetus, which especially occurs with an occiput posterior presentation. Abdominal effleurage is a gentle stroking of the abdomen in rhythm with breathing during contractions. Hydrotherapy, a back rub, and massage may be helpful, but counterpressure is most effective in relieving back discomfort.

 NCLEX® Connection: Basic Care and Comfort, Complementary and Alternative Therapies

3. A nurse anesthetist is explaining an epidural procedure to a client who agrees that this is the best way to help suppress her pain. What is the role of the nurse before, during, and after administration of an epidural? (Select all that apply.)

   __X__   **Administer a bolus of IV fluids prior to epidural insertion.**

   _____   Position the client in the lithotomy position for epidural catheter insertion.

   __X__   **Have oxygen and suction ready in the event of respiratory depression.**

   __X__   **Palpate the client's bladder for distention and insert indwelling Foley catheter if necessary.**

   _____   Encourage the client to ambulate to the bathroom every 1 to 2 hr to void.

An IV bolus of fluids may be administered prior to epidural anesthesia to compensate for hypotension. The client is either in a sitting position or modified Sims' position to widen the intervertebral space for catheter insertion. Maternal vital signs are monitored for hypotension and respiratory depression. Oxygen and suction should be available for respiratory depression or aspiration. Epidural anesthesia diminishes the client's ability to recognize the urge to void. Therefore, bladder palpation for distention with possible catheterization is necessary. The client should not ambulate to the bathroom without assistance while receiving epidural anesthesia.

(N) NCLEX® Connection: Pharmacological and Parenteral Therapies, Parenteral/Intravenous Therapy

4. A nurse is caring for a client who is primipara and in active labor. The client received meperidine (Demerol) 50 mg IV for pain 30 min prior to precipitous delivery. Which of the following medications should the nurse be prepared to administer?

A. Naloxone (Narcan) to the mother

B. Promethazine (Phenergan) to the mother

C. Naloxone (Narcan) to the neonate

D. Promethazine (Phenergan) to the neonate

Naloxone (Narcan) (an opioid antagonist) should be administered to the neonate for respiratory depression. Promethazine is administered as an adjunct to opioid medications to reduce the amount of opioid medication required or to counteract nausea.

(N) NCLEX® Connection: Pharmacological and Parenteral Therapies, Pharmacological Pain Management

5. A nurse is caring for a client who is in labor. Which of the following should the nurse assess for following placement of an epidural?

    A. Tachycardia in the fetus

    B. Hypotension in the mother

    C. Facial edema in the mother

    D. Irregular heartbeats in the fetus

    Monitor the mother for hypotension because it is an adverse effect of epidural analgesia. Epidural analgesia also causes fetal bradycardia, not irregular heartbeats. Epidurals do not affect maternal edema.

 NCLEX® Connection: Pharmacological and Parenteral Therapies, Parenteral/Intravenous Therapy

6. A client in the labor and delivery unit is in the second stage of labor. Her labor has been progressing well without complications and she is expected to deliver vaginally in 20 min. The primary care provider is preparing to administer lidocaine (Xylocaine) for pain relief and perform an episiotomy. The nurse knows that this type of regional anesthetic block that will likely be used with which of the following?

    A. Pudendal block

    B. Epidural block

    C. Spinal block

    D. Paracervical block

    A pudendal block is a transvaginal injection of a local anesthetic into the area in front of the pudendal nerve that anesthetizes the perineum, vulva, and rectal areas for episiotomy, expulsion of the fetus, and episiotomy repair. Epidural blocks are administered during labor and allow the client to participate in the labor process while remaining comfortable. Spinal blocks are administered late in the second stage, but most commonly preceding a cesarean birth. Paracervical blocks are used early in labor to block pain of uterine contractions and are rarely used today because of serious adverse effects.

 NCLEX® Connection: Pharmacological and Parenteral Therapies, Pharmacological Pain Management

7. A nurse is caring for a client in labor. The client experiences hypotension and fetal bradycardia. Which of the following nursing actions should the nurse implement? (Select all that apply.)

   __X__   **Administer an ephedrine IV bolus.**

   __X__   **Place the client in side-lying position.**

   __X__   **Increase IV fluids.**

   __X__   **Administer O$_2$ via face mask.**

   _____   Administer naloxone (Narcan).

The nurse should be prepared to administer ephedrine via an IV bolus, position the client laterally, increase IV fluids, and initiate oxygen. Naloxone will not correct the hypotension or fetal bradycardia. It is used to correct neonatal depression caused by maternal opioids.

(N) **NCLEX® Connection: Health Promotion and Maintenance, Ante/Intra/Postpartum and Newborn Care**

UNIT 2	INTRAPARTUM NURSING CARE
Section	Labor and Delivery
Chapter 13	Fetal Assessment During Labor

 Overview

- Describe fetal assessment during labor.

- The diagnostic procedures mentioned in this chapter include FHR pattern and uterine contraction monitoring, Leopold maneuvers, fetal scalp blood sampling, and fetal oxygen monitoring.

LEOPOLD MANEUVERS

- Description of Procedure

> **View Media Supplement:** Leopold Maneuvers (Video)

- ○ Leopold maneuvers consist of performing external palpations of the maternal uterus through the abdominal wall to determine the:

    - Number of fetuses.

    - Presenting part.

    - Fetal attitude.

    - Fetal lie.

    - Degree of fetal descent into the pelvis.

    - Expected location of the point of maximal impulse (PMI).

        □ PMI is the optimal location where the fetal heart tones are auscultated the loudest on the woman's abdomen. These tones are best heard directly over the fetal back.

        □ In vertex presentation, PMI is either in the right- or left-lower quadrant or below the maternal umbilicus.

        □ In breech presentation, PMI is either in the right- or left-upper quadrant above the maternal umbilicus.

- Nursing Actions
  - Preparation of the client
    - Ask the client to empty her bladder before beginning the assessment.
    - Place the client in the supine position with a pillow under her head and have her flex her knees slightly.
    - Place a wedge under her right hip to displace the uterus to the left and prevent supine hypotension/vena cava syndrome.
  - Ongoing care
    - Identify the fetal part occupying the fundus. The head should feel round, firm, and move freely The breech should feel irregular and soft.
    - Identify the fetal lie and presenting part.
    - Locate and palpate the smooth contour of the fetal back using the palm of one hand and the irregular small parts of the hands, feet, and elbows using the palm of the other hand.
    - Identify the fetal presentation.
    - Determine the fetal presenting part over the true pelvis inlet by gently grasping the lower segment of the uterus between the thumb and fingers. If the head is presenting and not engaged, determine whether the head is flexed or extended.
    - Identify the fetal attitude.
    - Face the client's feet and outline the fetal head using the palmar surface of the fingertips on both hands to palpate the cephalic prominence. If the cephalic prominence is on the same side as the small parts, the head is flexed with vertex presentation. If the cephalic prominence is on the same side as the back, the head is extended with a face presentation.
    - Identify the attitude of the head.
  - Interventions
    - If using an external ultrasound transducer, place the tocotransducer based on the findings obtained from the maneuvers for optimal auscultation of the FHR.
    - Auscultate the FHR postmaneuvers to assess the fetal tolerance to the procedure.
    - Document the findings from the maneuvers.

FHR PATTERN AND UTERINE CONTRACTION MONITORING

- Description of Procedure
  - Intermittent auscultation and uterine contraction palpation

- Intermittent auscultation of the FHR is a low-technology method that can be performed during labor using a hand-held Doppler ultrasound device, an ultrasound stethoscope, or fetoscope to assess FHR. In conjunction, palpation of contractions at the fundus for frequency, duration, and intensity is used to evaluate fetal well-being. During labor, uterine contractions compress the uteroplacental arteries, temporarily stopping maternal blood flow into the uterus and intervillous spaces of the placenta, decreasing fetal circulation and oxygenation. Circulation to the uterus and placenta resumes during uterine relaxation between contractions. For low-risk labor and delivery, this procedure allows the woman freedom of movement and can be done at home or a birthing center.

- Guidelines for intermittent auscultation or continuous electronic fetal monitoring

  □ Low-risk women

    ‣ During latent phase, every 60 min

    ‣ During active phase, every 30 min

    ‣ During second stage, every 15 min

  □ High-risk women

    ‣ During latent phase, every 30 min

    ‣ During active phase, every 15 min

    ‣ During second stage, every 5 min

- Indications

  ○ Potential diagnoses

    - Rule out labor

    - Active labor

  ○ Guidelines for intermittent auscultation following routine procedures

    - Rupture of membranes, either spontaneously or artificially

    - Preceding and subsequent to ambulation

    - Prior to and following administration of or a change in medication anesthesia

    - At peak action of anesthesia

    - Following vaginal examination

    - Following expulsion of an enema

    - After urinary catheterization

    - In the event of abnormal or excessive uterine contractions

- Interpretation of Findings

  ○ A normal, reassuring FHR is 110 to 160/min with increases and decreases from baseline.

- Nursing Actions
  - Preparation of the client
    - Perform Leopold maneuvers to determine point of maximum impulse (PMI).
    - Auscultate at PMI using listening device.
    - Palpate the client's abdomen at uterine fundus to assess uterine activity.
    - Count FHR for 30 to 60 seconds to determine baseline rate.
    - Auscultate FHR during a contraction and for 30 seconds following the completion of the contraction.
  - Ongoing care
    - Identify any nonreassuring FHR patterns and notify the primary care provider.
  - Interventions
    - It is the responsibility of the nurse to assess FHR patterns, implement nursing interventions, and report nonreassuring patterns to the primary care provider.
    - The emotional, educational, and comfort needs of the mother and the family must be incorporated into the plan of care while continuing to assess the FHR pattern's response to the labor process.
  - The method and frequency of fetal surveillance during labor will vary and depend on maternal-fetal risk factors as well as the preference of the facility, primary care provider, and client.
- Description of Procedure
  - Continuous electronic fetal monitoring
    - Continuous external fetal monitoring is accomplished by securing an ultrasound transducer over the client's abdomen to determine PMI, which records the FHR pattern, and a tocotransducer on the fundus that records the uterine contractions.
    - Advantages of external fetal monitoring
      - Noninvasive and reduces risk for infection
      - Membranes do not have to be ruptured
      - Cervix does not have to be dilated
      - Placement of transducers can be performed by the nurse
      - Records permanent record of FHR tracing
    - Disadvantages of external fetal monitoring
      - Contraction intensity is not measurable
      - Movement of the client requires frequent repositioning of transducers
      - Quality of recording is affected by client obesity and fetal position

- Indications for Monitoring
  - Potential diagnoses
    - Multiple gestations; oxytocin (Pitocin) infusion (augmentation or induction of labor)
    - Placenta previa
    - Fetal bradycardia
    - Maternal complications (diabetes mellitus, pregnancy-induced hypertension, renal disease)
    - Intrauterine growth restriction
    - Post dates
    - Active labor
    - Meconium-stained amniotic fluid
    - Abruption placenta – suspected or actual
    - Abnormal nonstress test or contraction stress test
    - Abnormal uterine contractions
    - Fetal distress
  - Interpretation of findings
    - A normal fetal heart rate baseline at term is 110 to 160/min excluding accelerations, decelerations, and periods of marked variability within a 10 min window. At least 2 min of baseline segments in a 10 min window should be present. A single number should be documented instead of a baseline range.
    - Fetal heart rate baseline variability is described as fluctuations in the FHR baseline that are irregular in frequency and amplitude. Classification of variability is as follows:
      - Absent or undetectable variability (considered nonreassuring)
      - Minimal variability (> undetectable but < 5/min)
      - Moderate variability (6 to 25/min)
      - Marked variability (> 25/min)
    - Changes in fetal heart rate patterns are categorized as episodic or periodic changes. Episodic changes are not associated with uterine contractions and periodic changes occur with uterine contractions. These changes include accelerations and decelerations.
    - According to a report from the 2008 National Institute of Child Health Human Development Workshop, current recommendations for fetal monitoring include a three-tier fetal heart rate interpretation system.
      - Category I: All of the following are included in the fetal heart rate tracing:
        - Baseline fetal heart rate of 110-160/min
        - Baseline fetal heart rate variability: moderate

- ▸ Accelerations: present or absent
- ▸ Early decelerations: present or absent
- ▸ Variable or late decelerations: absent
- ▫ Category II: Category II tracings include all fetal heart rate tracings not categorized as Category I or Category III. Examples of Category II fetal heart rate tracings contain any of the following:
  - ▸ Baseline rate
    - ▹ Tachycardia
    - ▹ Bradycardia not accompanied by absent baseline variability
  - ▸ Baseline FHR variability
    - ▹ Minimal baseline variability
    - ▹ Absent baseline variability not accompanied by recurrent decelerations
    - ▹ Marked baseline variability
  - ▸ Episodic or periodic decelerations
    - ▹ Prolonged fetal heart rate deceleration > 2 min but < 10 min
    - ▹ Recurrent late decelerations with moderate baseline variability
    - ▹ Recurrent variable decelerations with minimal or moderate baseline variability
    - ▹ Variable decelerations with additional characteristics, including "overshoots", "shoulders", or slow return to baseline fetal heart rate
  - ▸ Accelerations
    - ▹ Absence of induced accelerations after fetal stimulation
- ▫ Category III: Category III fetal heart rate tracings include either:
  - ▸ Sinusoidal pattern
  - ▸ Absent baseline fetal heart rate variability and any of the following:
    - ▹ Recurrent variable decelerations
    - ▹ Recurrent late decelerations
    - ▹ Bradycardia
- ■ Each uterine contraction is comprised of:
  - ▫ Increment – the beginning of the contraction as intensity is increasing.
  - ▫ Acme – the peak intensity of the contraction.
  - ▫ Decrement – the decline of the contraction intensity as the contraction is ending.
- ■ Nonreassuring FHR patterns are associated with fetal hypoxia and include:
  - ▫ Fetal bradycardia.
  - ▫ Fetal tachycardia.

□   Absence of FHR variability.

□   Late decelerations.

□   Variable decelerations.

FHR PATTERNS	CAUSES/COMPLICATIONS	NURSING INTERVENTIONS
Accelerations (variable transitory increase in the FHR above baseline)	• Healthy fetal/placental exchange • Intact fetal central nervous system (CNS) response to fetal movement • Vaginal exam • Fundal pressure	• Reassuring • No interventions required • Indicate reactive nonstress test
Fetal bradycardia (FHR <110/min for 10 min or more)	• Uteroplacental insufficiency • Umbilical cord prolapse • Maternal hypotension • Prolonged umbilical cord compression • Fetal congenital heart block • Anesthetic medications	• Discontinue oxytocin (Pitocin) if it is being infused. • Help the client into a side-lying position. • Administer oxygen (8 to 10 L/min by mask). • Start an IV line if one is not in place. • Administer a tocolytic medication as prescribed. • Notify the primary care provider.
Fetal tachycardia (FHR >160 beats/min for 10 min or more)	• Maternal infection, chorioamnionitis • Fetal anemia • Fetal heart failure • Fetal cardiac dysrhythmias • Maternal use of cocaine or methamphetamines • Maternal dehydration	• If maternal fever exists, administer antipyretics as prescribed. • Administer oxygen (8 to 10 L/min by mask). • Give bolus of IV fluids.
Decrease or loss of FHR variability (decrease or loss of irregular fluctuations in the baseline of the FHR)	• Medications that depress the CNS such as narcotics, barbiturates, tranquilizers, or general anesthetics • Fetal hypoxemia with resulting acidosis • Fetal sleep cycle • Congenital abnormalities	• Stimulate the fetal scalp. • Assist primary care provider with application of scalp electrode or fetal blood pH sampling. • Position the client into a left-lateral position.

FHR PATTERNS	CAUSES/COMPLICATIONS	NURSING INTERVENTIONS
Early deceleration of FHR (slowing of FHR with start of contraction with return of FHR to baseline at end of contraction)	• Compression of the fetal head resulting from uterine contraction • Vaginal exam • Fundal pressure	• No intervention required.
Late deceleration of FHR (slowing of FHR after contraction has started with return of FHR to baseline well after contraction has ended)	• Uteroplacental insufficiency causing inadequate fetal oxygenation • Maternal hypotension, abruptio placentae, uterine hyperstimulation with oxytocin (Pitocin)	• Change the client to a side-lying position. • Start an IV line if not in place or increase the IV rate. • Discontinue oxytocin (Pitocin) if being infused. • Administer oxygen 8 to 10 L/min per mask. • Notify the primary care provider. • Prepare for an assisted vaginal birth or cesarean birth.
Variable deceleration of FHR (transitory, abrupt slowing of FHR <110 beats/min, variable in duration, intensity, and timing in relation to uterine contraction)	• Umbilical cord compression • Short cord • Prolapsed cord • Nuchal cord (around fetal neck) • Oligohydramnios	• Change the client's position. • Discontinue oxytocin (Pitocin) if it is being infused. • Administer oxygen at 8 to 10 L/min per mask. • Perform or assist with a vaginal examination. • Assist with an amnioinfusion if ordered.

View Media Supplement:

- Early Decelerations (Image)
- Minimal Variability (Image)
- Late Decelerations (Image)
- Variable Decelerations (Image)

- Nursing Actions

  - Preparation of the Client

    - Use Leopold maneuvers to locate the fetal presenting part and the optimal location for placement of the ultrasound transducer for the best possible auscultation of FHR.

    - Palpate uterine activity at the fundus to identify proper placement location for the tocotransducer to monitor uterine contractions.

- Ongoing Care
  - Provide education regarding the procedure to the client and the client's partner during placement and adjustments of the fetal monitor equipment.
  - Encourage frequent maternal position changes. Explain to the client that adjustments of the monitor may be necessary with position changes.
  - If the client needs to void and can ambulate, and it is not contraindicated, the nurse can disconnect the external monitor for the client to use the bathroom.
  - If disconnecting of FHR monitor is contraindicated or internal FHR monitor is being used, the nurse can bring the client a bedpan.

- Description of Procedure
  - Continuous internal fetal monitoring
    - Continuous internal fetal monitoring with a scalp electrode is performed by attaching a small spiral electrode to the presenting part of the fetus to monitor the FHR. The electrode wires are then attached to a leg plate that is placed on the client's thigh and then attached to the fetal monitor.
    - Continuous internal fetal monitoring may be used in conjunction with an intrauterine pressure catheter (IUPC), which is a solid or fluid-filled transducer placed inside the client's uterine cavity to monitor the frequency, duration, and intensity of contractions. The average pressure is usually 50 to 85 mm Hg.
      - Advantages of internal fetal monitoring
        - Early detection of abnormal FHR patterns suggestive of fetal distress
        - Accurate measurement of uterine contraction intensity
        - Obesity or maternal and fetal movement does not affect recording
        - Accurate assessment of FHR variability
        - Allows greater maternal freedom of movement without compromising tracing
      - Disadvantages of internal fetal monitoring
        - Membranes must have ruptured to use internal monitoring
        - Cervix must be adequately dilated to a minimum of 2 to 3 cm
        - Presenting part must have descended enough to place electrode
        - Potential risk of injury to fetus if electrode is not properly applied
        - Contraindicated with vaginal bleeding
        - Potential risk of infection to the client and the fetus
        - A primary care provider, nurse practitioner/midwife, or specially trained registered nurse must perform this procedure

- Nursing Actions
  - Preparation of the client
    - Ensure electronic fetal monitoring equipment is functioning properly.
    - Continue to monitor FHR patterns.
    - Use aseptic techniques if assisting with procedures.
  - Ongoing care
    - Monitor maternal vital signs and obtain maternal temperature every 1 to 2 hr.
    - Encourage frequent repositioning of the client. If the client is lying supine, place a wedge under one of the client's hips to tilt her uterus.
- Complications
  - Misinterpretation of FHR patterns
  - Maternal or fetal infection
  - Fetal trauma if fetal monitoring electrode or IUPC are inserted into the vagina improperly
  - Supine hypotension secondary to internal monitor placement

FETAL SCALP BLOOD SAMPLING

- Description of Procedure
  - Fetal scalp blood sampling is performed by obtaining a sample of blood from the fetal scalp through the cervical opening once the cervix has sufficiently dilated and the membranes have ruptured.
    - This sampling is obtained to assess the fetal blood gases consisting of the pH, PO_2, and PCO_2.
- Indications
  - Potential diagnoses
    - Fetal distress
    - High-risk fetus
  - Client presentation
    - Nonreassuring FHR (to verify an ominous heart rate pattern on the monitor)
- Nursing Actions
  - Interventions
    - Continue to monitor FHR pattern.
    - Communicate nonreassuring FHR to primary care provider so that a decision can be made whether to perform a fetal scalp blood sampling.
    - Assist with swabbing the fetal scalp with disinfectant prior to the primary care provider performing the scalp puncture.
    - After the procedure, monitor contractions. Monitor for new scalp bleeding.

- Interpretation of Findings
  - The pH will decrease if fetal hypoxia is present. A normal fetal scalp blood pH is 7.25. A finding of < 7.20 is indicative of fetal distress and requires immediate intervention.

FETAL OXYGEN SATURATION MONITORING

- Description of Procedure

  - Fetal oxygen saturation monitoring/fetal pulse oximetry is performed by inserting a specially designed sensor next to the fetal cheek or temple area to assess fetal oxygen saturation ($FSpO_2$).
    - Criteria for use of fetal oxygen saturation
      - Nonreassuring FHR
      - Used in single fetus gestation
      - At least 36 weeks gestation
      - Vertex presentation
      - Ruptured membranes
      - Cervix dilated to at least 2 cm
      - Fetal station at least -2
    - Evaluation of fetal oxygen saturation provides further information to support the decision of whether to allow labor to continue or to intervene with augmentation or preparation of an emergency cesarean birth.

- Indications

  - Potential diagnoses
    - High-risk fetus
    - Fetal distress
  - Client presentation
    - Nonreassuring FHR

- Interpretation of Findings

  - Normal $FSpO_2$ is 30 to 70%

- Nursing Actions

  - Ongoing care
    - Identify potential candidates for fetal oxygen saturation monitoring.
    - Assist in interpreting data obtained from fetal oxygen saturation monitoring.
    - Assist the primary care provider during the procedure as needed.
    - Communicate findings to the primary care provider.
    - Document findings and interventions.

CHAPTER 13: FETAL ASSESSMENT DURING LABOR

(A) Application Exercises

1. A nurse is providing care for a client who is in active labor. Her cervix is dilated to 5 cm and her membranes are intact. The FHR and uterine contractions are being monitored by an external electronic fetal monitor. The nurse notes a FHR of 115 to 125/min with occasional increases up to 150 to 155/min that last for 25 seconds, and have beat-to-beat variability of 20/min. There is no slowing of FHR from the baseline. The nurse should recognize that this client is exhibiting signs of which of the following? (Select all that apply.)

_____ Moderate variability

_____ FHR accelerations

_____ No FHR decelerations

_____ Normal baseline FHR

_____ Fetal tachycardia

2. A nurse is caring for a client who is being induced for labor and is being monitored by an external electronic fetal monitor. The nurse notes that the FHR variability is decreased and resembles a straight line. The mother has not had any pain medication. Which of the following should occur first for an internal scalp electrode to be applied?

A. Dilation

B. Rupture of the membranes

C. Effacement

D. Engagement

3. A nurse is reviewing the fetal monitor tracing of a client who is in active labor. The nurse knows that a fetus receives more oxygen during which of the following?

A. Peak of the uterine contraction

B. Increment of the uterine contraction

C. Decrement of the uterine contraction

D. Relaxation between uterine contractions

4. A client who is delivering in a birthing center is in the second stage of labor and is having no complications. Intermittent auscultation of FHR and uterine palpation of contractions is being performed to monitor FHR patterns. The nurse should assess the FHR every

A. 60 min.

B. 30 min.

C. 15 min.

D. 5 min.

5. Which of the following is the initial nursing action the nurse should take when late decelerations appear on the fetal monitor?

    A. Reposition the client into the left-lateral position.

    B. Apply a fetal scalp electrode.

    C. Increase the IV fluid rate.

    D. Perform a vaginal exam to assess dilation.

6. Episodic accelerations of the FHR from baseline should be interpreted by the nurse as indicative of

    A. intact CNS response to fetal movement.

    B. fetal response to maternal fever.

    C. fetal distress requiring intervention.

    D. fetal hypoxia requiring maternal oxygen.

CHAPTER 13: FETAL ASSESSMENT DURING LABOR

 Application Exercises Answer Key

1. A nurse is providing care for a client who is in active labor. Her cervix is dilated to 5 cm and her membranes are intact. The FHR and uterine contractions are being monitored by an external electronic fetal monitor. The nurse notes a FHR of 115 to 125/min with occasional increases up to 150 to 155/min that last for 25 seconds, and have beat-to-beat variability of 20/min. There is no slowing of FHR from the baseline. The nurse should recognize that this client is exhibiting signs of which of the following? (Select all that apply.)

   __X__ **Moderate variability**

   __X__ **FHR accelerations**

   __X__ **No FHR decelerations**

   __X__ **Normal baseline FHR**

   _____ Fetal tachycardia

   There is a normal FHR baseline of 115 to 125/min (110 to 160/min is normal). Therefore, there is no evidence of fetal tachycardia. There is a moderate variability (6 to 25 beat/min) with FHR accelerations increasing to 150 to 155/min, lasting for 25 seconds. There are no FHR decelerations because the FHR does not slow down.

    NCLEX® Connection: Health Promotion and Maintenance, Ante/Intra/Postpartum and Newborn Care

2. A nurse is caring for a client who is being induced for labor and is being monitored by an external electronic fetal monitor. The nurse notes that the FHR variability is decreased and resembles a straight line. The mother has not had any pain medication. Which of the following should occur first for an internal scalp electrode to be applied?

   A. Dilation

   B. Rupture of the membranes

   C. Effacement

   D. Engagement

   Prior to the insertion of an internal fetal monitor and an intrauterine pressure catheter, the membranes must first have ruptured. Cervical dilation, effacement, and engagement of the fetus are also needed for the internal fetal scalp electrode application.

    NCLEX® Connection: NCLEX Connection: Health Promotion and Maintenance, Ante/Intra/Postpartum and Newborn Care

3. A nurse is reviewing the fetal monitor tracing of a client who is in active labor. The nurse knows that a fetus receives more oxygen during which of the following?

    A. Peak of the uterine contraction

    B. Increment of the uterine contraction

    C. Decrement of the uterine contraction

    D. Relaxation between uterine contractions

A fetus is most oxygenated during the relaxation period between contractions. During contractions, the arteries to the uteroplacental intervillous spaces are compressed, resulting in a decrease in fetal circulation and oxygenation. The constriction is most acute during the contraction acme (peak of the uterine contraction intensity), but is also present on the increment and decrement (incline and decline of the contraction).

 NCLEX® Connection: NCLEX Connection: Health Promotion and Maintenance, Ante/Intra/ Postpartum and Newborn Care

4. A client who is delivering in a birthing center is in the second stage of labor and is having no complications. Intermittent auscultation of FHR and uterine palpation of contractions is being performed to monitor FHR patterns. The nurse should assess the FHR every

    A. 60 min.

    B. 30 min.

    C. 15 min.

    D. 5 min.

With women who are low risk, the FHR should be assessed every 15 min in the second stage of labor. In women who are high risk, FHR should be assessed every 5 min in the second stage of labor. Every 60 min, FHR assessments are done during the latent phase for women who are low risk. Every 30 min, assessments are done in the active phase for women who are low risk and in the latent phase for women who are high risk.

 NCLEX® Connection: NCLEX Connection: Health Promotion and Maintenance, Ante/Intra/ Postpartum and Newborn Care

5. Which of the following is the initial nursing action the nurse should take when late decelerations appear on the fetal monitor?

A. Reposition the client in to left-lateral position.

B. Apply a fetal scalp electrode.

C. Increase the intravenous fluid rate.

D. Perform a vaginal exam to assess dilation.

The greatest risk to the fetus during late decelerations is uteroplacental insufficiency. The initial nursing action should be to reposition the client to the left-lateral position to increase uteroplacental perfusion. Increasing IV fluid rate is an intervention for late decelerations, but is not the initial nursing intervention that should be taken. In addition, the nurse may perform a vaginal exam to assess dilation. The application of a fetal scalp electrode will help in the assessment of fetal well-being.

 NCLEX® Connection: NCLEX Connection: Health Promotion and Maintenance, Ante/Intra/Postpartum and Newborn Care

6. Episodic accelerations of the FHR from baseline should be interpreted by the nurse as indicative of

A. intact CNS response to fetal movement.

B. fetal response to maternal fever.

C. fetal distress requiring intervention.

D. fetal hypoxia requiring maternal oxygen.

Occasional accelerations indicate that the fetal CNS is intact and responding to fetal movement. This is referred to as baseline variability. Lack of variable accelerations would indicate fetal distress, which requires intervention and oxygen via a face mask for the mother. Maternal fever causes tachycardia and prolonged, rather than transient, FHR accelerations.

 NCLEX® Connection: NCLEX Connection: Health Promotion and Maintenance, Ante/Intra/Postpartum and Newborn Care

UNIT 2	INTRAPARTUM NURSING CARE
Section	Labor and Delivery

Chapter 14   Nursing Care During Stages of Labor

Overview

- Labor occurs in four stages.

- It is the responsibility of a nurse to care, monitor, and provide interventions during each stage.

- Nursing responsibilities

    o   Assess the client by:

    - Orienting her and her partner to the unit during admission.

    - Assessing the client prior to admission to the birthing facility.

        □   Provide culturally-competent care that respects and is compatible with the client's culture.

        □   Conduct an admission history, review of antepartum care, and review of the birth plan.

        □   Obtain laboratory results.

        □   Monitor baseline fetal heart tones and uterine contraction patterns for 20 to 30 min.

        □   Obtain maternal vital signs.

        □   Check the status of the amniotic membranes.

    o   Perform maternal and fetal assessments continuously throughout the labor process and immediately after birth.

    o   Avoid vaginal examinations in the presence of vaginal bleeding or until placenta previa or placenta abruptio is ruled out. If necessary, vaginal examinations should be done by the primary care provider.

    o   Cervical dilation is the single most important indicator of the progress of labor.

    o   The progress of labor is affected by fetal lie, presentation, attitude, and fetal size in relationship to the mother's pelvis.

    o   The frequency, duration, and strength (intensity) of the uterine contractions cause fetal descent and cervical dilation.

First Stage

- Nursing Assessments During the First Stage

  - Leopold maneuvers will determine:

    - Number of fetuses.

    - Presenting part.

    - Fetal lie.

  - Perform a vaginal examination as indicated (only when signs indicate that progress has occurred or not contraindicated) to allow the examiner to assess if client is in true labor and if membranes have ruptured.

    - Encourage the client to take slow, deep breaths prior to the vaginal exam.

    - Monitor the cervical dilation and effacement.

    - Monitor the fetal station and presentation.

    - Prepare for an impending delivery as the presenting part moves into positive stations and begins to push against the pelvic floor (crowning).

  - Assessments related to possible rupture of membranes

    - When there is suspected rupture of membranes the nurse should first assess the FHR to assure there is no fetal distress from possible umbilical cord prolapse, which can occur with the gush of amniotic fluid.

    - Nitrazine paper will be used, which will turn blue in the presence of alkaline amniotic fluid (pH 6.5 to 7.5).

    - A sample of the fluid may be obtained and viewed on a slide under a microscope. Amniotic fluid will exhibit a frond-like ferning pattern. Additionally, assess the amniotic fluid for color and odor. The fluid should be a clear straw color and free of odor. Abnormal findings include the presence of meconium, abnormal color (yellow or port-wine), or a foul odor.

  - Perform bladder palpation on a regular basis to prevent bladder distention, which can impede fetal descent through the birth canal and cause trauma to the bladder.

    - Clients may experience the inability to feel the urge to void secondary to the labor process or anesthesia.

    - Encourage the client to engage in frequent voiding.

  - Blood pressure, pulse, and respiration measurements

    - Latent phase every 30 to 60 min

    - Active phase every 30 min

    - Transition phase every 15 to 30 min

  - Temperature assessment every 4 hr (every 1 to 2 hr if membranes have ruptured).

- o Contraction monitoring
  - Latent phase every 30 to 60 min
  - Active phase every 15 to 30 min
  - Transition phase every 10 to 15 min
- o FHR monitoring (normal range 110 to 160/min)
  - Latent phase every 30 to 60 min
  - Active phase every 15 to 30 min
  - Transitional phase every 15 to 30 min
- Nursing Interventions During the First Stage of Labor
  - o Provide the client and coach education about what to expect during labor and on implementing relaxation measures: breathing (deep cleansing breaths help divert focus away from contractions), effleurage (gentle circular stroking of the abdomen in rhythm with breathing during contractions), diversional activities (distraction, concentration on a focal point, or imagery).
  - o Encourage upright positions, application of warm/cold packs, ambulation, or hydrotherapy if not contraindicated to promote comfort.
  - o Encourage voiding every 2 hr.
    - During first stage, active phase of labor
      - □ Provide client/fetal monitoring.
      - □ Encourage frequent position changes.
      - □ Encourage voiding at least every 2 hr.
      - □ Encourage deep cleansing breaths.
      - □ Encourage relaxation.
      - □ Provide nonpharmacological comfort measures.
      - □ Provide pharmacological pain relief as prescribed.
    - During first stage, transition phase of labor
      - □ Continue to encourage voiding every 2 hr.
      - □ Continue to monitor and support the client and fetus.
      - □ Encourage a rapid pant-pant-blow breathing pattern if the client has not learned a particular breathing pattern prenatally.
      - □ Discourage pushing efforts until the cervix is fully dilated.
      - □ Listen for client statements expressing the need to have a bowel movement. This sensation is a sign of complete dilation and fetal descent.
      - □ Prepare the client for the birth.

      ☐   Observe for perineal bulging or crowning (appearance of the fetal head at the perineum).

      ☐   Encourage the client to begin bearing down with contractions once the cervix is fully dilated.

Second Stage

- Nursing Assessments During the Second Stage (begins with complete dilation and effacement)

  - Blood pressure, pulse, and respiration measurements every 5 to 30 min

  - Contractions

  - Each pushing effort made by client

  - Increase in bloody show

  - FHR every 15 min and immediately following birth

  - Assessment for perineal lacerations, which usually occur as the fetal head is expulsed. Perineal lacerations are defined in terms of depth.

    - First degree – laceration extends through the skin of the perineum and does not involve the muscles.

    - Second degree – laceration extends through the skin and muscles into the perineum.

    - Third degree – laceration extends through the skin, muscles, perineum, and anal sphincter muscle.

    - Fourth degree – laceration extends through skin, muscles, anal sphincter, and the anterior rectal wall.

- Nursing Interventions During the Second Stage

  - Continue to monitor the client/fetus.

  - Assist in positioning the client for effective pushing.

  - Assist in coaching pushing efforts and in encouraging bearing down efforts during contractions.

  - Promote rest between contractions.

  - Provide comfort measures such as cold compresses.

  - Cleanse the client's perineum as needed if fecal material is expelled during pushing.

  - Provide feedback on labor progress to the client.

  - It is imperative for the nurse to be prepared prior to the birth of the neonate. A nurse trained in neonatal resuscitation should attend all deliveries. All equipment should be checked prior to delivery, such as preheating the radiant warmer, testing the oxygen flow, resuscitation bag, and suction. Emergency medications, a stethoscope, and a laryngoscope should also be available and in working order.

Third Stage

- Nursing Assessments During the Third Stage

  - Blood pressure, pulse, and respiration measurements every 15 min

  - Signs of placental separation from the uterus as indicated by:

    - Fundus firmly contracting.

    - Swift gush from introitus of dark blood.

    - Umbilical cord appears to lengthen as placenta descends.

    - Vaginal fullness on exam.

  - Assignment of 1 and 5 min Apgar scores to the neonate.

- Nursing Interventions During the Third Stage

  - Instruct the client to push once signs of placental separation are indicated.

  - Promote bonding between the family and the newborn, which facilitates the release of endogenous oxytocics.

  - Administer analgesics as prescribed.

  - Administer oxytocics once the placenta is expulsed to stimulate the uterus to contract and thus prevent hemorrhage.

  - Gently cleanse the vulvar area with warm water or 0.9% sodium chloride, and apply a perineal pad or ice pack to the perineum.

Fourth Stage

- Nursing Assessments During the Fourth Stage

  - Maternal vital signs

  - Fundus

  - Lochia

  - Urinary output

  - Maternal newborn bonding activities

- Nursing Interventions During the Fourth Stage

  - Assess maternal vital signs every 15 min for the first hour and then according to facility protocol.

  - Assess fundus and lochia every 15 min for the first hour and then according to facility protocol.

  - Massage the uterine fundus and/or administer oxytocics as prescribed to maintain uterine tone and to prevent hemorrhage.

  - Encourage voiding to prevent bladder distention.

  - Promote an opportunity for maternal-infant bonding.

CHAPTER 14: NURSING CARE DURING STAGES OF LABOR

(A) Application Exercises

1. A client who is primigravida and at 39 weeks of gestation comes to the birthing unit with her partner because she has been having regular contractions. She states that her "water broke." Which of the following is the priority assessment the nurse should perform at this time?

   A. FHR monitoring

   B. Vaginal exam

   C. Nitrazine paper test

   D. Leopold maneuvers

2. A client and her partner have not taken prepared childbirth classes prior to labor. When should the nurse provide the client and coaching partner education during the labor process?

   A. The first stage, latent phase

   B. The first stage, active phase

   C. The first stage, transition phase

   D. The second stage of labor

3. A client is in the transition phase of labor and feels that she needs to have a bowel movement with the peak of contractions. Which of the following is an appropriate nursing intervention?

   A. Assist the client to the bathroom.

   B. Prepare for an impending delivery.

   C. Prepare to remove a fecal impaction.

   D. Encourage the client to take deep, cleansing breaths.

4. A nurse is caring for a client in active labor. Her vaginal exam 1 hr ago showed that she was 3 cm dilated, 50 percent effaced, and had a - 3 station. Her membranes ruptured spontaneously. The nurse should assess her for which of the following signs?

   A. Prolapsed cord

   B. Premature rupture of membranes

   C. Infection

   D. Fetal tachycardia

5. A nurse is palpating a client's bladder and is encouraging her to void every 1 to 2 hr during labor predominantly because a

   A. full bladder increases the risk for fetal trauma.

   B. full bladder increases the risk for bladder infections.

   C. distended bladder will be traumatized by frequent pelvic exams.

   D. distended bladder reduces pelvic space needed for birth.

CHAPTER 14: NURSING CARE DURING STAGES OF LABOR

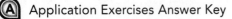 Application Exercises Answer Key

1. A client who is primigravida and at 39 weeks of gestation comes to the birthing unit with her partner because she has been having regular contractions. She states that her "water broke." Which of the following is the priority assessment the nurse should perform at this time?

   A. FHR monitoring

   B. Vaginal exam

   C. Nitrazine paper test

   D. Leopold maneuvers

   The initial assessment that is most important with suspected rupture of membranes is assessing the FHR to ensure there is no fetal distress as a result of possible prolapse of the umbilical cord during the escape of the amniotic fluid. A prolapsed cord could result in either compression of the cord or the cord wrapping around the neck of the fetus. The nurse should perform Leopold maneuvers to determine fetal lie, presentation, and attitude, and monitor contraction pattern in conjunction with FHR monitoring. However, these assessments would not be of initial concern. If the FHR rate was within normal limits, the nurse should then perform a Nitrazine and/or ferning test to assess for the rupture of membranes. The nurse would then perform a vaginal exam to assess cervical dilation, effacement, and fetal station after labor progress has been firmly established.

   NCLEX® Connection: Health Promotion and Maintenance: Ante/Intra/Postpartum and Newborn Care

2. A client and her partner have not taken prepared childbirth classes prior to labor. When should the nurse provide the client and coaching partner education during the labor process?

   A. The first stage, latent phase

   B. The first stage, active phase

   C. The first stage, transition phase

   D. The second stage of labor

   During the latent phase of the first stage the client is talkative and eager for the labor to progress and is not yet in a lot of pain. At this time, the client and her coaching partner will be most receptive to any educational information. As the labor progresses through the active and transition phases of the first stage and into the second stage of delivery, the client will be in too much pain from contractions to focus on educational information.

   NCLEX® Connection: Health Promotion and Maintenance: Ante/Intra/Postpartum and Newborn Care

3. A client is in the transition phase of labor and feels that she needs to have a bowel movement with the peak of contractions. Which of the following is an appropriate nursing intervention?

    A. Assist the client to the bathroom.

    B. Prepare for an impending delivery.

    C. Prepare to remove a fecal impaction.

    D. Encourage the client to take deep, cleansing breaths.

The urge to have a bowel movement is a sign of complete dilation and fetal descent. If there is fecal material present at the rectum, the nurse should cleanse the perineum rather than escorting the client to the bathroom. The nurse should not remove a fecal impaction. However, encouraging deep cleansing breaths is indicated, this has nothing to do with the client's sensation of needing to have a bowel movement.

 NCLEX® Connection: Health Promotion and Maintenance: Ante/Intra/Postpartum and Newborn Care

4. A nurse is caring for a client in active labor. Her vaginal exam 1 hr ago showed that she was 3 cm dilated, 50 percent effaced, and had a - 3 station. Her membranes ruptured spontaneously. The nurse should assess her for which of the following signs?

    A. Prolapsed cord

    B. Premature rupture of membranes

    C. Infection

    D. Fetal tachycardia

The nurse should always assess for signs of a prolapsed cord when membranes rupture. The client is in labor, so the rupture of membranes is not premature. Labor has not continued for 24 hr past rupture of membranes, so infection is not a concern at this point. An abrupt FHR is indicative of prolapsed cord decelerations, not tachycardia.

 NCLEX® Connection: Health Promotion and Maintenance: Ante/Intra/Postpartum and Newborn Care

5. A nurse is palpating the client's bladder and is encouraging her to void every 1 to 2 hr during labor predominantly because a

    A. full bladder increases the risk for fetal trauma.

    B. full bladder increases the risk for bladder infections.

    C. distended bladder will be traumatized by frequent pelvic exams.

    D. distended bladder reduces pelvic space needed for birth.

A distended bladder reduces pelvic space, impedes the fetal descent necessary for delivery, and places the bladder at risk for trauma during the labor process. Urinary stasis, which can occur with prolonged bladder distention due to a full bladder, does increase bladder infection risk. However, this is not the primary concern at this time. A full bladder does not place the fetus at risk for trauma.

 NCLEX® Connection: Health Promotion and Maintenance: Ante/Intra/Postpartum and Newborn Care

UNIT 2	INTRAPARTUM NURSING CARE
Section	Labor and Delivery

Chapter 15	Therapeutic Procedures to Assist with Labor and Delivery

Overview

- In this chapter the various methods of therapeutic procedures to assist with labor and delivery will be discussed.

- The following therapeutic procedures that will be covered include external cephalic version, Bishop score, cervical ripening, induction/augmentation of labor, amniotomy, amnioinfusion, episiotomy, vacuum-assisted delivery, forceps-assisted delivery, cesarean birth, and vaginal delivery after cesarean birth.

EXTERNAL CEPHALIC VERSION

Overview

- Description of Procedure

  ○ External cephalic version (ECV) is the attempt to manipulate the abdominal wall to direct a malpositioned fetus into a normal vertex cephalic presentation after 37 weeks of gestation. There is a high risk of prolapse of the umbilical cord surrounding this procedure. Contraindications to this procedure include uterine anomalies, previous cesarean birth, cephalopelvic disproportion, placenta previa, multifetal gestation, and/ or oligohydramnios.

- Indications

  ○ Potential diagnoses

    ▪ A malpositioned fetus in a breech or transverse position after 37 weeks of gestation.

- Client Outcomes

  ○ The client's labor will progress without complications.

  ○ Nursing actions

    ▪ Obtain an informed consent from the client.

    ▪ The primary care provider will perform ultrasound screening prior to the procedure to evaluate fetal position, locate the umbilical cord, assess placental placement to rule out placenta previa, determine the amount of amniotic fluid, determine fetal age, assess for the presence of anomalies, evaluate pelvic adequacy for delivery and/or guide the direction of the fetus during the procedure.

- Perform a nonstress test to evaluate fetal well-being.
- Ensure that $RH_o(D)$ immune globulin (RhoGAM) was administered at 28 weeks of gestation if the mother is Rh-negative prior to external version.
- Administer IV fluid and tocolytics to relax uterus to permit easier manipulation prior to external version.

○ Ongoing care

- Continuously monitor FHR patterns to assess for bradycardia and variable decelerations.
- Monitor maternal vital signs.
- Monitor the client's blood pressure to detect if vena cava compression with resulting hypotension is occurring.
- Monitor for maternal pain.
- Rh-negative clients require a Kleihauer-Betke test. The test detects for the presence and amount of fetal blood in the maternal circulation because manipulation can cause fetomaternal bleeding. If more than 15 mL of fetal blood is present, the dosage of Rh-immune globulin must be administered to suppress the maternal immune response to fetal Rh-positive blood.

○ Interventions

- Monitor the client for uterine activity, contraction frequency, duration, and intensity.
- Monitor the client for rupture of membranes.
- Monitor the client for bleeding until maternal condition is stable.
- Monitor the client for a decrease in fetal activity.

BISHOP SCORE

Overview

- Description of Procedure

  ○ A Bishop score is used to determine the maternal readiness for labor by evaluating if the cervix is favorable by rating the following:

  ○ Cervical dilation.

  ○ Cervical effacement.

  ○ Cervical consistency (firm, medium, or soft).

  ○ Cervical position (posterior, midposition, or anterior).

  ○ Presenting part station.

- The five factors are assigned a numerical value of 0 to 3, the total score is calculated, and a score of 9 for nulliparas and 5 or more for multiparas indicates readiness for labor induction.

- Indications

  o Potential diagnoses

    ▪ Any condition in which augmentation or induction of labor is indicated.

CERVICAL RIPENING

Overview

- Description of Procedure

  o Cervical ripening increases cervical readiness for labor by either a chemical or mechanical method to promote cervical softening, dilation, and effacement.

    ▪ Cervical ripening makes labor induction more successful.

    ▪ Cervical ripening lowers the dosage of oxytocin (Pitocin) needed for induction. For certain clients, cervical ripening is adequate to induce labor and eliminates the need for oxytocin administration.

  o Chemical agents consist of prostaglandin gel (Cytotec, Cervidil, Prepidil), which is used to "ripen" the cervix (soften and thin) and to increase cervical readiness prior to the induction of labor.

  o Mechanical methods ripen the cervix by using:

    ▪ Balloon catheters inserted into the intracervical canal to dilate the cervix.

    ▪ Hydroscopic dilators and sponges to absorb fluid from the surrounding tissues and then enlarge.

    ▪ Laminaria tents made from desiccated seaweed.

    ▪ Synthetic dilators and sponges containing magnesium sulfate (Lamicel) are inserted into the endocervix without rupture of the membranes. The dilators and sponges absorb fluid and expand causing cervical dilation.

  o Insertion of fresh dilators may be necessary for further dilation as required.

  o Membrane stripping and an amniotomy may also be used to ripen the cervix.

- Potential Diagnoses

  o Any condition in which augmentation or induction of labor is indicated.

- Client Presentation

  o Failure of the cervix to dilate and efface

  o Failure of labor to progress

- Client Outcomes

  o The client's labor will progress without complications.

- Nursing Actions
  - Ongoing care includes the nurse assessing for:
    - Urinary retention.
    - Rupture of membranes.
    - Uterine tenderness or pain.
    - Contractions.
    - Vaginal bleeding.
    - Fetal distress.
  - Interventions
    - Document the number of dilators and/or sponges inserted during the procedure.
    - The client should remain in a side-lying position.
    - Assist with augmentation or induction of labor as prescribed.
    - Monitor the client for potential side effects such as, hypertension, diarrhea, and vomiting.
    - The nurse should proceed with caution in clients who have glaucoma, asthma, cardiovascular, or renal disease.
- Complications
  - Hyperstimulation
    - Nursing actions
      - Administer terbutaline (Brethine) subcutaneously.
  - Fetal distress
    - Nursing actions
      - Apply O_2 via face mask at 10 L/min.
      - Position the client on her left side.
      - Increase IV fluids.
      - Notify the primary care provider.

INDUCTION OF LABOR

 Overview

- Description of Procedure
  - Induction of labor is the deliberate initiation of uterine contractions to stimulate labor before spontaneous onset to bring about the birth either by chemical or mechanical means.

- o Methods
  - Prostaglandins applied cervically
  - Administration of IV oxytocin (Pitocin)
  - Amniotomy or stripping of membranes.
  - Nipple stimulation to trigger the release of endogenous oxytocin
- Indications
  - o Any condition in which augmentation or induction of labor is indicated
- Client Presentation
  - o Postterm pregnancy (beyond 42 weeks of gestation)
  - o Dystocia (prolonged, difficult labor)
    - Inadequate uterine contractions
  - o Prolonged rupture of membranes
    - Predisposes the mother and fetus to risk of infection.
  - o Maternal medical complications
    - Rh-isoimmunization
    - Diabetes mellitus
    - Pulmonary disease
    - Pregnancy-induced hypertension
  - o Fetal demise
  - o Chorioamnionitis
- Client Outcomes
  - o The client will be free of injury.
  - o The client's labor will progress without complications.
- Nursing Actions
  - o Prepare the client for cervical ripening
    - Obtain the client's consent.
    - If cervical-ripening agents (Cytotec, Cervidil, and Prepidil) are used, baseline data on fetal and maternal well-being should be obtained.
    - The nurse may initiate oxytocin (Pitocin) 6 to 12 hr after administration of the prostaglandin.
    - The nurse should monitor FHR and uterine activity after administration of cervical-ripening agents.
    - The nurse should notify the primary care provider if uterine hyperstimulation or fetal distress is noted.

○ Prepare the client for an amniotomy or amniotic membrane stripping.

- When an amniotomy is performed, the nurse should record a baseline assessment of the FHR prior to the procedure and continuously during and after the procedure.

- The nurse should assess the amount, color, consistency, and odor of the amniotic fluid.

- The nurse should document the time of the amniotomy and the findings.

○ Prepare of the client for oxytocin (Pitocin).

- Prior to the administration of oxytocin, it is essential that the nurse confirm that the fetus is engaged in the birth canal at a minimum of station 0.

- Use the infusion port closest to the client for administration. Oxytocin should be connected "piggyback" to the main IV line and administered via an infusion pump.

- An intrauterine pressure catheter (IUPC) may be used to monitor frequency, duration, and intensity of contractions.

- When oxytocin is administered, assessments include maternal blood pressure, pulse, and respirations every 30 min and with every change in dose.

- Monitor FHR and contraction pattern every 15 min and with every change in dose.

- Assess fluid intake and urinary output.

- A Bishop score rating should be obtained prior to starting any labor induction protocol.

○ Ongoing care

- Assist with or perform administration of labor induction agents as prescribed.

  □ Increase oxytocin as prescribed until desired contraction pattern is obtained and then maintain the dose if there is a:

  □ Contraction frequency of 2 to 3 min.

  □ Contraction duration of 60 to 90 sec.

  □ Contraction intensity of 40 to 90 mm Hg on IUPC.

  □ Uterine resting tone of 10 to 15 mm Hg.

  □ Cervical dilation of 1 cm/hr.

  □ Reassuring FHR between 110 to 160/min.

- Discontinue oxytocin if uterine hyperstimulation occurs. Symptoms of uterine hyperstimulation include:

  □ Contraction frequency more often than every 2 min.

  □ Contraction duration longer than 90 seconds.

  □ Contraction intensity that results in pressures greater than 90 mm Hg as shown by IUPC.

□ Uterine resting tone greater than 20 mm Hg between contractions.

□ No relaxation of uterus between contractions

○ Complications

- A nonreassuring FHR is noted.

○ Description

□ An abnormal baseline less than 110 or greater than 160/min

□ Loss of variability

□ Late or prolonged decelerations

○ Interventions

- Notify the primary care provider.

- Position the client in a side-lying position to increase uteroplacental perfusion.

- Keep the IV line open and increasing fluid rate up to 200 mL/hr unless contraindicated.

- Administer oxygen by a face mask at 8 to 10 L/min as prescribed.

- Administer the tocolytic terbutaline (Brethine) 0.25 mg subcutaneously as prescribed to diminish uterine activity.

- Monitor FHR and patterns in conjunction with uterine activity.

- Document responses to interventions.

- If unable to restore reassuring FHR, an emergency cesarean birth should be performed.

AUGMENTATION OF LABOR

Overview

- Description of Procedure

  ○ Augmentation of labor is the stimulation of hypotonic contractions once labor has spontaneously begun, but progress is inadequate.

  ○ Certain primary care providers favor active management of labor to establish effective labor with the aggressive use of oxytocin (Pitocin) or rupture of membranes. This ensures that the client delivers within 12 hr of admission to the labor unit so that the risk of cesarean birth will be decreased.

- Risk factors requiring augmentation of labor, administration procedures, nursing assessments and interventions, and possible procedure complications are the same for labor induction.

AMNIOTOMY

Overview

- Description of Procedure

    o An amniotomy is the artificial rupture of the amniotic membranes (AROM) by the primary care provider using an Amnihook or other sharp instrument.

    o Labor typically begins within 12 hr after the membranes rupture.

    o The client is at an increased risk for cord prolapse or infection.

- Indications

    ▪ Labor progression is too slow and augmentation or induction of labor is indicated.

    ▪ An amnioinfusion is indicated for cord compression.

    o Client outcomes

    ▪ The client's labor will progress without complications.

- Nursing Actions

    o Ongoing care

    ▪ Assure that the presenting part of the fetus is engaged prior to an amniotomy to prevent cord prolapse.

    ▪ Monitor FHR prior to and following AROM to assess for cord prolapse as evidenced by variable or late decelerations.

    ▪ Assess and document characteristics of amniotic fluid including color, odor, and consistency.

    o Interventions

    ▪ Document the time of rupture.

    ▪ Obtain temperature every 2 hr.

AMNIOINFUSION

 Overview

- Description of Procedure

- An amnioinfusion of 0.9% sodium chloride or lactated Ringer's solution, as prescribed, is instilled into the amniotic cavity through a transcervical catheter introduced into the uterus to supplement the amount of amniotic fluid. The instillation will reduce the severity of variable decelerations caused by cord compression or dilute meconium-stained amniotic fluid.

- Indications

  o Potential diagnoses

    ▪ Oligohydramnios (scant amount or absence of amniotic fluid) caused by any of the following:

      □ Uteroplacental insufficiency.

      □ Premature rupture of membranes.

      □ Postmaturity of the fetus.

    ▪ Fetal cord compression secondary to:

      □ Postmaturity of fetus (macrosomic, large body), which places the fetus at risk for variable deceleration from cord compression.

- Client Outcomes

  o The client's labor will progress without complications.

- Nursing Actions

  o Interventions

    ▪ Assist with the amniotomy if membranes have not already ruptured. Membranes must have ruptured to perform an amnioinfusion.

    ▪ Warm fluid using a blood warmer prior to infusion.

    ▪ Perform nursing measures to maintain comfort and dryness because the infused fluid will continuously leak out.

    ▪ Monitor the client continuously to prevent uterine overdistention and increased uterine tone, which can initiate, accelerate, or intensify uterine contractions and cause nonreassuring FHR changes.

    ▪ Continually assess intensity and frequency of the client's uterine contractions.

    ▪ Continually monitor FHR.

    ▪ Monitor fluid output from vagina to prevent uterine overdistention.

VACUUM-ASSISTED DELIVERY

Overview

- Description of Procedure

    o A vacuum-assisted birth involves the use of a cuplike suction device that is attached to the fetal head. Traction is applied during contractions to assist in the descent and birth of the head, after which, the vacuum cup is released and removed preceding delivery of the fetal body.

    o Recommendations by the manufacturer should be followed for product use to ensure safety.

    o Conditions for use consist of a vacuum-assisted birth

        ▪ Vertex presentation

        ▪ Absence of cephalopelvic disproportion

        ▪ Ruptured membranes

    o Risks associated with vacuum-assisted births

        ▪ Scalp lacerations

        ▪ Subdural hematoma of the neonate

        ▪ Cephalohematoma

        ▪ Maternal lacerations to the cervix, vagina, or perineum

- Indications

        ▪ Maternal exhaustion and ineffective pushing efforts

        ▪ Fetal distress during second stage of labor

- Client Outcomes

    o The client's labor will progress without complications.

- Nursing Actions

    o Preparation of the client

        ▪ Provide the client and her partner with support and education regarding the procedure.

        ▪ Assist the client into the lithotomy position to allow for sufficient traction of the vacuum cup when it is applied to the fetal head.

        ▪ Assess and record FHR before and during vacuum assistance.

        ▪ Assessing for bladder distention and catheterize if necessary.

    o Ongoing care

        ▪ Prepare for a forceps-assisted birth if a vacuum-assisted birth is not successful.

    o Interventions

- Alert postpartum care providers that vacuum assistance was used.

- Observe the neonate for lacerations, cephalohematomas, or subdural hematomas, after delivery.

- Check the neonate for caput succedaneum. Caput succedaneum is a normal occurrence and should resolve within 24 hr.

FORCEPS-ASSISTED BIRTH

Overview

- Description of Procedure

  - A forceps-assisted birth consists of using an instrument with two curved spoon-like blades to assist in the delivery of the fetal head. Traction is applied during contractions.

- Indications

  - Client presentation

    - Fetal distress during labor

    - Abnormal presentations or a breech position requiring delivery of the head

    - Arrest of rotation

- Client Outcomes

  - The client's labor will progress without complications.

- Nursing Actions

  - Preparation of the client

    - Explain the procedure to the client and the client's support person.

    - Assist the client into the lithotomy position.

    - Assess to assure that the client's bladder is empty and catheterize if necessary.

    - Assess to ensure that the fetus is engaged and that membranes have ruptured.

    - Assess and record FHR before, during, and after forceps assistance.

  - Ongoing care

    - Assist with the procedure as necessary.

  - Interventions

    - Assess and record FHR before, during, and after forceps assistance.

      - Compression of the cord between the fetal head and forceps will cause a decrease in the FHR.

      - If a FHR decrease occurs, the forceps are removed and reapplied.

    - Observe the neonate for bruising and abrasions at the site of forceps application after delivery.

- Checking the mother for any possible injuries after birth.
  - Vaginal or cervical lacerations indicated by bleeding in spite of contracted uterus
  - Urine retention resulting from bladder or urethral injuries
  - Hematoma formation in the pelvic soft tissues resulting from blood vessel damage
  - Report to the postpartum nursing caregivers that forceps or vacuum-assisted delivery methods were used.
- Complications
  - Lacerations of the cervix
  - Lacerations of the vagina and perineum
  - Injury to the bladder
  - Facial nerve palsy of the neonate
  - Facial bruising on the neonate

EPISIOTOMY

Overview

- Description of Procedure
  - An episiotomy is an incision made into the perineum to enlarge the vaginal opening to more easily facilitate delivery and minimize soft tissue damage.
- Indications for an Episiotomy
  - Shorten the second stage of labor
  - Facilitate forceps-assisted or vacuum-assisted delivery
  - Prevent cerebral hemorrhage in a fragile preterm fetus
  - Facilitate birth of a macrosomic (large) infant
- The site and direction of the incision designates the type of episiotomy.
- A median (midline) episiotomy extends from the vaginal outlet toward the rectum, and is the most commonly used.
  - Much easier to repair
  - Less blood loss
  - Associated with a higher incidence of third- and fourth-degree lacerations
- A mediolateral episiotomy extends from the vaginal outlet posterolateral, either to the left or right of the midline, and is used when posterior extension is likely.
  - Third-degree laceration may occur

- ○ Blood loss is greater and the repair is more difficult

- ○ Local anesthetic is administered to the perineum prior to the incision

- Client Outcomes

  - ○ The client will deliver without complications and will be free of injury during the birthing process.

- Nursing Actions

  - ○ Ongoing care

    - Encourage alternate labor positions to reduce pressure on the perineum and promote perineal stretching to reduce the necessity for an episiotomy.

CESAREAN BIRTH

Overview

- Description of Procedure

  - ○ A cesarean birth is the delivery of the fetus through a transabdominal incision of the uterus to preserve the life or health of the mother and fetus when there is evidence of complications.

    - Incisions are currently made horizontally into the lower segment of the uterus.

    - Previously made as a classical vertical incision into the muscular body of the uterus.

- Indications

  - ○ Potential diagnoses

    - Malpresentation, particularly breech presentation

    - Cephalopelvic disproportion

    - Fetal distress

    - Placental abnormalities

      - □ Placenta previa

      - □ Abruptio placenta

    - High-risk pregnancy.

      - □ Positive HIV status

      - □ Hypertensive disorders such as preeclampsia and eclampsia

      - □ Maternal diabetes mellitus

      - □ Active genital herpes outbreak

    - Previous cesarean birth

    - Dystocia

- - Multiple gestations
  - Umbilical cord prolapse
- Client Outcomes
  - The client will be free of injury during the birthing process.
- Preprocedure
  - Nursing actions
    - Assess and record FHR, maternal vital signs, and blood pressure.
    - Assist with obtaining abdominal an ultrasound to assess if a cesarean birth is indicated.
    - Position the client in a supine position with a wedge under one hip to laterally tilt her and keep her off of the vena cava and descending aorta. This will help maintain optimal perfusion of oxygenated blood to the fetus during the procedure.
    - Insert an indwelling urinary catheter.
    - Administer any preoperative medications.
    - Prepare the surgical site.
    - Insert an IV line.
    - Obtain an informed consent form from the client.
    - Determine if the client has had nothing by mouth since midnight before the procedure. If the client has, notify the anesthesiologist.
    - Assure that preoperative diagnostic tests are complete including an Rh-factor test.
  - Client education
    - Prepare the client and the client's support person and explain the procedure to them.
    - Provide emotional support.
- Intraprocedure
  - Nursing actions
    - Assist in positioning the client on the operating table.
    - Continue to monitor FHR.
    - Continue to monitor vital signs, IV fluids, and urinary output.

- Postprocedure

  o Nursing actions

    - Monitor for signs of infection and excessive bleeding at the incision site.

    - Assess the uterine fundus for firmness or tenderness.

    - Assess the lochia for amount and characteristics.

      □ A tender uterus and foul-smelling lochia may indicate endometritis.

    - Assess for productive cough or chills, which could be symptoms of pneumonia.

    - Assess for signs and symptoms of thrombophlebitis, which include: tenderness, pain, and heat on palpation.

    - Monitor I&O.

    - Monitor vital signs per protocol.

    - Provide pain relief and antiemetics as prescribed.

    - Encourage the client to turn, cough, and deep breathe to prevent pulmonary complications.

    - Encourage splinting of the incision with pillows.

    - Encourage ambulation to prevent thrombus formation.

    - Assess the client for symptoms of burning and pain on urination, which could be suggestive of a urinary tract infection.

- Complications

  o Maternal

    - Aspiration

    - Amniotic fluid pulmonary embolism

    - Wound infection

    - Wound dehiscence

    - Severe abdominal pain

    - Thrombophlebitis

    - Hemorrhage

    - Urinary tract infection

    - Injuries to the bladder or bowel

    - Anesthesia associated complications

  o Fetal

    - Premature birth of fetus if gestational age is inaccurate

    - Fetal injuries during surgery

VAGINAL DELIVERY AFTER CESAREAN BIRTH

 Overview

- A vaginal birth after cesarean birth is when the client delivers vaginally after having had a previous cesarean birth.

- Indications

  - Client presentation

    - Previous documented low-segment transverse incision

    - No current contraindications.

      - Large for gestational age newborn

      - Malpresentation

      - Cephalopelvic disproportion

      - Previous classical vertical uterine incision

- Client Outcomes

  - The client will be free of injury during the birthing process.

- Nursing Actions

  - Preprocedure

    - Nursing actions

      - Review medical records for evidence of a previous low-segment transverse cesarean incision.

    - Client education

      - Explain the procedure to the client and the client's support person.

  - Intraprocedure

    - Nursing actions

      - Assess and record FHR during the labor.

      - Assess and record contraction patterns for strength, duration, and frequency of contractions.

      - Assess for signs of uterine rupture.

      - Promote relaxation and breathing techniques during labor.

      - Provide analgesia as prescribed and requested.

  - Postprocedure

    - Nursing actions

      - Nursing interventions for a vaginal delivery after a cesarean birth are the same as for a vaginal delivery.

CHAPTER 15: THERAPEUTIC PROCEDURES TO ASSIST WITH LABOR AND DELIVERY

(A) Application Exercises

1. Which of the following positions should a nurse place a client in prior to a cesarean birth?

   A. Trendelenburg with the lower extremities elevated

   B. Left-lateral side-lying with head elevated

   C. Prone with a wedge under the right hip

   D. Supine with a wedge under the right hip

2. A nurse is caring for a client who is at 42 weeks of gestation and is admitted to the labor and delivery unit. During an ultrasound, it is noted that the fetus is large for gestational age. The nurse reviews the prescription from the primary care provider to begin an amnioinfusion. The nurse knows that an amnioinfusion is indicated for which of the following reasons? (Select all that apply.)

   _____ Oligohydramnios

   _____ Hydramnios

   _____ Fetal cord compression

   _____ Hydration

   _____ Meconium in amniotic fluid

3. A nurse is caring for a client who has meconium stained fluid. Which of the following solutions does the nurse anticipate the provider to prescribe for an amnioinfusion? (Select all that apply).

   _____ Lactated Ringer's solution

   _____ Dextrose 5% in lactated Ringer's solution

   _____ Dextrose 5% in 0.9% sodium chloride

   _____ 0.45% sodium chloride

   _____ 0.9% sodium chloride

4. A client in the labor and delivery unit has been in labor for 12 hr. Her membranes are still intact. The primary care provider has decided to perform an amniotomy in an effort to facilitate the progress of labor. The nurse performs a sterile vaginal examination to ensure which of the following prior to the performance of the amniotomy?

   A. Fetal engagement

   B. Fetal lie

   C. Fetal attitude

   D. Fetal position

5. Which of the following medications should the nurse anticipate will be necessary to administer preceding an external version for a client who has Rh-negative blood and did not receive adequate prenatal care?

    A. Prostaglandin gel

    B. Magnesium sulfate

    C. $Rh_o(D)$ immune globulin (RhoGAM)

    D. Oxytocin (Pitocin)

6. A nurse is caring for a client who is receiving oxytocin (Pitocin) for induction of labor and has an intrauterine pressure catheter (IUPC) placed to monitor uterine contractions. For which of the following contraction patterns should the nurse discontinue the infusion of oxytocin?

    A. Frequency of every 2 min

    B. Duration of 90 to 120 seconds

    C. Intensity of 60 to 90 mm Hg

    D. Resting tone of 15 mm Hg

7. In addition to oxytocin (Pitocin) administration, what other methods of augmenting or inducing labor should a nurse anticipate?

    A. Cervical ripening

    B. Amnioinfusion

    C. Cesarean birth

    D. Episiotomy

CHAPTER 15: THERAPEUTIC PROCEDURES TO ASSIST WITH LABOR AND DELIVERY

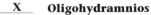 Application Exercises Answer Key

1. Which of the following positions should a nurse place a client in prior to a cesarean birth?

   A. Trendelenburg with the lower extremities elevated

   B. Left-lateral side-lying with head elevated

   C. Prone with a wedge under the right hip

   D. Supine with a wedge under the right hip

   The client will need to be positioned supine, on her back, for the cesarean birth. Placing a wedge under one of the client's hips, preferably the right, will tilt the client so she will not experience the pressure of her gravid uterus that is compressing on the inferior vena cava. This could possibly compromise circulation to the fetus. Trendelenburg position, on the back with legs elevated, still places pressure on the maternal descending aorta and vena cava, compromising uteroplacental circulation. Prone position, on the mother's stomach, would be contraindicated along with the side-lying position, both of which would make surgical approach inaccessible.

   NCLEX® Connection: Reduction of Risk Potential, Potential for Complications of Diagnostic Tests/Treatments/Procedures

2. A nurse is caring for a client who is at 42 weeks of gestation and is admitted to the labor and delivery unit. During an ultrasound, it is noted that the fetus is large for gestational age. The nurse reviews the prescription from the primary care provider to begin an amnioinfusion. The nurse knows that an amnioinfusion is indicated for which of the following reasons? (Select all that apply.)

X	**Oligohydramnios**
	Hydramnios
X	**Fetal cord compression**
	Hydration
X	**Meconium in amniotic fluid**

   Oligohydramnios is an inadequate amount of amniotic fluid, less than 300 mL, which can contribute to intrauterine growth restriction of the fetus, restrict fetal movement, and cause fetal distress during labor. Oligohydramnios can also lead to fetal cord compression, which decreases fetal oxygenation. Meconium staining of the amniotic fluid with thick fresh meconium places the fetus at risk for meconium aspiration syndrome. Hydramnios is excessive amniotic fluid. Amnioinfusion does not increase hydration. IV fluids or oral intake would provide this.

   NCLEX® Connection: Physiological Adaptation, Alterations in Body Systems

3. A nurse is caring for a client who has meconium stained fluid. Which of the following solutions does the nurse anticipate the provider to prescribe for an amnioinfusion? (Select all that apply).

__X__	**Lactated Ringer's solution**
_____	Dextrose 5% in lactated Ringer's solution
_____	Dextrose 5% in 0.9% sodium chloride
_____	0.45% sodium chloride
__X__	**0.9% sodium chloride**

An instillation of an isotonic solution, such as 0.9% sodium chloride or lactated Ringer's solution, is prescribed for an amnioinfusion. Dextrose 5% in lactated Ringer's solution, dextrose 5% in 0.9% sodium chloride, and 0.45% sodium chloride are not prescribed for an amnioinfusion.

 NCLEX® Connection: Health Promotion and Maintenance, Ante/Intra/Postpartum and Newborn Care

4. A client in the labor and delivery unit has been in labor for 12 hr. Her membranes are still intact. The primary care provider has decided to perform an amniotomy in an effort to facilitate the progress of labor. The nurse performs a sterile vaginal examination to ensure which of the following prior to the performance of the amniotomy?

A. Fetal engagement

B. Fetal lie

C. Fetal attitude

D. Fetal position

Prior to the performance of an amniotomy, the amniotic membranes should have ruptured. It is also imperative that the fetus is engaged at a level 0 station and at the level of the maternal ischial spines to prevent prolapse of the umbilical cord. Fetal lie pertains to the axis of the maternal spine in relation to the axis of the fetal spine. Fetal attitude is the relationship of the fetal extremities and chin to the fetal torso. Fetal position refers to the direction of a reference point in the fetal presenting part to the maternal pelvis.

 NCLEX® Connection: Health Promotion and Maintenance, Ante/Intra/Postpartum and Newborn Care

5. Which of the following medications should the nurse anticipate will be necessary to administer preceding an external version for a client who has Rh-negative blood and did not receive adequate prenatal care?

    A. Prostaglandin gel

    B. Magnesium sulfate

    C. Rh$_0$(D) immune globulin (RhoGAM)

    D. Oxytocin (Pitocin)

Rh$_0$(D) immune globulin (RhoGAM) is given to Rh-negative mothers at 28 weeks of gestation to prevent isoimmunization in which maternal antibodies attack the RBCs of an Rh-positive fetus. During the external version there is a risk of fetal blood entering the maternal circulation. Prostaglandin is a cervical ripening agent. Magnesium sulfate is a tocolytic medication used to decrease contractions or for seizure prevention in eclampsia, which is a severe form of pregnancy-induced hypertension. Magnesium sulfate or another tocolytic medication would be administered prior to external version to relax the uterus for easier manipulation, but these have nothing to do with the lack of prenatal care for a client who has Rh-negative blood. Oxytocin is administered to increase contraction frequency, intensity, and duration in labor augmentation and induction.

 NCLEX® Connection: Reduction of Risk Potential, Potential for Complications of Diagnostic Tests/Treatments/Procedures

6. A nurse is caring for a client who is receiving oxytocin (Pitocin) for induction of labor and has an intrauterine pressure catheter (IUPC) placed to monitor uterine contractions. For which of the following contraction patterns should the nurse discontinue the infusion of oxytocin?

    A. Frequency of every 2 min

    B. Duration of 90 to 120 seconds

    C. Intensity of 60 to 90 mm Hg

    D. Resting tone of 15 mm Hg

Discontinue oxytocin if uterine hyperstimulation occurs with contraction frequency more often than every 2 min; contraction duration longer than 90 seconds; contraction intensity results with pressures greater than 90 mm Hg as shown by IUPC; and a uterine resting tone greater than 20 mm Hg between contractions showing no relaxation of uterus between contractions. The other contraction patterns do not require discontinuing oxytocin.

 NCLEX® Connection: Health Promotion and Maintenance, Ante/Intra/Postpartum and Newborn Care

7. In addition to oxytocin (Pitocin) administration, what other methods of augmenting or inducing labor should a nurse anticipate?

A. Cervical ripening

B. Amnioinfusion

C. Cesarean birth

D. Episiotomy

Cervical ripening increases cervical readiness for labor by either chemical or mechanical means to promote the softening, dilation, and effacement of the cervix. In some instances, cervical ripening alone is enough to induce labor. An amnioinfusion instills fluid into the uterine cavity, but is not intended to initiate labor. However, overdistention of the uterus can increase uterine activity. Cesarean birth is a method of delivery, not an induction method. Episiotomy extends the vaginal outlet, but does not induce labor.

NCLEX® Connection: Health Promotion and Maintenance: Ante/Intra/Postpartum and Newborn Care

Overview

- Complications occurring during the labor process are emergent and require immediate intervention in order to improve maternal fetal outcomes. This chapter will explore prolapsed umbilical cord, meconium-stained amniotic fluid, fetal distress, dystocia, precipitous labor, uterine rupture, and amniotic fluid embolus. Assessment findings, interventions and therapeutic outcomes will be discussed.

PROLAPSED UMBILICAL CORD

Overview

- A prolapsed umbilical cord occurs when the umbilical cord is displaced, preceding the presenting part of the fetus, or protruding through the cervix. This results in cord compression and compromised fetal circulation.

 View Media Supplement: Prolapsed Cord (Image)

Risk Factors

- Rupture of amniotic membranes

  ○ It is necessary to check FHR immediately following rupture of membranes.

- Abnormal fetal presentation is any presentation other than vertex (occiput is the presenting part) is abnormal.

- Transverse lie

  ○ The presenting part is high in the pelvis and not yet engaged when the membranes rupture. This leaves room for the cord to descend and precede the presenting part.

- Small-for-gestational-age newborn

- Unusually long umbilical cord

- Multifetal pregnancy

- Cephalopelvic disproportion

    o This can result in a loose fit between fetal presenting part and maternal pelvis, leaving room for the cord to slip down.

- Placenta previa

- Intrauterine tumor preventing the presenting part from engaging.

- Hydramnios or polyhydramnios

    o Hydramnios or polyhydramnios is excessive amniotic fluid of more than 2,000 mL.

Assessment

- Subjective Data

    o The client states that she can feel something coming through her vagina.

- Objective Data

    o Physical assessment findings

        ▪ Visualization or palpation of the umbilical cord protruding from the introitus

        ▪ Assessment that shows FHR to have variable or prolonged decelerations

        ▪ Extreme increase in fetal activity that occurs and then ceases; suggestive of severe fetal hypoxia

Collaborative Care

- Nursing Care

    ▪ Call for assistance immediately.

    ▪ Notify the primary care provider of the prolapsed cord.

    ▪ Use a sterile-gloved hand, insert two fingers into the vagina, and apply finger pressure on either side of the cord to the fetal presenting part to elevate it off of the cord.

    ▪ Reposition the client in a knee-chest, Trendelenburg, or a side-lying position with a rolled towel under the client's right or left hip to relieve pressure on the cord.

    ▪ Apply a sterile saline-soaked towel to the cord to prevent drying and to maintain blood flow if it is protruding from the vaginal introitus.

    ▪ Closely monitor the FHR with an electronic fetal monitor for variable decelerations, which are indicative of fetal asphyxia and hypoxia from cord compression.

- Administer oxygen at 8 to 10 L via a face mask. This will improve fetal oxygenation.

- Initiate IV infusion or administer a bolus.

- Prepare the client for a cesarean birth if other measures fail.

- Inform and educate the client and her support person about the interventions.

  o Client outcomes

  - The client and fetus will be free from injury.

MECONIUM-STAINED AMNIOTIC FLUID

Overview

- Meconium passage in the amniotic fluid during the antepartum period prior to the start of labor is typically not associated with an unfavorable fetal outcome.

- The fetus has had an episode of loss of sphincter control, allowing meconium to pass into amniotic fluid.

Risk Factors

- There is an increased incidence for meconium in the amniotic fluid after 38 weeks of gestation.

- Umbilical cord compression results in fetal hypoxia that stimulates the vagal nerve in mature fetuses.

- Hypoxia stimulates the vagal nerve, which induces peristalsis of the fetal gastrointestinal tract and relaxation of the anal sphincter, which results in release of meconium (the first stool of the fetus or neonate) as well as fetal bradycardia.

Assessment

- Objective Data

  o Physical assessment findings

  - The presence of meconium in the amniotic fluid can be determined by visual inspection.

  - The fluid may vary in color from black to greenish, yellow or brown, and it will have a thick fresh consistency.

  - Criteria for evaluation of meconium-stained amniotic fluid

    □ Consistency that is thick and fresh, which indicates of fetal stress

    □ Meconium is first passed in later labor with variable or late FHR decelerations (ominous sign)

        □ Meconium alone in the amniotic fluid is not a sign of fetal distress; it must be accompanied by variable or late FHR decelerations with or without acidosis, which is confirmed by scalp blood sampling to be considered ominous

- Diagnostic Procedures
  - Intrapartal meconium requires further careful evaluation if birth is not imminent to determine necessary interventions.
    - □ Electronic fetal monitoring
    - □ Fetal scalp blood sampling

Collaborative Care

- Nursing Care
  - Document the meconium-stained amniotic fluid and its color.
  - An amnioinfusion of 0.9% sodium chloride or lactated Ringer's solution should be instilled into the amniotic cavity through a transcervical cavity into the uterus to thin meconium-stained fluid.
  - At the time of birth, the nurse should be prepared to suction the nasopharynx of the neonate.
  - Suctioning reduces the incidence and severity of meconium aspiration syndrome in the neonate.
- Client Outcomes
  - The client and fetus will be free from injury.

FETAL DISTRESS

 Overview

- Fetal distress is present when:
  - The FHR is below 110/min or above 160/min.
  - The FHR shows decreased or no variability.
  - There is fetal hyperactivity or no fetal activity.
  - The fetal blood pH is less than 7.2.

Risk Factors

- Fetal anomalies
- Uterine anomalies
- Complications of labor and birth

Assessment

- Objective Data

    o Nonreassuring FHR pattern with decreased or no variability

    o Diagnostic procedures

        ▪ Monitor uterine contractions.

        ▪ Monitor FHR.

        ▪ Monitor findings of ultrasound and any other prescribed diagnostics.

Collaborative Care

- Nursing Care

    o Monitor maternal vital signs and FHR.

    o Position the client in a left side-lying reclining position with legs elevated.

    o Administer 8 to 10 L of oxygen via a face mask.

    o Discontinue oxytocin (Pitocin) if being administered.

    o Increase IV fluid rate to treat hypotension if indicated.

    o Prepare the client for an emergency cesarean birth.

- Client Outcomes

    o The client and fetus will be free from injury.

DYSTOCIA (DYSFUNCTIONAL LABOR)

Overview

- Dystocia, or dysfunctional labor, is a difficult or abnormal labor related to the five powers of labor (powers, passenger, passageway, psyche, and position).

- Atypical uterine contraction patterns prevent the normal process of labor. These contractions can be hypotonic (weak, inefficient, or completely absent) or hypertonic (excessively frequent, uncoordinated, and of strong intensity with inadequate uterine relaxation) with failure to efface and dilate the cervix for the progression of labor.

- Risk factors for dysfunctional labor

    o Short stature, overweight status

    o Age greater than 40 years

    o Uterine abnormalities

    o Pelvic soft tissue obstructions or pelvic contracture

    o Cephalopelvic disproportion (fetal head is larger than maternal pelvis)

    o Fetal macrosomia

- ○ Fetal malpresentation, malposition
- ○ Multifetal pregnancy
- ○ Hypertonic or hypotonic uterus
- ○ Maternal fatigue, fear, or dehydration
- ○ Inappropriate timing of anesthesia or analgesics

Assessment

- • Objective Data
  - ○ Physical assessment findings
    - ■ Note a lack of progress in dilatation, effacement, or fetal descent during labor.
      - □ A hypotonic uterus is easily indentable, even at peak of contractions.
      - □ A hypertonic uterus cannot be indented, even between contractions.
    - ■ Observe the client as having ineffective pushing with no voluntary urge to bear down.
      - □ Persistent occiput posterior presentation is when the fetal occiput is directed toward the posterior maternal pelvis rather than the anterior pelvis.
      - □ Persistent occiput posterior position prolongs labor and the client has a great deal of back pain as the fetus presses against the maternal sacrum.
  - ○ Diagnostic Procedures
    - ■ Ultrasound
    - ■ Amniotomy or stripping of membranes if not ruptured
    - ■ Oxytocin (Pitocin) infusion
    - ■ Vacuum-assisted birth
    - ■ Cesarean birth

Collaborative Care

- • Nursing Care Dysfunctional Labor
  - ○ Assist with the application of a fetal scalp electrode and/or intrauterine pressure catheter.
  - ○ Assist with an amniotomy (artificial rupture of membranes).
  - ○ Encourage the client to engage in regular voiding to empty her bladder.
  - ○ Encourage position changes to aid in fetal descent or to open up the pelvic outlet.
  - ○ Encourage ambulation to enhance the progression of labor
  - ○ Encourage hydrotherapy and other relaxation techniques to aid in the progression of labor

- ○ Assist the mother into a beneficial position for pushing and coaching her about how to bear down with contractions.

- ○ Prepare for a possible forceps-assisted, vacuum-assisted, or cesarean birth.

- ○ Continue assessing FHR in response to labor.

  - ■ The client should be positioned on her hands and knees to help the fetus to rotate from a posterior to anterior position.

  - ■ Counterpressure should be applied with the fist or heel of the hand to the sacral area. This technique can help to alleviate discomfort.

- • Medications

  - ○ Oxytocin (Pitocin)

    - ■ Therapeutic intent

      - □ Used to augment labor and strengthen uterine contractions

    - ■ Nursing considerations

      - □ Administer oxytocin if prescribed to augment labor. Oxytocin is not administered for hypertonic contractions.

- • Nursing Care for Hypertonic Contractions

  - ○ Maintain hydration.

  - ○ Promote rest and relaxation and provide comfort measures between contractions.

  - ○ Place the client in a lateral position and provide oxygen by mask.

- • Medications

  - ○ Administer analgesics if prescribed (for rest from hypertonic contractions).

- • Client Outcomes

  - ○ The client will experience labor without complications or injury.

PRECIPITOUS LABOR

Overview

- • Precipitous labor is defined as labor that lasts 3 hr or less from the onset of contractions to the time of delivery.

Risk Factors

- ○ Hypertonic uterine dysfunction

  - ■ Nonproductive, uncoordinated, painful, uterine contractions during labor that are too frequent and too long in duration and do not allow for relaxation of the uterine muscle between contractions (uterine tetany).

- Hypertonic contractions do not contribute to the progression of labor (cervical effacement, dilation, and fetal descent).

- Hypertonic contractions can result in uteroplacental insufficiency leading to fetal hypoxia.

  ○ Oxytocin (Pitocin) stimulation may be administered to augment or induce labor by increasing intensity and duration of contractions.

- Oxytocin stimulation can lead to hypertonic uterine contractions.

  ○ Multiparous client

- May move through the stages of labor more rapidly

Assessment

- Subjective Data (during labor)

  ○ Low backache

  ○ Abdominal pressure and cramping

- Objective Data

  ○ Increased or bloody vaginal discharge

  ○ Palpable uterine contractions

  ○ Progress of cervical dilation and effacement

  ○ Diarrhea

  ○ Fetal presentation, station, and position

  ○ Status of amniotic membranes (membranes can be intact or ruptured)

- Physical Assessment Findings (postbirth)

  - Assess maternal perineal area for signs of trauma or lacerations.

  - Assess the neonate's color and for signs of hypoxia.

  - Assess for signs of trauma to presenting part of neonate, especially on cephalic presentation.

Collaborative Care

- Nursing Care

  ○ Do not leave the mother unattended.

  - Provide reassurance and emotional support to help the mother remain calm.

  - Prepare for emergency delivery of the neonate.

  ○ Encourage the mother to pant with an open mouth between contractions to control the urge to push.

- Encourage the client to maintain a side-lying position to optimize uteroplacental perfusion and fetal oxygenation.

- Prepare for the rupturing of membranes upon crowning (fetal head visible at perineum) if not already ruptured.

- Do not attempt to stop delivery.

- Control the rapid delivery by applying light pressure to the perineal area and fetal head, gently pressing upward toward the vagina. This will ease the rapid expulsion of the fetus and help to prevent cerebral damage to the newborn and perineal lacerations to the mother.

  - Deliver the fetus between contractions assuring the cord is not around the fetal neck.

  - If the cord is around the fetal neck, attempt to gently slip it over the head. If not possible, clamp the cord with two clamps and cut between the clamps.

- Suction mucus from the neonate's mouth and nose with a bulb syringe when the head appears.

- Next, deliver the anterior shoulder located under the maternal symphysis pubis: next, the posterior shoulder; and then allow the rest of the fetal body to slip out.

- Assess for complications of precipitous labor.

- Maternal

  - Cervical, vaginal, and/or perineal lacerations

  - Resultant tissue trauma secondary to rapid birth

  - Uterine rupture

  - Amniotic fluid embolism

  - Postpartum hemorrhage

- Fetal/neonate

  - Fetal hypoxia

    - Fetal hypoxia can be caused by uteroplacental insufficiency resulting from hypertonic uterus.

    - An umbilical cord around the fetal neck can result in asphyxia and cause a decrease in fetal oxygenation.

  - Fetal intracranial hemorrhage

    - Resulting from cephalic trauma during rapid birth

- Client outcomes

  - The client and fetus will be free from injury.

RUPTURE OF THE UTERUS

Overview

- Rupture of the uterus may extend through the entire uterine wall muscle into the peritoneal cavity or broad ligament, which is a complete rupture of the uterus. Extension into the peritoneum, but not into the peritoneal cavity or broad ligament, is an incomplete rupture of the uterus.

  - Partial separation can occur at an old cesarean scar.

  o Bleeding uterine rupture is usually internal

Risk Factors

  o Separation of the scar from a previous classic vertical cesarean incision through the uterus

  o Congenital uterine abnormality

  o Uterine trauma from an accident or surgery

  o Overdistention of the uterus from a newborn who is large for gestational age, a multifetal gestation, or polyhydramnios

  o Hyperstimulation of the uterus, either spontaneous or from oxytocin (Pitocin) administration

  o External or internal fetal version done to correct malposition of the fetus

  o Forceps-assisted birth

- Rupture of the uterus occurs more often in clients who are multigravida

Assessment

- Subjective Data

  o The client reports of something tearing inside or sharp pain.

- Objective Data

  o Physical assessment findings

    - Assess the FHR for signs of distress, bradycardia, late decelerations, tachycardia, and absent variability.

    - Contractions stop and pain is relieved.

    - Fetal parts are palpable though the abdomen.

    - The client is vomiting.

    - The client is bleeding.

    - Assess for symptoms of shock: tachypnea, hypotension, pallor, and cool clammy skin.

Collaborative Care

- Nursing Care

    o   Administer IV fluids.

    o   Administer blood product transfusions if prescribed.

    o   Assist with a laparotomy and blood transfusions for an incomplete uterine rupture.

    o   Assist with a hysterectomy and blood transfusion for a complete uterine rupture.

    o   Prepare the client for an immediate cesarean birth.

    o   Inform the client and her support system about the treatment.

- Client Outcomes

    o   Schedule an emergency cesarean birth to minimize maternal fetal injury.

AMNIOTIC FLUID EMBOLUS

Overview

- An amniotic fluid embolism is caused by a rupture in the amniotic sac or maternal uterine veins accompanied by a high intrauterine pressure that causes infiltration of the amniotic fluid and its contents into the maternal circulation. This infiltrated amniotic fluid then travels to and obstructs pulmonary vessels and causes respiratory distress and circulatory collapse.

- Meconium-stained amniotic fluid or fluid containing other particulate matter can cause more maternal damage because it more readily clogs the pulmonary veins completely.

- Serious coagulation problems such as disseminated intravascular coagulopathy can occur.

- Risk factors for amniotic fluid embolism

    o   Multiparity

    o   Tumultuous labor

    o   Abruptio placentae

    o   Oxytocin (Pitocin) administration

    o   Fetal macrosomia

    o   Hydramnios

    o   Fetal demise

    o   Meconium-stained amniotic fluid

Assessment

- Subjective Data

  o Complaint of sudden chest pain.

- Objective Data

  o Physical assessment findings

  o Nursing assessments for a client with amniotic fluid embolism

  - Client is exhibiting signs of respiratory distress, which include:
    - □ Restlessness
    - □ Cyanosis
    - □ Dyspnea
    - □ Pulmonary edema
    - □ Respiratory arrest
  - Client is exhibiting signs of coagulation failure
    - □ Bleeding from incisions and venipuncture sites
    - □ Petechiae and ecchymosis
    - □ Uterine atony
  - Client is exhibiting signs of circulatory collapse
    - □ Tachycardia
    - □ Hypotension
    - □ Shock
    - □ Cardiac arrest

Collaborative Care

- Nursing Care

  o Administer oxygen via a mask at 8 to 10 L.

  o Assist with intubation and mechanical ventilation as indicated.

  o Perform cardiopulmonary resuscitation if necessary.

  o Administer IV fluids.

  o Position the client on her side with her pelvis tilted at a 30° angle to displace the uterus.

  o Administer blood products as prescribed to correct coagulation failure.

     ○   Insert an indwelling urinary catheter and measure hourly urine output.

     ○   Monitor maternal and fetal status.

     ○   Prepare the client for an emergency cesarean birth if the fetus is not yet delivered.

● Client Outcomes

     ○   The client and fetus will be free from injury.

CHAPTER 16: COMPLICATIONS RELATED TO THE LABOR PROCESS

(A) Application Exercises

1. If contractions are of too long a duration or do not have complete relaxation or uterine tone in between contractions, the adverse effect will be

    A. prolonged labor.

    B. reduced fetal oxygen supply.

    C. impairment of cervical dilation.

    D. increased maternal stress.

2. A nurse is caring for a client who is in active labor and reports severe back pain. During assessment, the fetus is noted to be in the occiput posterior position. Which of the following maternal positions should the nurse suggest to the client to help facilitate normal labor progress?

    A. Hands and knees

    B. Lithotomy

    C. Trendelenburg

    D. Supine with a rolled towel under one hip

3. A nurse is caring for a client who is admitted to the labor and delivery unit. With the use of Leopold maneuvers, it is noted that the fetus is in a breech presentation. For which of the following possible complications should the nurse observe?

    A. Precipitous labor

    B. Premature rupture of membranes

    C. Postmaturity syndrome

    D. Prolapsed umbilical cord

4. A nurse should be aware that which of the following are risk factors for dysfunctional labor?

    _____ Short stature

    _____ Cephalopelvic disproportion

    _____ Fetal microsomia

    _____ Fetal malpresentation

    _____ Maternal fatigue

5. A nurse is caring for a client who is at 42 weeks of gestation and in active labor. The nurse should understand that the fetus is at risk for which of the following?

    A. Intrauterine growth restriction

    B. Hyperglycemia

    C. Meconium aspiration

    D. Polyhydramnios

6. A nurse is caring for a client in active labor. When last examined 2 hr ago, the client's cervix was 3 cm dilated, 100% effaced, membranes intact, and the fetus was at a -2 station. The client suddenly states "my water broke." The monitor reveals a FHR of 80 to 85/min and the nurse performs a vaginal examination, noticing clear fluid and a pulsing loop of umbilical cord in the client's vagina. Which of the following actions should the nurse perform first?

    A. Place the client in the Trendelenburg position.

    B. Apply pressure to the presenting part with her fingers.

    C. Give the client 10 L of oxygen via a face mask.

    D. Call for assistance.

CHAPTER 16: COMPLICATIONS RELATED TO THE LABOR PROCESS

 Application Exercises Answer Key

1. If contractions are of too long a duration or do not have complete relaxation or uterine tone in between contractions, the adverse effect will be

   A. prolonged labor.

   B. reduced fetal oxygen supply.

   C. impairment of cervical dilation.

   D. increased maternal stress.

   When the uterus contracts there is a constriction of the blood vessels that provide oxygenation and nutrients to the fetus. If there is inadequate relaxation between contractions, there is a reduction of oxygenation to the fetus. These contractions, referred to as hypertonic contractions, can produce maternal stress, but are not an adverse effect. Hypertonic contractions usually cause precipitous labor, not prolonged labor. Hypertonic contractions do not usually impede cervical dilation.

   (N) NCLEX® Connection: Physiological Adaptation, Alterations in Body Systems

2. A nurse is caring for a client who is in active labor and reports severe back pain. During assessment, the fetus is noted to be in the occiput posterior position. Which of the following maternal positions should the nurse suggest to the client to help facilitate normal labor progress?

   A. Hands and knees

   B. Lithotomy

   C. Trendelenburg

   D. Supine with a rolled towel under one hip

   Having the client assume a position on her hands and knees may help the fetus rotate from a posterior to an anterior position. The lithotomy position is when the client lies on her back with her knees elevated. The Trendelenburg and supine positions both require the client to lie on her back. None of these positions put the client in a position that would assist in the rotation of the fetus.

   (N) NCLEX® Connection: Physiological Adaptation, Alterations in Body Systems

3. A nurse is caring for a client admitted to the labor and delivery unit. With the use of Leopold maneuvers, it is noted that the fetus is in a breech presentation. For which of the following possible complications should the nurse observe?

    A. Precipitous labor

    B. Premature rupture of membranes

    C. Postmaturity syndrome

    D. Prolapsed umbilical cord

A prolapsed umbilical cord is a potential complication for a fetus in a breech presentation. Breech presentation would most likely cause dystocia (prolonged, difficult labor) rather than a precipitous labor. It has no effect on the rupture of membranes and is not associated with postmaturity syndrome.

 NCLEX® Connection: Physiological Adaptation, Alterations in Body Systems

4. The nurse should be aware that which of the following are risk factors for dysfunctional labor?

    __X__   **Short stature**

    __X__   **Cephalopelvic disproportion**

    _____   Fetal microsomia

    __X__   **Fetal malpresentation**

    __X__   **Maternal fatigue**

Factors such as short stature, cephalopelvic disproportion, fetal malpresentation, and maternal fatigue are risk factors for dysfunctional labor. Fetal microsomia is not a risk factor.

 NCLEX® Connection: Physiological Adaptation, Alterations in Body Systems

5. A nurse is caring for a client who is at 42 weeks of gestation and in active labor. The nurse should understand that the fetus is at risk for which of the following?

    A. Intrauterine growth restriction

    B. Hyperglycemia

    C. Meconium aspiration

    D. Polyhydramnios

Postterm neonates are at risk for aspiration of meconium. Intrauterine growth restriction should occur earlier in the pregnancy and not at this point. A postterm neonate is at risk for hypoglycemia, not hyperglycemia. Postterm pregnancies result in oligohydramnios, not polyhydramnios.

 NCLEX® Connection: Physiological Adaptation, Alterations in Body Systems

6. A nurse is caring for a client in active labor. When last examined 2 hr ago, the client's cervix was 3 cm dilated, 100% effaced, membranes intact, and the fetus was at a -2 station. The client suddenly states "my water broke." The monitor reveals a FHR of 80 to 85/min and the nurse performs a vaginal examination, noticing clear fluid and a pulsing loop of umbilical cord in the client's vagina. Which of the following actions should the nurse perform first?

    A. Place the client in the Trendelenburg position.

    B. Apply pressure to the presenting part with her fingers.

    C. Give the client 10 L of oxygen via a face mask.

    D. Call for assistance.

    Calling for assistance is the first action the nurse should take. All of the other interventions should be performed after calling for assistance.

NCLEX® Connection: Physiological Adaptation, Alterations in Body Systems

UNIT 3: POSTPARTUM NURSING CARE

- Routine Postpartum Care

- Complications of the Postpartum Period

NCLEX® CONNECTIONS

When reviewing the chapters in this unit, keep in mind the relevant sections of the NCLEX® outline, in particular:

CLIENT NEEDS: HEALTH PROMOTION AND MAINTENANCE	**CLIENT NEEDS: PHARMACOLOGICAL AND PARENTERAL THERAPIES**	**CLIENT NEEDS: REDUCTION OF RISK POTENTIAL**
Relevant topics/tasks include:	Relevant topics/tasks include:	Relevant topics/tasks include:
• Ante/Intra/Postpartum and Newborn Care ○ Provide postpartum care and education. • Developmental Stages and Transitions ○ Assist the client to cope with life transitions. • Health Promotion/Disease Prevention ○ Provide information about healthy behaviors and health promotion/ maintenance recommendations.	• Adverse Effects/ Contraindications/Side Effects/Interactions ○ Notify the provider of side effects, adverse effects, and contraindications of medications and parenteral therapy. • Expected Actions/ Outcomes ○ Evaluate therapeutic effect of medications. • Medication Administration ○ Review pertinent data prior to medication administration.	• Changes/Abnormalities in Vital Signs ○ Assess and respond to changes in the client's vital signs. • Laboratory Values ○ Educate the client about the purpose and procedure of prescribed laboratory tests. • Potential for Complications from Surgical Procedures and Health Alterations ○ Apply knowledge of pathophysiology to monitoring for complications.

UNIT 3	POSTPARTUM NURSING CARE
Section	Routine Postpartum Care
Chapter 17	**Postpartum Physiological Adaptations**

Overview

- It is important for a nurse to provide comfort measures for a client during the fourth stage of labor. This maternal recovery period starts with the delivery of the placenta and lasts from 1 to 4 hr. Also during this stage, parent-newborn bonding should begin to occur.

- The main goal during the immediate postpartum period is to prevent postpartum hemorrhage. Other goals include assisting in a client's recovery, identifying any deviations from the norm, providing comfort measures and pharmacologic pain relief as prescribed, providing client education about newborn and self-care, and promoting family-infant bonding.

- The postpartum period includes physiological and psychological adjustments, also known as the puerperium. This period begins after the delivery of the placenta and ends when the body returns to the prepregnant state. This process takes approximately 6 weeks.

  ○ Physiological maternal changes consist of uterine involution, lochia flow, cervical involution, decrease in vaginal distention, changes in ovarian function and menstruation, breast changes, urinary tract changes, gastrointestinal tract changes, and cardiovascular changes.

  ○ The greatest risks during the postpartum period are hemorrhage, shock, and infection.

  ○ Oxytocin, a hormone released from the pituitary gland, coordinates and strengthens uterine contractions.

    ▪ Breastfeeding stimulates the release of endogenous oxytocin from the pituitary gland.

    ▪ Pitocin (exogenous oxytocin) may be administered postpartum to improve the quality of the uterine contractions.

    ▪ A firm and contracted uterus prevents excessive bleeding and hemorrhage.

    ▪ Uncomfortable uterine cramping is referred to as afterpains.

  ○ After delivery of the placenta, hormones (estrogen, progesterone, and placental enzyme insulinase) decrease, thus resulting in decreased blood glucose, estrogen, and progesterone levels.

    ▪ Decreased estrogen is associated with breast engorgement, diaphoresis (profuse perspiration), and diuresis (increased formation and excretion of urine) of excess extracellular fluid accumulated during pregnancy.

- Decreased estrogen diminishes vaginal lubrication. Local dryness and intercourse discomfort may persist until ovarian function returns and menstruation resumes.

- Decreased progesterone results in an increase in muscle tone throughout the body.

- Decreased placental enzyme insulinase results in reversal of the diabetogenic effects of pregnancy resting in lower blood glucose levels immediately puerperium.

○ Lactating and nonlactating women differ in the timing of the first ovulation and the resumption of menstruation.

- In lactating women, prolactin levels remain elevated postpartum. In nonlactating women, prolactin levels decrease postpartum.

○ Therapeutic and diagnostic procedures and nursing implementations

- Laceration and/or episiotomy repair is performed by the primary care provider. The nurse should assist as necessary during the procedure.

- For Rh-negative mothers:

  □ $RH_o(D)$ immune globulin (RhoGAM) is administered within 72 hr to women who are Rh-negative and gave birth to infants who are Rh-positive to prevent sensitization in future pregnancies.

  □ Kleihauer-Betke test determines the amount of fetal blood in maternal circulation if a large fetomaternal transfusion is suspected. If 15 mL or more of fetal blood is detected, the mother should receive an increased RhoGAM dose.

  □ A CBC may be ordered and will monitor Hgb and Hct, WBC count, and platelet counts.

○ Nursing assessments and interventions

- Postpartum assessments immediately following delivery include monitoring the client's vital signs, uterine firmness and its location in relation to the umbilicus, uterine position in relation to the midline of the abdomen, and amount of vaginal bleeding.

  □ If the client is stable, vital signs will be monitored every 15 min x 4 for the first hour, every 30 min x 2 for the second hr, hourly x 2 for at least 2 hr, then every 4 to 8 hr depending on the prescriptions set forth by the primary care provider.

 View Media Supplement: Postpartum Assessment (Video)

- A focused physical assessment should include assessing the client's
  - □ B-reasts.
  - □ U-terus (fundal height, uterine placement, and consistency).
  - □ B-owel and GI function.
  - □ B-bladder function.
  - □ L-ochia (color, odor, consistency, and amount [COCA]).
  - □ E-pisiotomy (edema, ecchymosis, approximation).
  - □ Vital signs to include in the pain assessment.
  - □ Teaching needs.

Thermoregulation

- Postpartum chill, which occurs in the first 2 hr puerperium, is an uncontrollable shaking chill experienced by the client immediately following birth. Postpartum chill is possibly related to a nervous system response, vasomotor changes, a shift in fluids, and/or the work of labor. This is a normal occurrence unless accompanied by an elevated temperature.

  - ○ Provide the client with warm blankets and fluids.
  - ○ Assure the client that these chills are a self-limiting common occurrence that will only last a short while.

Fundus

- Physical changes of the uterus include involution of the uterus. Involution occurs with contractions of the uterine smooth muscle, whereby the uterus returns to its prepregnant state. The uterus also rapidly decreases in size from approximately 1,000 g (2.2 lb) to 50 to 60 g (< 2 oz) over a period of 6 weeks with the fundal height steadily descending into the pelvis approximately one fingerbreadth (1 cm) per day.

 View Media Supplement: Fundal Height (Image)

  - ○ Immediately after delivery the fundus should be firm, midline with the umbilicus, and approximately at the level of the umbilicus. At 12 hr postpartum the fundus may be palpated at 1 cm above the umbilicus.
  - ○ Every 24 hr the fundus should descend approximately 1 to 2 cm. It should be halfway between the symphysis pubis and the umbilicus by the sixth postpartum day.
  - ○ By day 10, the uterus should lie within the true pelvis and should not be palpable.

- The nurse should assess the fundal height, uterine placement, and uterine consistency at least once a shift after the recovery period has ended.

  - ○ Explain the procedure to the client.
  - ○ Apply clean gloves, a lower perineal pad, and observe lochia flow as the fundus is palpated.

- o Cup one hand just above the symphysis pubis to support the lower segment of the uterus, and with the other hand, palpate the client's abdomen to locate the fundus.

- o Document the fundal height, location, and uterine consistency.

  - ■ Determine the fundal height by placing fingers on the abdomen and measuring how many fingerbreadths (centimeters) fit between the fundus and the umbilicus above, below, or at the umbilical level.

  - ■ Determine if the fundus is midline in the pelvis or displaced laterally (caused by a full bladder).

  - ■ Determine if the fundus is firm or boggy. If the fundus is boggy (not firm), lightly massage the fundus in a circular motion.

- • Nursing interventions related to uterine involution

  - o Administer oxytocics intramuscularly or IV as prescribed after the placenta is delivered to promote uterine contractions and to prevent hemorrhage.

    - ■ Oxytocics include oxytocin (Pitocin), methylergonovine maleate (Methergine), and carboprost tromethamine (Hemabate).

  - o Monitor for adverse affects of the oxytocics.

    - ■ Oxytocin may cause hypotension.

    - ■ Methylergonovine maleate, ergonovine maleate, and carboprost tromethamine may cause hypertension.

  - o Encourage early breastfeeding for a mother who is lactating. This will stimulate the production of natural oxytocin and will help prevent hemorrhage.

  - o Encourage frequent emptying of the bladder every 2 to 3 hr to prevent possible uterine displacement and atony.

Lochia

- • Physical changes in vaginal discharge include lochia, which is the blood flow from the uterus during puerperium.

  - o Three stages of lochia

    - ■ Lochia rubra – bright red color, bloody consistency, fleshy odor, may contain small clots, transient flow increases during breastfeeding and upon rising. Lasts 1 to 3 days after delivery.

    - ■ Lochia serosa – pinkish brown color and serosanguineous consistency. Lasts from approximately day 4 to day 10 after delivery.

    - ■ Lochia alba – yellowish, white creamy color, fleshy odor. Lasts from approximately day 11 up to and beyond 6 weeks postpartum.

- Lochia amount is assessed by the quantity of saturation on the perineal pad as being either:

  - Scant (< 2.5 cm)

  - Light (< 10 cm)

  - Moderate (> 10 cm)

  - Heavy (one pad saturated within 2 hr)

  - Excessive blood loss (one pad saturated in 15 min or less or pooling of blood under buttocks)

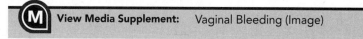

View Media Supplement: Vaginal Bleeding (Image)

- The nurse should assess the lochia flow for normal color, amount, and consistency.

  - Lochia typically trickles from the vaginal opening but flows more steadily during uterine contractions.

  - Massaging the uterus or ambulation may result in a gush of lochia with the expression of clots and dark blood that has pooled in the vagina, but should soon decrease back to a trickle of bright red lochia when in the early puerperium.

- Nursing interventions for abnormal lochia include notifying the primary care provider and performing prescribed interventions based on the cause of the abnormality.

  - Abnormal lochia is evidenced by:

    - Excessive spurting of bright red blood from the vagina, possibly indicating a cervical or vaginal tear.

    - Numerous large clots and excessive blood loss (saturation of one pad in 15 min or less), which may be indicative of a hemorrhage.

    - Foul odor, which is suggestive of an infection.

    - Persistent lochia rubra in the early postpartum period beyond day 3, which may indicate retained placental fragments.

    - Continued flow of lochia serosa or alba beyond the normal length of time may indicate endometritis, especially if it is accompanied by a fever, pain, or abdominal tenderness.

Cervix, Vagina, and Perineum

- Physical changes of the cervix, vagina, and perineum are as follows:

  - The cervix is soft directly after birth and may be edematous, bruised, and have some small lacerations. Within 2 to 3 days postpartum, it shortens and regains its form becoming firm with the os gradually closing.

    - Lacerations can delay the production of estrogen-influenced cervical mucus and are a predisposing factor to infection.

   ○ The vagina, which has distended, gradually returns to its prepregnancy size with the reappearance of rugae and a thickening of the vaginal mucosa. However, muscle tone is never restored completely.

   ○ The soft tissues of the perineum may be erythematous and edematous, especially in areas of an episiotomy or lacerations. Hematomas or hemorrhoids may be present. The pelvic floor muscles may be overstretched and weak.

- The nurse should assess for cervical, vaginal, and perineal healing.

   ○ Observe for perineal erythema, edema, and hematoma.

   ○ Assess episiotomy and lacerations for approximation, drainage, quantity, and quality.

     ■ A bright red trickle of blood from the episiotomy site in the early postpartum period is a normal finding.

- Nursing interventions for perineal tenderness, laceration, and episiotomy

   ○ Promote measures for the client to help to soften her stools.

   ○ Educate the client about proper cleansing to prevent infection.

     ■ The client should wash her hands thoroughly before and after voiding.

     ■ The client should use a squeeze bottle filled with warm water or antiseptic solution after each voiding to cleanse the perineal area.

     ■ The client should clean her perineal area from front to back (urethra to anus).

     ■ The client should blot dry, not wipe.

     ■ The client should sparingly use a topical application of antiseptic cream or spray.

     ■ The client's perineal pad should be changed from front to back after voiding or defecating.

   ○ Promote comfort measures.

     ■ Apply ice packs to the client's perineum for the first 24 to 48 hr to reduce edema and provide anesthetic effect.

     ■ Encourage sitz baths at a temperature of 38 to 40° C (100 to 104° F) or cooler at least twice a day.

     ■ Administer analgesia such as nonopioids (acetaminophen [Tylenol]), nonsteroidal anti-inflammatories (ibuprofen [Advil]), and opioids (codeine, hydrocodone) as prescribed for pain and discomfort.

     ■ Opioid analgesia may be administered via a PCA (patient controlled analgesia) pump after cesarean births. Continuous epidural infusions may also be used for pain control after cesarean births.

     ■ Apply topical anesthetics (Americaine spray or Dermoplast) to the client's perineal area as needed or witch hazel compresses (Tuck's) to the rectal area for hemorrhoids.

Breasts

- Physical changes of the breasts include the secretion of colostrum, which occurs during pregnancy and 2 to 3 days immediately after birth. Milk is produced 2 to 3 days after the delivery of the newborn.

- The nurse should assess the client's breasts as well as her ability to assist the newborn with latching on if breastfeeding.

  o Colostrum secretion in lactating and non-lactating clients

  o Engorgement of the breast tissue as a result of lymphatic circulation, milk production, and temporary vein congestion

  o Redness and tenderness of the breast

  o Cracked nipples and indications of mastitis (infection in a milk duct of the breast with concurrent flu-like symptoms)

  o Ascertain that the newborn who is breastfeeding has latched on correctly to prevent sore nipples

  o Ineffective newborn feeding patterns related to maternal discomfort, newborn positioning, or difficulty with the newborn latching onto the breast

- Nursing interventions pertaining to the client's breasts and breastfeeding

  o Encourage early demand breastfeeding for the mother who is lactating, which will also stimulate the production of natural oxytocin and help prevent uterine hemorrhage.

  o Assist the client into a comfortable position and have her try various positions during breastfeeding (cradle hold, side-lying, and football hold) and explaining how varying positions can prevent nipple soreness.

  o Teach the client the importance of proper latch techniques (the newborn takes in part of the areola and nipple, not just the tip of the nipple) to prevent nipple soreness.

  o Inform the client that breastfeeding causes the release of oxytocin, which stimulates uterine contractions. This is a normal occurrence and beneficial to uterine tone.

Cardiovascular System and Fluid and Hematologic Status

- Physical changes in the cardiovascular system during the postpartum period

  o The cardiovascular system undergoes a decrease in blood volume during the postpartum period related to:

    ▪ Blood loss during childbirth (average blood loss is 500 mL in an uncomplicated vaginal delivery and 1,000 mL for a cesarean birth).

    ▪ Diaphoresis and diuresis of the excess fluid accumulated during the last part of the pregnancy. Loss occurs within the first 2 to 3 days postdelivery.

- o Hypovolemic shock does not usually occur in response to the normal blood loss of labor and birth, because:
  - ▪ Readjustments in the maternal vasculature occur in response to the following:
    - ▫ Elimination of the placenta diverting 500 to 750 mL of blood into the maternal systemic circulation.
    - ▫ Rapid reduction in the size of the uterus putting more blood into the maternal systemic circulation.

- Physical changes in blood values, coagulation factors, and fibrinogen levels during the puerperium

  - o Increased Hct and Hgb values are present immediately after delivery for up to 72 hr. Leukocytosis (white blood cell count elevation) of up to 20,000 to 25,000/mm³ occurs for the first 10 to 14 days without the presence of infection and then returns to normal.

  - o Coagulation factors and fibrinogen levels increase during pregnancy and remain elevated for 2 to 3 weeks postpartum. Hypercoagulability predisposes the postpartum woman to thrombus formation and thromboembolism.

- Vital sign changes

  - o Blood pressure is usually unchanged with an uncomplicated pregnancy, but may have an insignificant slight transient increase.

  - o Possible orthostatic hypotension within the first 48 hr postpartum may occur immediately after standing up with feelings of faintness or dizziness resulting from splanchnic (viscera/internal organs) engorgement that can occur after birth.

  - o Elevation of pulse, stroke volume, and cardiac output for the first hour postpartum occurs and then gradually decreases to a prepregnant state baseline by 8 to 10 weeks.

  - o Elevation of temperature to 38° C (100° F) resulting from dehydration after labor during the first 24 hr may occur, but should return to normal after 24 hr postpartum.

- The nurse should assess for cardiovascular and vital sign changes and monitor blood component changes.

  - o The nurse should also inspect the client's legs for redness, swelling, and warmth, which are additional signs of venous thrombosis.

- Nursing interventions for abnormal findings include notifying the primary care provider and performing prescribed interventions based on the cause of the abnormality.

  - o Encourage early ambulation to prevent venous stasis and thrombosis.

  - o Apply antiembolism hose to the client's lower extremities if she is at high-risk for developing venous stasis and thrombosis. The hose should be removed as soon as the client is ambulating.

  - o Administer medications as prescribed.

Gastrointestinal System and Bowel Function

- Physical changes in the gastrointestinal system

  o An increased appetite following delivery

  o Constipation with bowel evacuation delayed until 2 to 3 days after birth

  o Hemorrhoids

- The nurse should assess the gastrointestinal system including bowel function.

  o Assess the client for reports of hunger. The nurse should expect the client to have a good appetite.

  o Assess the client for bowel sounds and the return of normal bowel function.

    ▪ Spontaneous bowel movement may not occur for 2 to 3 days after delivery secondary to decreased intestinal muscle tone during labor and puerperium and prelabor diarrhea and dehydration. The client may also anticipate discomfort with defecation because of perineal tenderness, episiotomy, lacerations, or hemorrhoids.

  o Assess the client's rectal area for varicosities (hemorrhoids).

  o Operative vaginal birth (forceps-assisted and vacuum-assisted) and anal sphincter lacerations increase the risk of temporary postpartum anal incontinence that usually resolves within 6 months.

- Nursing interventions for gastrointestinal and bowel function

  o Encourage the client to take measures to soften her stools and promote bowel function (early ambulation, increased fluids, and high-fiber food sources).

  o Administer stool softeners (docusate sodium) as prescribed to prevent constipation.

    ▪ Enemas and suppositories are contraindicated.

Urinary System and Bladder Function

- The urinary system may show evidence of:

  o Urinary retention secondary to loss of bladder elasticity and tone and/or loss of bladder sensation resulting from trauma, medications, or anesthesia.

    ▪ A distended bladder as a result of urinary retention can cause uterine atony and displacement to one side, usually to the right. The ability of the uterus to contract is also lessened.

  o Postpartal diuresis with increased urinary output begins within 12 hr of delivery.

- The nurse should assess the urinary system and bladder function.

  o Assess the client's ability to void every 2 to 3 hr (perineal/urethral edema may cause pain and difficulty in voiding during the first 24 to 48 hr).

- Assess the client's bladder elimination pattern (client should be voiding every 2 to 3 hr). Excessive urine diuresis (1,500 to 3,000 mL/day) is normal within the first 2 to 3 days after delivery.

- Assess for signs of a distended bladder

  - Fundal height above the umbilicus or baseline level

  - Fundus displaced from the midline over to the side

  - Bladder bulges above the symphysis pubis

  - Excessive lochia

  - Tenderness over the bladder area

  - Frequent voiding of less than 150 mL of urine is indicative of urinary retention with overflow

- Nursing interventions for the urinary system and bladder function

  - Encourage the client to empty her bladder frequently (every 2 to 3 hr) to prevent possible displacement of the uterus and atony.

  - Measure the client's first few voidings after delivery to assess for bladder emptying.

  - Encourage the client to increase her oral fluid intake to replace fluids lost at delivery and to prevent or correct dehydration.

  - Catheterize if necessary for bladder distention if the client is unable to void to ensure complete emptying of the bladder and allow uterine involution.

Musculoskeletal System

- Physical changes of the musculoskeletal system involve a reversal of the musculoskeletal adaptations that occurred during pregnancy. By 6 to 8 weeks after birth:

  - The joints return to their pregnant state and are completely restabilized. The feet however, may remain permanently increased in size.

  - Muscle tone begins to be restored throughout the body with the removal of progesterone's effect following delivery of the placenta.

    - The rectus abdominis muscles of the abdomen and the pubococcygeal muscle tone are restored following placental expulsion.

- The nurse should assess the musculoskeletal system for changes.

  - Assess the client's abdominal wall for diastasis recti (a separation of the rectus muscle) anywhere from 2 to 4 cm. It usually resolves within 6 weeks.

- Nursing interventions pertaining to the musculoskeletal system

  o Teach the client postpartum strengthening exercises, advising her to start with simple exercises, and then gradually progressing to more strenuous ones.

  o Instruct clients who have had a cesarean birth to postpone abdominal exercises until about 4 weeks after delivery or follow recommendations of her health care provider.

  o Advise the client on good body mechanics and proper posture.

Immune System

- Review rubella status – a client who has a titer of less than 1:8 is administered a subcutaneous injection of rubella vaccine or an measles, mumps and rubella vaccine during the postpartum period to protect a subsequent fetus from malformations. The client should not get pregnant for 4 weeks following the vaccination.

- Review hepatitis B status – newborns born to infected mothers should receive the hepatitis B vaccine and the hepatitis B immune globulin within 12 hr of birth.

- Review the Rh status – all Rh-negative mothers who have newborns who are Rh-positive must be given RH_o (D) immune globulin (RhoGAM) administered IM within 72 hr of the newborn being born to suppress antibody formation in the mother.

- Test the client who receives both the rubella vaccine and RhoGAM after 3 months to determine if immunity to rubella has been developed.

Comfort Level

- Nursing assessments and interventions for the client's comfort level

  o Assess pain related to episiotomy, lacerations, incisions, afterpains, and sore nipples.

  o Assess location, type, and quality of the pain to guide nursing interventions and client education.

  o Administer pain medications as prescribed.

CHAPTER 17: POSTPARTUM PHYSIOLOGICAL ADAPTATIONS

(A) Application Exercises

1. After delivery, the uterus contracts and gradually returns to its prepregnant state. This is referred to as uterine

    A. inversion.

    B. subinvolution.

    C. involution.

    D. exfoliation.

2. A nurse is performing a fundal assessment for a client in her second postpartum day and observes the client's perineal pad for lochia. She notes the pad to be saturated approximately 12 cm with lochia that is bright red in color and contains small clots. The nurse knows that this finding is

    A. moderate lochia rubra.

    B. excessive lochia rubra.

    C. light lochia rubra.

    D. scant lochia serosa.

3. During ambulation to the bathroom, a postpartum client experiences a gush of dark red blood that soon stops. On assessment, a nurse finds the client's uterus to be firm and midline and at the level of the umbilicus. The nurse interprets this finding as

    A. a sign of a possible vaginal hematoma.

    B. an indication of a cervical or perineal laceration.

    C. a normal postural discharge of lochia.

    D. abnormally excessive lochia rubra flow.

4. A nurse is assessing a postpartum client for fundal height, location, and consistency. The fundus is found to be displaced laterally to the right and there is uterine atony. Which of the following is the cause of the uterine atony?

    A. Poor involution

    B. Urinary retention

    C. Hemorrhage

    D. Infection

5. A client is in the fourth stage of labor, has just delivered her newborn, and is stable. A nurse knows that during the maternal recovery period vital signs should be assessed at regular intervals. How often should vital sign intervals be assessed during the fourth stage of labor?

6. Which of the following nursing interventions will promote comfort for a client who has a small hematoma of the perineal area? (Select all that apply.)

_____ Apply ice to the perineal area for the first 24 to 48 hr.

_____ Encourage use of donut- shaped pillow for sitting.

_____ Encourage sitz baths at least twice a day.

_____ Use a topical antiseptic cream or spray on the perineal area.

_____ Obtain an order for an indwelling urinary catheter.

CHAPTER 17: POSTPARTUM PHYSIOLOGICAL ADAPTATIONS

(A) Application Exercises Answer Key

1. After delivery, the uterus contracts and gradually returns to its prepregnant state. This is referred to as uterine

    A. inversion.

    B. subinvolution.

    C. involution.

    D. exfoliation.

    Uterine involution is the return of the uterus to the prepregnant state, and postpartum contractions aid in this occurring. Uterine inversion is a condition in which the uterus turns inside out and can be caused by the placenta being removed too vigorously prior to its natural detachment process. Uterine subinvolution is the delay of the uterus in returning to the prepregnancy state. Uterine exfoliation is the shedding of the decidua tissue layers.

    (N) NCLEX® Connection: Physiological Adaptation, Alterations in Body Systems

2. A nurse is performing a fundal assessment for a client in her second postpartum day and observes the client's perineal pad for lochia. She notes the pad to be saturated approximately 12 cm with lochia that is bright red in color and contains small clots. The nurse knows that this finding is

    A. moderate lochia rubra.

    B. excessive lochia rubra.

    C. light lochia rubra.

    D. scant lochia serosa.

    The client has moderate lochia rubra containing small clots with a fleshy odor, which is a normal finding for the second day postpartum. There are three stages of lochia. Lochia rubra is bright red in color, with a bloody consistency that may have small clots, and lasts 1 to 3 days after birth. Lochia serosa is pinkish brown in color with a serosanguineous consistency, and lasts approximately from day 4 to day 10 after delivery. Lochia alba is yellowish white in color, and lasts from approximately day 11 up to and beyond 6 weeks postpartum. The amount of lochia is assessed by the quantity of saturation on the perineal pad with scant being less than 2.5 cm, light less than 10 cm, moderate, more than 10 cm, heavy, one pad within 2 hr, and excessive, one pad within 15 min.

    (N) NCLEX® Connection: Health Promotion and Maintenance, Ante/Intra/Postpartum and Newborn Care

3. During ambulation to the bathroom, a postpartum client experiences a gush of dark red blood that soon stops. On assessment, a nurse finds the client's uterus to be firm and midline and at the level of the umbilicus. The nurse interprets this finding as

    A. a sign of a possible vaginal hematoma.

    B. an indication of a cervical or perineal laceration.

    C. a normal postural discharge of lochia.

    D. abnormally excessive lochia rubra flow.

Lochia typically trickles from the vaginal opening, but flows more steadily during uterine contractions. Massaging the uterus or ambulation may result in a gush of lochia with the expression of clots and dark blood that has been pooled in the vagina, but should soon decrease back to a trickle of bright red lochia in the early puerperium. Excessive blood loss consists of one pad saturated in 15 min or less or the pooling of blood under the buttocks, which is not affected by the client's postural changes. A client who has a vaginal hematoma may report excessive pain or vaginal pressure. Excessive spurting of bright red blood from the vagina indicates a possible cervical or perineal laceration.

(N) NCLEX® Connection: Health Promotion and Maintenance, Ante/Intra/Postpartum and Newborn Care

4. A nurse is assessing a postpartum client for fundal height, location, and consistency. The fundus is found to be displaced laterally to the right and there is uterine atony. Which of the following is the cause of the uterine atony?

    A. Poor involution

    B. Urinary retention

    C. Hemorrhage

    D. Infection

Urinary retention can result in a distention of the bladder. A distended bladder can cause uterine atony and lateral displacement from the midline, usually to the right. Poor involution and hemorrhage are results of uterine atony; they do not cause it. Infection does not cause uterine displacement or atony and would be characterized by foul-smelling vaginal discharge and elevated temperature.

(N) NCLEX® Connection: Health Promotion and Maintenance, Ante/Intra/Postpartum and Newborn Care

5. A client is in the fourth stage of labor, has just delivered her newborn, and is stable. A nurse knows that during the maternal recovery period vital signs should be assessed at regular intervals. How often should vital sign intervals be assessed during the fourth stage of labor?

Every 15 min x 4, every 30 min x 2, hourly x 2

The fourth stage of labor is referred to as the maternal recovery period, which lasts from 1 to 4 hr. If all factors are stable, postpartum assessments of vital signs as well as uterine firmness, location, and position should be done every 15 min x 4 for the first hour, every 30 min x 2 for the second hour, hourly x 2 for at least 2 hr, and then every 4 to 8 hr for the remainder of the client's hospitalization.

 NCLEX® Connection: Health Promotion and Maintenance, Ante/Intra/Postpartum and Newborn Care

6. Which of the following nursing interventions will promote comfort for a client who has a small hematoma of the perineal area? (Select all that apply.)

__X__	**Apply ice to the perineal area for the first 24 to 48 hr.**
_____	Encourage the use of a donut-shaped pillow for sitting.
__X__	**Encourage sitz baths at least twice a day.**
__X__	**Use a topical antiseptic cream or spray on the perineal area.**
_____	Obtain an order for an indwelling urinary catheter.

To promote perineal comfort for a small hematoma, ice should be applied for the first 24 to 48 hr to reduce swelling and provide anesthetic effects. Sitz baths and use of a topical antiseptic cream or spray should be encouraged. Donut-shaped pillows should be avoided because they result in an increase in pain and discomfort. Use of indwelling urinary catheters is not indicated and can lead to infection.

 NCLEX® Connection: Health Promotion and Maintenance, Ante/Intra/Postpartum and Newborn Care

UNIT 3	POSTPARTUM NURSING CARE
Section	Routine Postpartum Care
Chapter 18	Bonding and Integration of Infant into Family System

Overview

- Bonding and integration of an infant into the family structure should start during pregnancy, continue into the fourth stage of labor, and throughout hospitalization.

- Assessment of bonding and integration of an infant into the family structure requires that a nurse understand the normal postpartum psychological changes the mother undergoes in the attainment of the maternal role and the recognition of deviations. Bonding behaviors can be promoted by delaying nursing procedures during the first hour after birth to allow for immediate parent-infant contact.

  ○ A mother's emotional and physical condition (unwanted pregnancy, adolescent pregnancy, history of depression, difficult pregnancy and delivery) and the infant's physical condition (prematurity, congenital anomalies) after birth can affect the family's bonding process.

  ○ Culture, age, and socioeconomic level are factors that can influence the bonding process.

- Miscellaneous Relevant Information

  ○ Bonding can be delayed secondary to maternal or neonatal factors.

Psychosocial and Maternal Adaptation

- Psychosocial adaptation and maternal adjustment begin during pregnancy as the client goes through commitment, attachment, and preparation for the birth of the newborn. During the first 2 to 6 weeks after birth, the client goes through a period of acquaintance with her newborn, as well as physical restoration. During this time she also focuses on competently caring for her newborn. Finally, the act of achieving maternal identity is accomplished around 4 months following birth. It is important to note that these stages may overlap, and are variable based on maternal, infant, and the environmental factors.

- Nursing assessments include noting the mother's condition after birth, observing the maternal adaptation process, assessing maternal emotional readiness to care for the infant, and assessing how comfortable the mother appears in providing infant care.

  ○ Assess for behaviors that facilitate and indicate mother-infant bonding.

    ▪ Considers the infant a family member

    ▪ Holds the infant face to face (en face) maintaining eye contact

- Assigns meaning to the infant's behavior and views positively

- Identifies the infant's unique characteristics and relates them to those of other family members

- Touches the infant and maintains close physical proximity and contact

- Provides physical care for the infant such as feeding and diapering

- Responds to the infant's cries

- Smiles at, talks to, and sings to the infant

○ Assess for behaviors that impair and indicate a lack of mother-infant bonding.

- Apathy when the infant cries

- Disgust when the infant voids, stools, or spits up

- Expresses disappointment in the infant

- Turns away from the infant

- Does not seek close physical proximity to the infant

- Does not talk about the infant's unique features

- Handles the infant roughly

- Ignores the infant entirely

○ Assess for signs of mood swings, conflict about maternal role, and/or personal insecurity.

- Feelings of being "down"

- Feelings of inadequacy

- Feelings of anxiety related to ineffective breastfeeding

- Emotional labiality with frequent crying

- Flat affect and being withdrawn

- Feeling unable to care for the infant

- Nursing interventions to assist with maternal-infant bonding

○ Provide a quiet and private environment that enhances the family bonding process.

○ Facilitate the bonding process by placing the infant skin-to-skin with the mother soon after birth in an en face position.

○ Encourage the parents to bond with their infant through cuddling, feeding, diapering, and inspection.

○ Provide frequent praise, support, and reassurance to the mother as she moves toward independence in caring for her infant and adjusting to her maternal role.

○ Encourage the mother/parents to express their feelings, fears, and anxieties about caring for their infant.

Paternal Adaptation

- Paternal adaptation takes place as the father develops a parent-infant bond.

    ○ The father may touch, hold, and maintain eye-to-eye contact with the infant.

    ○ The father should observe the infant for features similar to his own to validate his claim of the infant.

    ○ The father should talk and sing to the infant.

- Paternal transition to fatherhood consists of a predictable three-stage process during the first few weeks of transition.

    ○ Expectations – the father has preconceived ideas about what it will be like to be a father.

    ○ Reality – the father discovers that his expectations may not be met. Commonly expressed emotions include feeling sad, frustrated, and jealous. He embraces the need to be actively involved in parenting.

    ○ Transition to mastery – the father decides to become actively involved in the care of the infant.

- The development of the father-infant bond consists of three stages.

    ○ Making a commitment – the father takes the responsibility of parenting.

    ○ Becoming connected – experiences feelings of attachment to the infant.

    ○ Making room for the infant – the father modifies his life to include the care of the infant.

- Nursing assessment of paternal adaptation includes observing for the characteristics of father-infant bonding.

- Nursing interventions to assist in the father-infant bonding process

    ○ Provide education about infant care when the father is present.

    ○ Assist the father in his transition to fatherhood by providing guidance and involving him as a full partner rather than just a helper.

    ○ Encourage couples to verbalize their concerns and expectations related to infant care.

Sibling Adaptation

- The addition of an infant into the family unit affects everyone in the family including siblings who may experience a temporary separation from the mother. Siblings become aware of changes in the parents' behavior because the infant requires much more of the parents' time.

- Nursing assessment of sibling adaptation to the infant

    ○ Assess for positive responses from the sibling.

        ▪ Interest and concern for the infant

        ▪ Increased independence

- o   Assess for adverse responses from the sibling.

    - ▪   Signs of sibling rivalry and jealousy

    - ▪   Regression in toileting and sleep habits

    - ▪   Aggression toward the infant

    - ▪   Increased attention-seeking behaviors and whining

- ●   Nursing interventions to facilitate sibling acceptance of the infant

    - o   Take the sibling on a tour of the obstetric unit.

    - o   Encourage the parents to:

        - ▪   Let the sibling be one of the first to see the infant.

        - ▪   Provide a gift from the infant to give the sibling.

        - ▪   Arrange for one parent to spend time with the sibling while the other parent is caring for the infant.

        - ▪   Allow older siblings to help in providing care for the infant.

        - ▪   Provide the preschooler with a doll to care for.

Complications and Nursing Implications

- ●   Impaired parenting may include:

    - o   Emotional detachment and inability to care for the infant, thus placing the infant at risk for neglect and failure to thrive. Failure to bond with the infant increases the risk of physical and/or emotional abuse.

- ●   Nursing interventions for impaired parenting

    - o   Emphasize verbal and nonverbal communication skills between the mother, caregivers, and the infant.

    - o   Provide continued assessment of the new mother's parenting abilities as well as any other caregivers for the infant.

    - o   Encourage the continued support of grandparents and other family members.

    - o   Provide home visits by a nurse and group sessions for discussion regarding infant care and parenting problems.

    - o   Give the mother/caregivers information about social networks that provide a support system where the mother and caregivers can seek assistance.

    - o   Involve outreach programs concerned with self-care, parent-child interactions, child injuries, and failure to thrive.

    - o   Notify programs that provide prompt and effective community interventions to prevent more serious problems from occurring.

- Desired Client Outcomes

  ○ The client will demonstrate positive bonding with infant.

  ○ Paternal attachment and bonding will be observed.

  ○ Siblings will demonstrate positive bonding behaviors with infant.

CHAPTER 18: BONDING AND INTEGRATION OF INFANT INTO FAMILY SYSTEM

(A) Application Exercises

1. A nurse concludes that the father of an infant is not showing positive signs of parent-infant bonding and appears to be very anxious and nervous when the infant's mother asks him to bring her the infant. Which of the following is an appropriate nursing intervention to promote father-infant bonding?

   A. Hand the father the infant and insist that he change the diaper.

   B. Ask the father why he is so anxious and nervous.

   C. Tell the father that he will get used to the infant in time.

   D. Provide education about infant care when the father is present.

2. A client in the early postpartum period is very excited and talkative. She is repeatedly telling the nurse every detail of her labor and birth. Because the woman will not stop talking, the nurse is having difficulty completing her postpartum assessments. The appropriate response of the nurse is to

   A. come back later when the client is more cooperative.

   B. give the client time to express her feelings.

   C. tell the that client she needs to be quiet so the assessment can be completed.

   D. redirect the client's focus so that she will become quiet.

3. A nurse is caring for a client who is 1-day postpartum. The nurse is assessing for maternal adaptation and mother-infant bonding. Which of the following behaviors by the mother indicates a need for the nurse to intervene? (Select all that apply.)

   _____ Demonstrates apathy when the infant cries

   _____ Touches the infant and maintains close physical proximity

   _____ Views the infant's behavior as uncooperative during diaper changing

   _____ Identifies and relates infant's characteristics to those of family members

   _____ Interprets the infant's behavior as meaningful and a way of expressing needs

4. A home-health nurse is conducting a visit to the home of a client who has a 2-month-old infant and a 4-year-old son. The mother expresses frustration about the behavior of the 4-year-old who was previously toilet trained and is now frequently wetting himself. The nurse provides client education and explains to the mother that

   A. her son was probably not ready for toilet training and should wear training pants.

   B. this is an adverse sibling response to the infant.

   C. this is abnormal and counseling should be sought for the child.

   D. this can be resolved by sending the child to preschool.

CHAPTER 18: BONDING AND INTEGRATION OF INFANT INTO FAMILY SYSTEM

(A) Application Exercises Answer Key

1. A nurse concludes that the father of an infant is not showing positive signs of parent-infant bonding and appears to be very anxious and nervous when the infant's mother asks him to bring her the infant. Which of the following is an appropriate nursing intervention to promote father-infant bonding?

   A. Hand the father the infant and insist that he change the diaper.

   B. Ask the father why he is so anxious and nervous.

   C. Tell the father that he will get used to the infant in time.

   D. Provide education about infant care when the father is present.

   Nursing interventions to assist the father in bonding with the infant include providing education about infant care when the father is present. It would not be helpful to push the father into providing care such as changing a diaper without first providing education. Asking the father why he is anxious and nervous, and telling him he will get used to the infant, are both nontherapeutic responses.

   (N) NCLEX® Connection: Health Promotion and Maintenance, Developmental Stages and Transitions

2. A client in the early postpartum period is very excited and talkative. She is repeatedly telling the nurse every detail of her labor and birth. Because the woman will not stop talking, the nurse is having difficulty completing her postpartum assessments. The appropriate response of the nurse is to

   A. come back later when the client is more cooperative.

   B. give the client time to express her feelings.

   C. tell the client that she needs to be quiet so the assessment can be completed.

   D. redirect the client's focus so that she will become quiet.

   The nurse should recognize that the client in is the taking-in phase, which begins immediately following birth and lasts a few hours to a couple of days. The woman is excited and talkative during this phase and repeatedly reviews the labor and birth experience. It is important for the nurse to allow her the time to express her feelings. The nurse must complete vital signs and focused assessments per the postpartum protocol and cannot delay the assessments. It is not necessary for the client to stop talking for the nurse to complete her assessment.

   (N) NCLEX® Connection: Health Promotion and Maintenance, Developmental Stages and Transitions

3. A nurse is caring for a client who is 1-day postpartum. The nurse is assessing for maternal adaptation and mother-infant bonding. Which of the following behaviors by the mother indicates a need for the nurse to intervene? (Select all that apply.)

__X__	**Demonstrates apathy when the infant cries**
_____	Touches the infant and maintains close physical proximity
__X__	**Views the infant's behavior as uncooperative during diaper changing**
_____	Identifies and relates infant's characteristics to those of family members
_____	Interprets the infant's behavior as meaningful and a way of expressing needs

Behaviors that facilitate and indicate mother-infant bonding include viewing the characteristics of the infant, face to face (en face) with the infant maintaining eye contact, considering the infant a family member, identifying the infant's unique characteristics and relating them to those of other family members, touching the infant and maintaining close physical proximity and contact, providing physical care such as feeding and diapering, smiling, talking, cooing, and singing to the infant, and assigning a meaning to the infant's behavior and viewing behaviors positively. Behaviors that impair and show lack of mother-infant bonding include apathy when the infant cries, disgust when the infant voids, stools, or spits up, an expression of disappointment in the infant, not seeking a close physical proximity with the infant, not talking about the infant's unique features, ignoring the infant entirely, and viewing the infant's behaviors as being deliberately uncooperative or disruptive.

 NCLEX® Connection: Health Promotion and Maintenance, Developmental Stages and Transitions

4. A home-health nurse is conducting a visit to the home of a client who has a 2-month-old infant and a 4-year-old son. The mother expresses frustration about the behavior of the 4-year-old who was previously toilet trained and is now frequently wetting himself. The nurse provides client education and explains to the mother that

A. her son was probably not ready for toilet training and should wear training pants.

B. this is an adverse sibling response to the infant.

C. this is abnormal and counseling should be sought for the child.

D. this can be resolved by sending the child to preschool.

Adverse responses from the sibling to a new infant can include signs of sibling rivalry and jealousy, regression in toileting and sleep habits, aggression toward the infant, increased attention-seeking behaviors, and whining. Some nursing interventions to facilitate sibling acceptance of the infant include encouraging the parents to have a gift from the infant to give the sibling, arranging for one parent to spend time with the sibling while the other parent is caring for the infant, and giving preschool and school-age children a doll as their "baby." Providing instructions to seek counseling, sending the child to preschool, and informing the mother of the child's readiness for toilet training are not appropriate nursing interventions.

NCLEX® Connection: Health Promotion and Maintenance, Developmental Stages and Transitions

UNIT 3	POSTPARTUM NURSING CARE
Section	Routine Postpartum Care

Chapter 19   Client Education and Discharge Teaching

Overview

- Discharge teaching is an important aspect of postpartum care. It is important for a mother to be able to perform self-care and recognize signs and symptoms of possible complications prior to discharge.

- Discharge planning should be initiated at admission with time spent during the hospitalization on providing client education regarding postpartum self-care.

- A nurse should use a variety of teaching strategies to promote learning. Return demonstrations are important to ensure that adequate learning has taken place.

Assessing A Client's Knowledge of Postpartum Care

- Inquire about the mother's current knowledge regarding self-care.

- Assess the mother's home support system and who will be there to assist her. Include support persons in the educational process.

- Determine the mother's readiness for learning and her ability to verbalize or demonstrate what she has been instructed to do by the nurse.

Nursing Interventions for Postpartum Care

- Provide client teaching on self-care

  - Perineal care

    - Cleanse the perineal area with warm water after each voiding and bowel movement.

    - Wipe perineal area from front to back.

    - Remove and apply perineal pads from front to back.

  - Breast care

    - Wear a well-fitting bra continuously for the first 72 hr after birth.

    - Provide breast care for women who are lactating.

      - Emphasize the importance of hand hygiene prior to breastfeeding to prevent infection.

        □   To relieve breast engorgement, have the client completely empty her breasts at each feeding. Allow the infant to nurse every 2 hr. Massaging the breasts during feeding can help with emptying. Allow the infant to feed 15 to 20 min per breast, or until the breast softens. If the second breast does not soften after the infant's feeding, the breast may be emptied with a breast pump.

        □   For breast engorgement, apply cool compresses between feedings and apply warm compresses or take a warm shower prior to breastfeeding. These actions will increase milk flow and promote the letdown reflex. Cold cabbage leaves may also be applied to the breasts to decrease swelling and relieve discomfort.

        □   For flat nipples, suggest to the client that she roll the nipples between her fingers just before breastfeeding to help them become more erect and make it easier for the infant to latch on.

        □   For sore nipples, the client should apply a small amount of breast milk to her nipple and allow it to air dry after breastfeeding.

        □   Have the client apply breast creams as prescribed and wear breast shields in her bra to soften her nipples if they are irritated and cracked.

        □   Promote adequate fluid intake in the client, because it is important to replace fluid lost from breastfeeding as well as produce an adequate amount of milk for the infant.

    ■   Breast care for nonlactating women

        □   Suppression of lactation is necessary for women who are not breastfeeding. Avoid breast stimulation and running warm water over the breasts for prolonged periods until no longer lactating.

        □   For breast engorgement, which may occur on the third or fifth postpartum day, apply cold compresses 15 min on and 45 min off. Fresh cabbage leaves can be placed inside the bra. Mild analgesics may be taken for pain and discomfort of breast engorgement.

  ○ Rest/sleep

    ■   Plan at least one daily rest period; rest when the infant naps.

  ○ Activity

    ■   Do not perform housework requiring heavy lifting for at least 3 weeks.

    ■   Do not lift anything heavier than the infant.

    ■   Avoid sitting for prolonged periods of time with legs crossed (to prevent thrombophlebitis).

    ■   Limit stair climbing for the first few weeks postpartum.

    ■   Clients who have had a cesarean birth should wait until the 6-week follow-up visit before performing strenuous exercise, heavy lifting, or excessive stair climbing.

    ■   Instruct the client not to drive for the first 2 weeks postpartum, or while taking opioids for pain control.

- ○ Nutrition
  - ▪ Teach the client the importance of eating a nutritious diet including all food groups. Encourage a diet high in protein, which will aid in tissue repair. The client should also consume 2,000 to 3,000 mL (2 to 3 L) of water each day from food and beverage sources.
  - ▪ Encourage women who are lactating to add an additional 500 calories/day to their prepregnancy diet. This includes calcium-enriched foods.
- ○ Postpartum exercises
  - ▪ The client can regain pelvic floor muscle control by performing Kegel exercises. The same muscles are used when starting and stopping the flow of urine. Have the client relax and contract the pelvic floor muscles 10 times 8 times a day.
  - ▪ Teach the client how to perform pelvic tilt exercises to strengthen back muscles and relieve strain on the lower back. These exercises involve alternately arching and straightening the back.
- ○ Sexual intercourse
  - ▪ Teach the client to avoid sexual intercourse until the episiotomy/laceration is healed and vaginal discharge has turned white (lochia alba). This usually takes 2 to 4 weeks or until the client is seen by her primary care provider. Over-the-counter lubricants may be needed during the first 6 weeks.
  - ▪ Physiological reactions to sexual activity may be slower and less intense for the first 3 months following birth.
- ○ Contraception
  - ▪ Advise clients to begin using contraception upon resumption of sexual activity and that pregnancy can occur while breastfeeding even though menses has not returned.
  - ▪ Menses for nonlactating mothers may not resume until around 4 to 10 weeks.
  - ▪ Menses for lactating mothers may not resume for 3 months or until cessation of breastfeeding.
- • Provide client education on danger signs to report to her primary care provider.
  - ○ Chills or fever greater than 38° C (100.4° F) for 2 or more days
  - ○ Change in vaginal discharge with increased amount, large clots, change to a previous lochia color such as bright red bleeding, and a foul odor
    - ▪ Normal lochial flow pattern shows:
      - □ Bright red vaginal drainage for 2 to 3 days.
      - □ Blood-tinged serous vaginal drainage from days 4 to 10.
      - □ White vaginal discharge from day 11 to 6 weeks.
  - ○ Episiotomy, laceration, or incision pain, that does not resolve with analgesics, foul-smelling drainage, redness, and/or edema

- o Pain or tenderness in the abdominal or pelvic areas that does not resolve with analgesics

- o Breast(s) with localized areas of pain and tenderness with redness and swelling and/or nipples with cracks or fissures

- o Calves with localized pain and tenderness, redness, and swelling. A lower extremity with either areas of redness and warmth or coolness and paleness

- o Urination with burning, pain, frequency, urgency; urine that is cloudy or has blood

- Postpartum depression is when the client feels apathy toward the infant, cannot provide self- or infant-care, or has feelings that she might hurt herself or her infant.

- The client should be discharged with an appointment set for a postpartum follow-up visit or a number to call and schedule an appointment. Following a vaginal delivery the follow up visit should take place in 6 weeks and following a cesarean birth the visit should take place in 2 weeks.

- Date and time of the follow-up appointment should be written and discussed in the discharge instructions.

Desired Client Outcomes

- The client will verbalize signs and symptoms of when to contact the primary care provider.

- The client will demonstrate appropriate breastfeeding techniques.

- The client will demonstrate appropriate perineal care.

CHAPTER 19: CLIENT EDUCATION AND DISCHARGE TEACHING

Ⓐ Application Exercises

1. A nurse is conducting a home visit for a client who is 2 weeks postpartum and breastfeeding. The client reports breast engorgement. Which of the following recommendations should the nurse make?

    A. "Apply cold compresses between feedings."

    B. "Take a warm shower right after feedings."

    C. "Apply breast milk to the nipples and allow them to air dry."

    D. "Use the various infant positions for feedings."

2. A nurse is providing discharge instructions for a client. At 4 weeks postpartum, the client should contact her primary care provider for which of the following client findings?

    A. Scant, nonodorous white vaginal discharge

    B. Uterine cramping during breastfeeding

    C. Sore nipple with cracks and fissures

    D. Decreased response with sexual activity

3. A nurse is conducting a home visit with a client who is 3 months postpartum and breastfeeding. Menses has not yet resumed. The client is discussing contraception with the nurse stating that she does not want to have another child for a couple of years. The nurse understands that this client needs further instruction if the client makes which of the following statements?

    A. "I have already started using the mini pill for oral protection."

    B. "Because of our beliefs, we are going to use the rhythm method."

    C. "I am being refitted for a diaphragm with my doctor next week."

    D. "I will not need birth control until I stop breastfeeding."

4. A nurse is providing care to multiple clients on the postpartum unit. Which of the following clients is at greatest risk for developing a puerperal infection?

    A. A client who has an episiotomy that is erythematous and has extended into a third-degree laceration

    B. A client who does not wash her hands between perineal care and breastfeeding

    C. A client who is not breastfeeding and is using measures to suppress lactation

    D. A client who has a cesarean incision that is well-approximated with no drainage

5. A nurse is providing discharge instructions to a postpartum client following a cesarean birth. The client reports leaking urine every time she sneezes or coughs. The nurse suggests the client perform which of the following to help alleviate this problem?

    A. Sit-ups

    B. Pelvic tilt

    C. Kegel exercises

    D. Crunches

CHAPTER 19: CLIENT EDUCATION AND DISCHARGE TEACHING

(A) Application Exercises Answer Key

1. A nurse is conducting a home visit for a client who is 2 weeks postpartum and breastfeeding. The client reports breast engorgement. Which of the following recommendations should the nurse make?

    A. "Apply cold compresses between feedings."

    B. "Take a warm shower right after feedings."

    C. "Apply breast milk to the nipples and allow them to air dry."

    D. "Use the various infant positions for feedings."

    Cold compresses applied to the breasts between feedings can help with breast engorgement. Taking a warm shower prior to feedings, not immediately after, can assist with the letdown reflex and milk flow. Breast milk applied to the nipples with air drying and using various positions for feedings help with preventing nipple soreness, but have no effect on breast engorgement.

    (N) NCLEX® Connection: Health Promotion and Maintenance, Ante/Intra/Postpartum and Newborn Care

2. A nurse is providing discharge instructions for a client. At 4 weeks postpartum, the client should contact her primary care provider for which of the following client findings?

    A. Scant, nonodorous white vaginal discharge

    B. Uterine cramping during breastfeeding

    C. Sore nipple with cracks and fissures

    D. Decreased response with sexual activity

    A sore nipple that has cracks and fissures is an indication of mastitis. Lochia alba, a white vaginal discharge, is normal from the 11th day postpartum to approximately 6 weeks following birth. Oxytocin, which is released with breastfeeding, causes the uterus to contract and may cause discomfort. Physiological reactions to sexual activity may be slower and less intense for the first 3 months following birth.

    (N) NCLEX® Connection: Health Promotion and Maintenance, Ante/Intra/Postpartum and Newborn Care

3. A nurse is conducting a home visit with a client who is 3 months postpartum and breastfeeding. Menses has not yet resumed. The client is discussing contraception with the nurse stating that she does not want to have another child for a couple of years. The nurse understands that this client needs further instruction if the client makes which of the following statements?

    A. "I have already started using the mini pill for protection."

    B. "Because of our beliefs, we are going to use the rhythm method."

    C. "I am being refitted for a diaphragm with my doctor next week."

    D. "I will not need birth control until I stop breastfeeding."

Lactating does not prevent pregnancy, even if menses has not yet resumed. Progesterone-only oral contraceptives (mini pills) are a good form of birth control once lactation has been established. The rhythm method is not as effective, but if that is what the couple chooses because of their belief system, this is their option. The client is correct in having her diaphragm refitted by her primary care provider, which should be done after a pregnancy and birth or a 7 kg (15 lb) weight change.

 NCLEX® Connection: Health Promotion and Maintenance, Family Planning

4. A nurse is providing care to multiple clients on the postpartum unit. Which of the following clients is at greatest risk for developing a puerperal infection?

    A. A client who has an episiotomy that is erythematous and has extended into a third-degree laceration

    B. A client who does not wash her hands between perineal care and breastfeeding

    C. A client who is not breastfeeding and is using measures to suppress lactation

    D. A client who has a cesarean incision that is well-approximated with no drainage

The client who does not wash her hands between perineal care and breastfeeding is at an increased risk for developing mastitis; therefore, she is most at risk for developing a puerperal infection. An episiotomy, lacerations, cesarean incisions, and suppression of lactation (increases the risk of milk stasis), places the other clients at risk for infection; however, they are not at greatest risk for developing a puerperal infection.

 NCLEX® Connection: Physiological Adaptation, Alterations in Body Systems

5. A nurse is providing discharge instructions to a postpartum client following a cesarean birth. The client reports leaking urine every time she sneezes or coughs. The nurse suggests the client perform which of the following to help alleviate this problem?

    A. Sit-ups

    B. Pelvic tilt

    C. Kegel exercises

    D. Crunches

Kegel exercises consist of the voluntary contraction and relaxation of the pubococcygeal muscle as if to start and stop the urine flow. This strengthens the pelvic muscles, which will assist the client in decreasing the stress incontinence that occurs with sneezing and coughing. Sit-ups and crunches are both abdominal exercises that should not be performed until the client's 6-week postpartum follow-up appointment. Pelvic tilt exercises consist of the alternate arching and straightening of the back to strengthen the back muscles and relieve back discomfort.

NCLEX® Connection: Health Promotion and Maintenance, Ante/Intra/Postpartum and Newborn Care

UNIT 3	POSTPARTUM NURSING CARE
Section	Complications of the Postpartum Period
Chapter 20	Postpartum Disorders

Overview

- Postpartum disorders are unexpected events or occurrences that may happen during the postpartum period. They include:

  ○ Superficial and deep vein thrombosis, pulmonary embolus, coagulopathies (idiopathic thrombocytopenic purpura and disseminated intravascular coagulation), postpartum hemorrhage, uterine atony, subinvolution of the uterus, inversion of the uterus, retained placenta, and lacerations and/or hematomas. It is imperative for a nurse to have a thorough understanding of each disorder and initiate appropriate nursing interventions to achieve positive outcomes.

DEEP VEIN THROMBOSIS

Overview

- Thrombophlebitis refers to a thrombus that is associated with inflammation.

- Thrombophlebitis of the lower extremities may be of superficial veins or of the deep veins, which are most often of the femoral, saphenous, or popliteal veins.

  ○ The postpartum client is at greatest risk for a deep vein thrombosis (DVT) that may lead to a pulmonary embolism.

Risk Factors

- Pregnancy

- Immobility

- Obesity

- Smoking

- Cesarean birth

- Multiparity

- Greater than 35 years of age

- Previous thromboembolism

- Diabetes mellitus

Assessment

- Subjective Data
  - Leg pain
  - Chills
- Objective Data
  - Physical assessment findings
    - Unilateral swelling, warmth, and redness
    - Warm extremity
    - Calf tenderness
    - Elevated temperature
    - Cough
    - Tachycardia
  - Diagnostic procedures
    - Noninvasive methods
      - Doppler ultrasound scanning
      - Computed tomography
      - Magnetic resonance imaging

Collaborative Care

- Nursing Care
  - Prevention of thrombophlebitis
    - Provide the client with education and encouragement pertaining to measures for prevention of DVT.
      - Initiate early and frequent ambulation postpartum.
      - Avoid prolonged periods of standing, sitting, or immobility.
      - Have the client elevate her legs when sitting.
      - Tell the client to avoid crossing her legs, which will reduce the circulation and exacerbate venous stasis.
      - Maintain fluid intake of 2 to 3 L of water each day from food and beverage sources to prevent dehydration, which causes circulation to be sluggish.
      - Tell the client to discontinue smoking, which is known to be a risk factor.
      - Measure the client's lower extremities for fitted elastic thromboembolic hose to lower extremities.

- ○ Management of thrombophlebitis
  - Encourage the client to rest.
  - Facilitate bedrest and elevation of the client's extremity above the level of her heart as prescribed (avoid using a knee gatch or pillow under knees).
  - Administer intermittent or continuous warm moist compresses as prescribed.
  - Do NOT massage the affected limb to prevent thrombus from dislodging and becoming an embolus.
  - Measure the client's leg circumferences.
  - Provide thigh-high antiembolism stockings for the client at high risk for venous insufficiency.
  - Administer analgesics (nonsteroidal anti-inflammatory agents).
  - Administer anticoagulants for DVT.
- Medications
  - ○ Heparin
    - Classification
      - □ Anticoagulant
    - Therapeutic intent
      - □ Heparin is given IV to prevent formation of other clots and to prevent enlargement of the existing clot.
    - Nursing considerations
      - □ Initially, IV heparin is administered by continuous infusion for 5 to 7 days with doses adjusted according to coagulation studies. Protamine sulfate, the heparin antidote, should be readily available to counteract the development of heparin-induced antiplatelet antibodies.
      - □ Monitor aPTT.
    - Client education
      - □ Instruct the client to report bleeding from the gums or nose, increased vaginal bleeding, blood in the urine, and frequent bruising.
  - ○ Warfarin (Coumadin)
    - Classification
      - □ Anticoagulant

- Therapeutic intent
  - Warfarin is used for treatment of clots. It is administered orally and is continued by the client for approximately 3 months.
- Nursing considerations
  - Phytonadione (vitamin K), the warfarin antidote, should be readily available for prolonged clotting times.
  - Monitor PT and aPTT.
- Client education
  - Instruct the client to watch for bleeding from the gums or nose, increased vaginal bleeding, blood in the urine, and frequent bruising.

- Health Promotion and Disease Prevention
  - Client education
    - Provide client teaching about precautions to take while receiving anticoagulants.
      - Avoid taking aspirin or ibuprofen (increases bleeding tendencies).
      - Use an electric razor for shaving.
      - Avoid alcohol use (inhibits warfarin).
      - Brush teeth gently.
      - Avoid rubbing or massaging legs.
      - Avoid periods of prolonged sitting or crossing legs.

- Client outcomes
  - The client will have restored venous patency.
  - The client will not develop pulmonary embolus.

PULMONARY EMBOLUS

Overview

- An embolus occurs when fragments or an entire clot dislodges and moves into circulation.
- A pulmonary embolism is a complication of DVT that occurs if the embolus moves into the pulmonary artery or one of its branches and lodges in a lung, occluding the vessel and obstructing blood flow to the lungs.

Risk Factors

- Risk factors for pulmonary embolism are the same as those for DVT.

Assessment

- Subjective Data
  - Chills
  - Apprehension
  - Pleuritic chest pain
- Objective Data
  - Dyspnea
  - Tachypnea
  - Hemoptysis
  - Heart murmurs
  - Peripheral edema
  - Distended neck veins
  - Elevated temperature
  - Hypotension
  - Hypoxia
- Diagnostic Procedures
  - Diagnostic studies to determine pulmonary embolism
    - Ventilation/perfusion lung scan
    - Chest radiographic study
    - Radioisotope lung scan
    - Pulmonary angiogram
  - Embolectomy surgically removes the embolus.

Collaborative Care

- Nursing Care
  - Place the client in a semi-Fowler's position with the head of the bed elevated to facilitate breathing.
  - Administer oxygen to the client by mask.
  - Medications prescribed include the medications listed under DVT.
    - Thrombolytic therapy may be prescribed.
    - Alteplase (Activase), Streptokinase (Streptase).
      - Used to break up blood clots.
    - Similar side effects and contraindications as anticoagulants.

○ Client outcomes

- The client will be compliant with anticoagulant therapy.

- The client maintains adequate gas exchange.

- The client is free from severe bleeding incidences.

- The client will be free of pain.

COAGULOPATHIES (IDIOPATHIC THROMBOCYTOPENIC PURPURA AND DISSEMINATED INTRAVASCULAR COAGULATION)

Overview

- Idiopathic thrombocytopenic purpura (ITP) is a coagulopathy that is an autoimmune disorder in which the life span of platelets is decreased by antiplatelet antibodies. This can result in severe hemorrhage following a cesarean birth or lacerations.

- Disseminated intravascular coagulation (DIC) is a coagulopathy in which clotting and anticlotting mechanisms occur at the same time.

- The client is at risk for both internal and external bleeding as well as damage to organs resulting from ischemia caused by microclots.

- Coagulopathies are suspected when the usual measures to stimulate uterine contractions fail to stop vaginal bleeding.

Risk Factors

- Risk factors for ITP are genetic factors inherited from parents.

- Risk factors for DIC that occur secondary to other complications

  ○ Abruptio placenta

  ○ Amniotic fluid embolism

  ○ Missed abortion

  ○ Fetal death in utero (fetus has died but is retained in the uterus for at least 6 weeks)

  ○ Severe preeclampsia or eclampsia (gestational hypertension)

  ○ Septicemia

  ○ Cardiopulmonary arrest

  ○ Hemorrhage

  ○ Hydatidiform mole

Assessment

- Objective Data

  - Physical assessment findings

    - Unusual spontaneous bleeding from the client's gums and nose (epistaxis)

    - Oozing, trickling, or flow of blood from incision, lacerations, or episiotomy

    - Petechiae and ecchymoses

    - Excessive bleeding from venipuncture, injection sites, or slight traumas

    - Tachycardia, hypotension, and diaphoresis

    - Oliguria

- Laboratory Tests

  - CBC with differential

  - Blood typing and crossmatch

  - Clotting factors

    - Platelet levels (thrombocytopenia)

    - Fibrinogen levels (decreased)

    - PT (increased)

    - Fibrin split product levels (increased)

- Diagnostic Procedures

  - A splenectomy may be performed by the primary care provider if ITP does not respond to medical management.

  - Surgical intervention (hysterectomy) for DIC is performed by the primary care provider as indicated.

Collaborative Care

- Nursing Care

  - Nursing assessments for ITP and DIC

    - Skin, venipuncture, injection sites, lacerations, and episiotomy for bleeding

    - Vital signs and hemodynamic status

    - Urinary output usually by insertion of an indwelling urinary catheter

    - Transfuse platelets

    - Assist in preparing the client for a splenectomy if ITP does not respond to medical management and provide postsurgical care

- Nursing interventions for DIC focus on assessing for and correcting the underlying cause (removal of dead fetus or placental abruption, treatment of infection, preeclampsia, or eclampsia).

  - Administer fluid volume replacement, which may include blood and blood products.

  - Administer pharmacologic interventions including antibiotics, vasoactive medications, and uterotonic agents as prescribed.

  - Administer supplemental oxygen.

  - Provide protection from injury.

- Client Outcomes

  - The client is injury free.

POSTPARTUM HEMORRHAGE

Overview

- Postpartum hemorrhage is considered to occur if the client loses more than 500 mL of blood after a vaginal birth or more than 1,000 mL of blood after a cesarean birth. Two complications that can occur following postpartum hemorrhage include hypovolemic shock and anemia.

Risk Factors

- Uterine atony

- Complications during pregnancy (e.g., placenta previa, abruptio placenta)

- Precipitous delivery

- Administration of magnesium sulfate therapy during labor

- Lacerations and hematomas

- Inversion of uterus

- Subinvolution of the uterus

- Retained placental fragments

- Coagulopathies (DIC)

Assessment

- Subjective Data

  - Increased vaginal bleeding

- Objective Data
  - Physical assessment findings
    - Uterine atony
    - Blood clots larger than a quarter
    - Perineal pad saturation in 15 min or less
    - Return of lochia rubra once lochia has progressed to serosa or alba
    - Constant oozing, trickling, or frank flow of bright red blood from the vagina
    - Tachycardia and hypotension
    - Skin that is pale, cool, and clammy with poor turgor and pale mucous membranes
    - Oliguria
  - Laboratory tests
    - Hgb and Hct
    - Coagulation profile (PT)
    - Blood type and crossmatch

Collaborative Care

- Nursing Care
  - Monitor vital signs.
  - Assess the client for the source of bleeding.
    - Assess fundus for height, firmness, and position.
    - Assess lochia for color, quantity, and clots.
    - Assess for signs of bleeding from lacerations, episiotomy site, or hematomas.
  - Assess bladder for distention.
    - Insert an indwelling urinary catheter to assess the client's kidney function and obtain an accurate measurement of urinary output.
  - Maintain or initiate IV fluids to replace fluid volume loss with IV isotonic solutions, such as lactated Ringer's solution or 0.9% sodium chloride, colloid volume expanders, such as albumin and blood products (packed RBCs and fresh frozen plasma).
  - Provide oxygen to the client at 2 to 3 L per nasal cannula as prescribed to increase RBC saturation and monitor oxygen saturation with a pulse oximeter.
  - Elevate the client's legs to a 20 to 30° angle to increase venous return.

- Medications
  - Oxytocin (Pitocin)
    - Classification
      - Uterine stimulant
    - Therapeutic intent
      - Promotes uterine contractions
    - Nursing considerations
      - Assess uterine tone and vaginal bleeding.
        - Monitor the client for adverse reactions of water intoxication, such as lightheadedness, nausea, vomiting, headache, and malaise. These reactions can progress to cerebral edema with seizures, coma, and death.
  - Methylergonovine (Methergine)
    - Classification
      - Uterine stimulant
    - Therapeutic intent
      - Controls postpartum hemorrhage
    - Nursing considerations
      - Assess uterine tone and vaginal bleeding. Do not administer to clients who have hypertension.
      - Monitor the client for adverse reactions including hypertension, nausea, vomiting, and headache.
  - Misoprostol (Cytotec)
    - Classification
      - Uterine stimulant
    - Therapeutic intent
      - Controls postpartum hemorrhage.
    - Nursing considerations
      - Assess uterine tone and vaginal bleeding.
  - Carboprost tromethamine (Hemabate)
    - Classification
      - Uterine stimulant
    - Therapeutic intent
      - Controls postpartum hemorrhage.

- Nursing considerations
  - Assess uterine tone and vaginal bleeding.
    - Monitor for adverse reactions including fever, chills, headache, nausea, vomiting, and diarrhea.

- Health Promotion and Disease Prevention
  - Client education
    - Provide discharge instructions to a client who has had a postpartum hemorrhage. Instruct the client to limit physical activity to conserve strength and to increase iron and protein intake to promote the rebuilding of RBC volume.

- Client Outcomes
  - The client's vaginal bleeding will be controlled with employed interventions.
  - The client's vital signs and laboratory results will be within normal limits.
  - The client will not experience complications or injury related to postpartum hemorrhage.

UTERINE ATONY

Overview

- Uterine atony results from the inability of the uterine muscle to contract adequately after birth. This can lead to postpartum hemorrhage.

Risk Factors

- Retained placental fragments

- Prolonged labor

- Oxytocin (Pitocin) induction or augmentation of labor

- Overdistention of the uterine muscle (multiparity, multiple gestations, polyhydramnios [hydramnios], macrosomic fetus)

- Precipitate labor

- Magnesium sulfate administration as a tocolytic

- Anesthesia and analgesia administration

- Trauma during labor and birth from operative delivery (forceps-assisted or vacuum-assisted birth, cesarean birth)

Assessment

- Subjective Data
  - Increased vaginal bleeding
- Objective Data
  - Physical assessment findings
    - A uterus that is larger than normal and boggy with possible lateral displacement on palpation
    - Prolonged lochial discharge
    - Irregular or excessive bleeding
    - Tachycardia and hypotension
    - Skin that is pale, cool, and clammy with poor turgor and pale mucous membranes
  - Diagnostic procedures
    - Bimanual compression or manual exploration of the uterine cavity for retained placental fragments by the primary care provider
    - Surgical management such as a hysterectomy

Collaborative Care

- Nursing Care
  - Ensure that the client's urinary bladder is empty.
  - Monitor:
    - Fundal height, consistency, and location.
    - Lochia for quantity, color, and consistency.
    - Perform fundal massage if indicated.
    - If the uterus becomes firm, continue assessing maternal hemodynamic status.
    - If uterine atony persists, anticipate surgical intervention, such as a hysterectomy.
  - Express clots that may have accumulated in the uterus, but only after the uterus is firmly contracted.
    - It is critical not to express clots prior to the uterus becoming firmly contracted because pushing on an uncontracted uterus can invert the uterus and result in extensive hemorrhage.
  - Monitor vital signs.
  - Maintain or initiate IV fluids.
  - Provide oxygen to the client at 2 to 3 L per nasal cannula.

- Medications (as noted above for postpartum hemorrhage)

- Health Promotion and Disease Prevention

    ○ Client education

        ▪ Provide discharge instructions to a client who has had a postpartum hemorrhage. Instruct the client to limit physical activity to conserve strength and to increase iron and protein intake to promote the rebuilding of RBC volume.

- Client Outcomes

    ○ The client's vital signs and laboratory results will be within normal limits.

        ▪ The client will be free of complications or injury related to postpartum hemorrhage.

SUBINVOLUTION OF THE UTERUS

Overview

- Subinvolution is when the uterus remains enlarged with continued lochial discharge and may result in postpartum hemorrhage.

Risk Factors

- Pelvic infection and endometritis

- Retained placental fragments not completely expelled from the uterus

Assessment

- Subjective Data

    ○ Increased vaginal bleeding

- Objective Data

    ○ Physical assessment findings

        ▪ A uterus that is enlarged and higher than normal in the abdomen relative to the umbilicus

        ▪ A boggy uterus

        ▪ Prolonged lochia discharge with irregular or excessive bleeding

    ○ Laboratory tests

        ▪ Blood, intracervical, and intrauterine bacterial cultures check for evidence of infection and/or endometritis.

    ○ Diagnostic procedures

        ▪ Dilation and curettage (D&C) is performed by the primary care provider to remove retained placental fragments if indicated.

Collaborative Care

- Nursing Care

    o Monitor fundal position and consistency.

    o Monitor lochia for color, amount, consistency, and odor.

    o Monitor vital signs.

    o Encourage the client to use factors that can enhance uterine involution

        ▪ Breastfeeding

        ▪ Early and frequent ambulation

        ▪ Frequent voiding

- Medications

    o Oxytocin (Pitocin)

- Classification

    o Uterine stimulant

- Therapeutic Intent

    o To promote uterine contractions and expel the retained fragments of placenta

- Nursing Considerations

    o Assess uterine tone and vaginal bleeding.

    o Monitor for adverse reactions of water intoxication, such as lightheadedness, nausea, vomiting, headache, and malaise, which can progress to cerebral edema with seizures, coma, and death.

    o Antibiotic therapy

        ▪ May be prescribed to prevent or treat infection

- Client Outcomes

    o The client will be free of complications or injury related to subinvolution.

INVERSION OF THE UTERUS

Overview

- Inversion of the uterus is the turning inside out of the uterus and may be partial or complete. Uterine inversion is an emergency situation that can result in postpartum hemorrhage and requires immediate intervention.

Risk Factors

- Retained placenta

- Uterine atony

- Excessive fundal pressure

- Abnormally adherent placental tissue

- Multiparity

- Fundal implantation of the placenta

- Extreme traction applied to the umbilical cord

- Leiomyomas (a benign uterine fibroid tumor)

Assessment

- Subjective Data

  - Pain in lower abdomen

- Objective Data

  - Physical assessment findings

    - Vaginal bleeding

      - Complete inversion as evidenced by a large, red, rounded mass that protrudes 20 to 30 cm outside the introitus

      - Partial inversion as evidenced by the palpation of a smooth mass through the dilated cervix

    - Dizziness

    - Low blood pressure

    - Pallor

  - Diagnostic procedures

    - Manual replacement of the uterus into the uterine cavity and repositioning of the uterus by the primary care provider

Collaborative Care

- Nursing Care

  - Assess for an inverted uterus by:

    - Visualizing the introitus.

    - Performing a pelvic exam.

    - Maintaining IV fluids.

    - Administering oxygen.

- ○ Stop oxytocin (Pitocin) if it is being administered at the time uterine inversion occurred.

- ○ Avoid strong pulls on the umbilical cord.

- ○ Anticipate surgery if nonsurgical interventions and management are unsuccessful.

- ○ Medications
  - ■ Terbutaline (Brethine)

- ○ Classification
  - ■ Tocolytic

- ○ Therapeutic intent
  - ■ To relax the uterus prior to the primary care provider's attempt at replacement of the uterus into the uterine cavity and uterus repositioning

- ○ Nursing considerations
  - ■ Following replacement of the uterus into the uterine cavity
    - □ Closely observe the client's response to treatment and assess for stabilization of hemodynamic status.
    - □ Avoid aggressive fundal massage.
    - □ Administer oxytocics as prescribed.
    - □ Administer broad-spectrum antibiotics for infection prophylaxis.

- ○ Client education
  - ■ Inform the client that a cesarean birth will be needed for subsequent pregnancies.

- ● Client Outcomes
  - ■ The client's vital signs and laboratory results will be within normal limits.

RETAINED PLACENTA

Overview

- ● When the placenta or fragments of the placenta remain in the uterus it prevents the uterus from contracting, which can lead to uterine atony or subinvolution.

Risk Factors

- ● Partial separation of a normal placenta

- ● Entrapment of a partially or completely separated placenta by a constricting ring of the uterus

- ● Excessive traction on the umbilical cord prior to complete separation of the placenta

- ● Placental tissue that is abnormally adherent to the uterine wall

- ● Common in preterm births between 20 and 24 weeks gestation

Assessment

- Objective Data
  - Physical assessment findings
    - Uterine atony, subinvolution, or inversion
    - Excessive bleeding or blood clots larger than a quarter
    - The return of lochia rubra once lochia has progressed to serosa alba
    - Malodorous lochia or vaginal discharge
    - Elevated temperature
  - Laboratory tests
    - Hgb and Hct
  - Diagnostic procedures
    - Manual separation and removal of the placenta is done by the primary care provider.
    - D&C if oxytocics are ineffective in expelling the placental fragments

Collaborative Care

- Nursing Care
  - Monitor the uterus for fundal height, consistency, and position.
  - Monitor lochia for color, amount, consistency, and odor.
  - Monitor vital signs.
  - Maintain or initiate IV fluids.
  - Provide oxygen to the client at 2 to 3 L per nasal cannula.
  - Anticipate surgical interventions, such as a hysterectomy, if postpartum bleeding is present and continues.
- Medications
  - Oxytocin (Pitocin)
    - To expel retained fragments of the placenta
  - Classification
    - Uterine stimulant
  - Therapeutic intent
    - Promotes uterine contractions and expel the retained fragments of placenta

- o Nursing considerations
  - ▪ Assess uterine tone and vaginal bleeding.
  - ▪ Monitor for adverse reactions of water intoxication, such as lightheadedness, nausea, vomiting, headache, malaise, which can progress to cerebral edema with seizures, coma, and death.
- o Terbutaline (Brethine)
- o Classification
  - ▪ Tocolytic
- o Therapeutic intent
  - ▪ Relaxes the uterus prior to D&C if placental expulsion with oxytocics is unsuccessful

- ● Health Promotion and Disease Prevention
  - o Client education
    - ▪ Instruct the client to limit physical activity to conserve strength and to increase iron and protein intake to promote the rebuilding of RBC volume.

- ● Desired Client Outcomes
  - o The client will experience minimal bleeding.
  - o The client's vital signs and laboratory results will be within normal limits.

LACERATIONS AND/OR HEMATOMAS

Overview

- ● Lacerations that occur during labor and birth consist of the tearing of soft tissues in the birth canal and adjacent structures including the cervical, vaginal, vulvar, perineal, and/or rectal areas.

- ● An episiotomy may extend and become a third- or fourth-degree laceration.

- ● A hematoma is a collection of 250 to 500 mL of clotted blood within tissues that may appear as a bulging bluish mass.
  - o Hematomas may occur in the pelvic region or higher up in the vagina or broad ligament.

- ● Hematomas will present with pain rather than visible bleeding. Pain is the distinguishable symptom of hematomas rather than noticeable bleeding.

- ● The client is at risk for hemorrhage or infection due to a laceration or hematoma.

Risk Factors

- Operative vaginal birth (forceps-assisted, vacuum assisted birth)

- Precipitate birth

- Cephalopelvic disproportion

- Size (macrosomic infant) and abnormal presentation or position of the fetus

- Prolonged pressure of the fetal head on the vaginal mucosa

- Previous scarring of the maternal birth canal from infection, injury, or operation

- Clients who are nulliparous are at a greater risk for injury due to firmer and less resistant tissue

- Women who have light skin, especially those with reddish hair, have less distensible tissue than women who are dark skin.

Assessment

- Subjective Data

  - Feelings of an urge to defecate

  - Difficulty voiding due to pressure on the urethra from a hematoma

- Objective Data

  - Physical assessment findings

    - Vaginal bleeding even though the uterus is firm and contracted

    - A continuous slow trickle of bright red blood from the vagina, laceration, or episiotomy

    - Severe perineal or rectal pain or a feeling of pressure in the vagina

  - Diagnostic procedures

    - Repair and suturing of the episiotomy or lacerations is done by the primary care provider.

    - Ligation of the bleeding vessel or surgical incision for evacuation of the clotted blood from the hematoma is done by the primary care provider.

Collaborative Care

- Nursing Care

  - Visually or manually inspect the cervix, vagina, perineum, and rectum for lacerations and/or hematomas.

  - Assess an episiotomy for extension into a third- or fourth-degree laceration.

  - Evaluate lochia.

- ○ Continue to assess the client's vital signs and hemodynamic status.

- ○ Attempt to identify the source of the bleeding.

- ○ Assist the primary care provider with repair procedures.

- ○ Use ice packs to treat small hematomas.

- ○ Administer prescribed pain medication.

- ○ Encourage sitz baths.

  - ■ Encouraging cleansing of the perineal area with a water bottle filled with warm tap water after voiding and defecation.

- Client Outcomes

  - ○ The client's bleeding will be controlled with employed interventions.

  - ○ The client's vital signs and laboratory results will be within normal limits.

CHAPTER 20: POSTPARTUM DISORDERS

(A) Application Exercises

1. A nurse is caring for a postpartum client. The nurse understands that which of the following findings are the earliest indication of hypovolemia caused by hemorrhage?

    A. Increasing pulse and decreasing blood pressure

    B. Dizziness and increasing respiratory rate

    C. Cool, clammy skin, and pale mucous membranes

    D. Altered mental status and level of consciousness

2. Which of the following are risk factors for postpartum hemorrhage? (Select all that apply.)

    _____ Precipitous delivery

    _____ Lacerations

    _____ Inversion of the uterus

    _____ Oligohydramnios

    _____ Retained placental fragments

3. A postpartum nurse is caring for a client who has deep vein thrombosis (DVT). Which of the following clinical findings should the nurse anticipate the client will exhibit? (Select all that apply.)

    _____ Calf tenderness

    _____ Calf swelling

    _____ Elevated temperature

    _____ Warm extremity

    _____ Nausea

4. A client with a deep vein thrombus is being cared for by a postpartum nurse. Which of the following nursing interventions should the nurse include in the client's plan of care?

    A. Apply cold compresses to the affected extremity.

    B. Massage the affected extremity.

    C. Allow the client to ambulate.

    D. Measure leg circumferences.

5. A nurse is caring for a client who has disseminated intravascular coagulation (DIC). Which of the following antepartum complications should the nurse understand is a risk factor for this client?

    A. Preeclampsia

    B. Thrombophlebitis

    C. Placenta previa

    D. Hyperemesis gravidarum

6. A nurse is caring for a client who is experiencing postpartum hemorrhage. Which of the following should the nurse use to replace fluid volume in this client? (Select all that apply.)

_____ Lactated Ringer's

_____ Albumin

_____ 0.9% sodium chloride

_____ Packed RBCs

_____ D$_5$LR

CHAPTER 20: POSTPARTUM DISORDERS

 Application Exercises Answer Key

1. A nurse is caring for a postpartum client. The nurse understands that which of the following findings are the earliest indication of hypovolemia caused by hemorrhage?

   A. Increasing pulse and decreasing blood pressure

   B. Dizziness and increasing respiratory rate

   C. Cool, clammy skin, and pale mucous membranes

   D. Altered mental status and level of consciousness

   A rising pulse rate and decreasing blood pressure are often the first signs of inadequate blood volume. Skin that is cool, clammy, and pale along with pale mucous membranes are changes that occur in the physical status of a client who has decreased blood volume, but they are not the first sign of inadequate blood volume. Dizziness and increased respiratory rate are findings that occur in hypovolemia, but they are not the earliest indicator. Altered mental status and changes in level of consciousness are later signs of decreased blood volume which leads to hypoxia and low oxygen saturation.

    NCLEX® Connection: Physiological Adaptation, Alterations in Body Systems

2. Which of the following are risk factors for postpartum hemorrhage? (Select all that apply.)

   __X__ **Precipitous delivery**

   __X__ **Lacerations**

   __X__ **Inversion of the uterus**

   _____ Oligohydramnios

   __X__ **Retained placental fragments**

   Precipitous delivery, lacerations, inversion of the uterus, and retained placental fragments are all risk factors associated with postpartum hemorrhage. Oligohydramnios does not place the client at risk for hemorrhage.

   NCLEX® Connection: Physiological Adaptation, Alterations in Body Systems

3. A postpartum nurse is caring for a client who has deep vein thrombosis (DVT). Which of the following clinical findings should the nurse anticipate the client will exhibit? (Select all that apply.)

   __X__ **Calf tenderness**

   __X__ **Calf swelling**

   __X__ **Elevated temperature**

   __X__ **Warm extremity**

   _____ Nausea

   Calf tenderness, swelling, warm extremity and elevated temperature are clinical findings in clients who have DVT. Nausea is not an expected finding.

   NCLEX® Connection: Physiological Adaptation, Alterations in Body Systems

4. A client with a deep vein thrombus is being cared for by a postpartum nurse. Which of the following nursing interventions should the nurse include in the client's plan of care?

    A. Apply cold compresses to the affected extremity.

    B. Massage the affected extremity.

    C. Allow the client to ambulate.

    D. Measure leg circumferences.

Nursing interventions for a client diagnosed with deep vein thrombosis include measuring leg circumferences, applying warm moist compresses to the affected extremity, and instructing the client to remain on bed rest with the affected extremity elevated. The nurse should not massage the affected extremity. This action may result in dislodgement of the clot.

 NCLEX® Connection: Health Promotion and Maintenance, Ante/Intra/Postpartum and Newborn Care

5. A nurse is caring for a client who has disseminated intravascular coagulation (DIC). Which of the following antepartum complications should the nurse understand is a risk factor for this client?

    A. Preeclampsia

    B. Thrombophlebitis

    C. Placenta previa

    D. Hyperemesis gravidarum

DIC may occur secondary in a client who has preeclampsia. Thrombophlebitis, placenta previa, and hyperemesis gravidarum are not risk factors for the development of DIC.

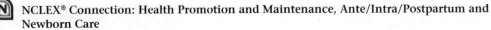 **NCLEX® Connection: Physiological Adaptation, Alterations in Body**

6. A nurse is caring for a client who is experiencing postpartum hemorrhage. Which of the following should the nurse use to replace fluid volume in this client? (Select all that apply.)

    __X__   **Lactated Ringer's**

    __X__   **Albumin**

    __X__   **0.9% sodium chloride**

    __X__   **Packed RBCs**

    _____ D_5LR

Fluid volume replacement should be with IV isotonic solutions such as lactated Ringer's solution or 0.9% sodium chloride, colloid volume expanders, such as albumin and blood products (packed RBCs and fresh frozen plasma). D_5LR is not an appropriate fluid to provide fluid volume replacement.

 NCLEX® Connection: Physiological Adaptation, Alterations in Body Systems

UNIT 3	POSTPARTUM NURSING CARE
Section	Complications of the Postpartum Period
Chapter 21	Postpartum Infections

Overview

- Postpartum infections are complications that may occur up to 28 days following childbirth, or a spontaneous or induced abortion. Fever of 38° C (100.4° F) or higher for 2 consecutive days during the first 10 days of the postpartum period is indicative of a postpartum infection and requires further investigation. The infection may be present in the bladder, uterus, wound, or breast of a postpartum client. The major complication of puerperal infection is septicemia.

- Uterine infection, wound infection, mastitis, and a urinary tract infection are examples of postpartum infections. Early identification and prompt treatment are imperative to promote positive outcomes.

INFECTIONS (ENDOMETRITIS, MASTITIS, AND WOUND INFECTIONS)

Overview

- Uterine infection is also referred to as endometritis. Endometritis is an infection of the uterine lining or endometrium. It is the most frequently occurring puerperal infection.

- Endometritis usually begins on the second to fifth postpartum day, generally starting as a localized infection at the placental attachment site and spreading to include the entire uterine endometrium.

- Sites of wound infections include cesarean incisions, episiotomies, lacerations, and/or any trauma wounds present in the birth canal following labor and birth.

- Mastitis is an infection of the breast involving the interlobular connective tissue and is usually unilateral. Mastitis may progress to an abscess if untreated.

  - It occurs most commonly in mothers breastfeeding for the first time and well after the establishment of milk flow, which is usually 2 to 4 weeks after delivery.

  - *Staphylococcus aureus* is usually the infecting organism.

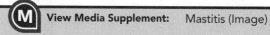
View Media Supplement: Mastitis (Image)

Risk Factors

- The immediate postpartum period following birth is a time of increased risk for all women for microorganisms entering the reproductive tract and migrating into the blood and other parts of the body, which could result in life-threatening septicemia.

    o Risk factors

        ■ Cervical dilation that provides the uterus with exposure to the external environment through the vagina

        ■ Well-supplied exposed blood vessels

        ■ Wounds from lacerations, incisions, and/or hematomas

        ■ Alkalinity of amniotic fluid, blood, and lochia during pregnancy and the early postpartum period, decreasing the acidity of the vagina

- Risk factors for endometritis

    o Cesarean birth

    o Retained placental fragments and manual extraction of the placenta

    o Prolonged rupture of membranes

    o Chorioamnionitis

    o Internal fetal/uterine pressure monitoring

    o Multiple vaginal examinations after rupture of membranes

    o Prolonged labor

    o Postpartum hemorrhage

- Risk factors for mastitis

    o Milk stasis from a blocked duct

    o Nipple trauma and cracked or fissured nipples

    o Poor breastfeeding technique with improper latching of the infant onto the breast, which can lead to sore and cracked nipples

    o Decrease in breastfeeding frequency due to supplementation with bottle feeding

    o Poor hygiene with inadequate hand hygiene between handling perineal pads and breasts

Assessment

- Subjective Data

    ■ Puerperal infections

        □ Flu-like symptoms such as body aches, chills, fever, and malaise

        □ Anorexia and nausea

- Endometritis
  - Pelvic pain
  - Chills
  - Fatigue
  - Loss of appetite
- Mastitis
  - Painful or tender, localized hard mass, and reddened area usually on one breast
  - Chills
  - Fatigue

- Objective Data
  - Physical assessment findings
    - Puerperal infections
      - Elevated temperature of at least 38° C (100° F) for 2 or more consecutive days.
      - Tachycardia
    - Endometritis
      - Uterine tenderness and enlargement
      - Dark profuse lochia
      - Lochia that is either malodorous or purulent
      - Fever > 38° C (100.4° F) typically on the third to fourth postpartum day
      - Tachycardia
    - Wound infection
      - Wound warmth, erythema, tenderness, pain, edema, seropurulent drainage, and wound dehiscence (separation of wound or incision edges) or evisceration (protrusion of internal contents through the separated wound edges)
      - Fever
    - Mastitis
      - Axillary adenopathy in the affected side (enlarged tender axillary lymph nodes) with an area of inflammation that may be red, swollen, warm, and tender
  - Laboratory tests
    - Blood, intracervical, or intrauterine bacterial cultures to reveal the offending organism
    - WBC count (leukocytosis)

- ■ RBC sedimentation rate (distinctly increased)
- ■ RBC count (anemia)
  - ○ Diagnostic procedures
    - ■ The primary care provider may need to open and drain the wound or perform wound debridement if indicated.

Collaborative Care

- Nursing Care
  - ○ Obtain frequent vital signs and temperature.
  - ○ Assess fundal height, position, and consistency.
  - ○ Assess the client's pain level.
  - ○ Observe lochia for color, quantity, and consistency.
  - ○ Inspect incisions, episiotomy, and lacerations.
  - ○ Inspect the client's breasts.
    - ■ Nursing interventions for puerperal infections
      - □ Provide client education about preventative measures.
        - ▸ Use aseptic techniques with proper hand hygiene and gloves for labor and birth.
        - ▸ Emphasize to the client thorough hand hygiene and good maternal perineal hygiene.
      - □ Maintain or initiate IV access.
      - □ Administer IV broad-spectrum antibiotic therapy (penicillins or cephalosporins) as prescribed.
      - □ Provide the client with comfort measures such as warm blankets or cool compresses, depending on the symptoms.
      - □ Educate the client about the signs of worsening conditions to report and the importance of adherence to the treatment plan with the completion of a full course of antibiotics.
      - □ Encourage the client to consume a diet high in protein to promote tissue healing.
  - Nursing interventions for endometritis
    - □ Collect vaginal and blood cultures.
    - □ Administer IV antibiotics as prescribed.
    - □ Administer analgesics as prescribed.
    - □ Teach the client hand hygiene techniques.
    - □ Encourage a mother to maintain interaction with her infant to facilitate bonding.

- Nursing interventions for wound infection

  □ Perform wound care.

  □ Provide or encourage comfort measures such as sitz baths, perineal care, and warm or cold compresses.

  □ Teach the client good hand hygiene techniques (changing perineal pads from front to back, performing thorough hand hygiene prior to and after perineal care).

- Nursing interventions for mastitis

  - Provide the client with education regarding breast hygiene to prevent mastitis.

    ▸ Instruct the client to thoroughly wash her hands prior to breastfeeding.

    ▸ Instruct the client to maintain cleanliness of her breasts with frequent changes of breast pads.

    ▸ Tell the client to allow her nipples to air-dry.

    ▸ Teach the client about proper infant positioning and latching-on techniques, including both the nipple and the areola. The mother should release the infant's grasp on the nipple prior to removing the infant from the breast.

    ▸ Instruct the client about how to completely empty her breasts during each feeding for prevention of milk stasis, which provides a medium for bacterial growth.

    ▸ Encourage the client to use ice packs or warm packs on her affected breasts for discomfort.

    ▸ Instruct the client to continue breastfeeding frequently (at least every 2 to 4 hr), especially on the affected side. Instruct the client to manually express breast milk or use a breast pump if breastfeeding is too painful.

    ▸ Instruct the client to begin breastfeeding from the unaffected breast first to initiate the letdown reflex in the affected breast that is distended or tender.

    ▸ Encourage rest, analgesics, and a fluid intake of at least 3,000 mL per day.

    ▸ Encourage the client to wear a well-fitting bra for support.

    ▸ Tell the client to report redness and fever.

    ▸ Administer antibiotics and teach the client the importance of completing the entire course of antibiotics as prescribed.

- Medications for endometritis
  - Clindamycin (Cleocin)
    - Classification and therapeutic intent
      - It is an antibiotic used in the treatment of bacterial infections.
    - Client education
      - Educate the client to take all the medication as prescribed.
      - Notify the provider of the development of watery, bloody diarrhea.
      - Notify the provider if the client is breastfeeding.
- Desired Client Outcomes
  - The client will be free of signs of infection as evidenced by vital signs and a WBC that is within normal limits, negative blood, and cultures.
  - The client's breast will be nontender and without redness.
    - The client's wound will be free of erythema, tenderness, pain, edema, and seropurulent.

URINARY TRACT INFECTION

Overview

- Urinary tract infections (UTI) are a common postpartum infection secondary to bladder trauma incurred during the delivery or a break in aseptic technique during bladder catheterization.
- A potential complication of a UTI is the progression to pyelonephritis with permanent renal damage leading to acute or chronic renal failure.

Risk Factors

- Postpartal hypotonic bladder and/or urethra (urinary stasis and retention)
- Epidural anesthesia
- Urinary bladder catheterization
- Frequent pelvic examinations
- Genital tract injuries
- History of UTIs
- Cesarean birth

Assessment

- Subjective Data

  - Reports of urgency, frequency, dysuria, and discomfort in the pelvic area

  - Fever

  - Chills

  - Malaise

- Objective Data

  - Physical assessment findings

    - Change in vital signs, elevated temperature

    - Urine (cloudy, blood-tinged, malodorous, sediment)

    - Urinary retention, hematuria, and pyuria

    - Pain in the suprapubic area

    - Pain at the costovertebral angle (pyelonephritis)

  - Diagnostic procedures

    - A urinalysis checks for WBCs, RBCs, protein, and bacteria.

Collaborative Care

- Nursing Care

  - Obtain either a random or clean-catch urine sample.

  - Administer antibiotics and teach the client the importance of completing the entire course of antibiotics as prescribed.

  - Teach the client proper perineal hygiene, such as wiping from front to back.

  - Encourage the client to increase her fluid intake to 3,000 mL/day to dilute the bacteria and flush her bladder.

  - Recommend that the client drink cranberry juice to promote urine acidification, which inhibits bacterial multiplication.

- Desired Therapeutic Outcomes

  - The client will be free of infection.

CHAPTER 21: POSTPARTUM INFECTIONS

(A) Application Exercises

1. A client who is at the greatest risk for postpartum infection is the client who

    A. experienced a precipitous labor less than 3 hr in duration.

    B. has premature rupture of membranes and prolonged labor.

    C. delivered a large for gestational age infant.

    D. has a boggy uterus that is not well-contracted.

2. A nurse is caring for a client who is breastfeeding and has mastitis. Which of the following should the nurse teach the client?

    A. "Limit the amount of time the infant nurses on each breast."

    B. "Nurse the infant only on the unaffected breast until resolved."

    C. "Completely empty each breast at each feeding or with a pump."

    D. "Wear a tight-fitting bra until lactation has ceased."

3. A postpartum client who is being discharged 2 days after delivery has been diagnosed with a urinary tract infection. The nurse reviews discharge instructions with the client. Which of the following statements by the client indicates a need for further teaching? (Select all that apply.)

    _____ "I will perform peri care and apply a perineal pad in a back-to-front direction."

    _____ "I will drink cranberry and prune juices to make my urine more acidic."

    _____ "I will drink large amounts of fluids to flush the bacteria from my urinary tract."

    _____ "I will not nurse my baby until I have finished taking the antibiotic."

    _____ "I will take Tylenol for any discomfort."

4. A nurse is caring for a client who has mastitis. Which of the following is the typical causative agent of mastitis?

    A. *Staphylococcus aureus*

    B. *Chlamydia trachomatis*

    C. *Klebsiella pneumonia*

    D. *Clostridium perfringens*

CHAPTER 21: POSTPARTUM INFECTIONS

(A) Application Exercises Answer Key

1. A client who is at the greatest risk for postpartum infection is the client who

   A. experienced a precipitous labor less than 3 hr in duration.

   B. has premature rupture of membranes and prolonged labor.

   C. delivered a large for gestational age infant.

   D. has a boggy uterus that is not well-contracted.

   All of the choices present a risk for postpartum infection. However, premature rupture of membranes with a prolonged labor poses the greatest risk because the uterus is open, thus allowing pathogens to enter. Precipitate labor and a large-for-gestational age infant place the client at risk for trauma and lacerations during delivery. A boggy uterus places the client at risk for hemorrhage and infection.

   (N) NCLEX® Connection: Health Promotion and Maintenance, Ante/Intra/Postpartum and Newborn Care

2. A nurse is caring for a client who is breastfeeding and has mastitis. Which of the following should the nurse teach the client?

   A. "Limit the amount of time the infant nurses on each breast."

   B. "Nurse the infant only on the unaffected breast until resolved."

   C. "Completely empty each breast at each feeding or with a pump."

   D. "Wear a tight-fitting bra until lactation has ceased."

   Instruct the client to completely empty each breast at each feeding for the prevention of milk stasis, which provides a medium for bacterial growth. Frequent breastfeeding should be encouraged to promote milk flow. The client should be instructed to continue breastfeeding, especially on the affected side. The client should wear a well-fitting bra, not one that is too tight or a binder.

   (N) NCLEX® Connection: Health Promotion and Maintenance, Ante/Intra/Postpartum and Newborn Care

3. A postpartum client who is being discharged 2 days after delivery has been diagnosed with a urinary tract infection. The nurse reviews discharge instructions with the client. Which of the following statements by the client indicates a need for further teaching? (Select all that apply.)

   X   **"I will perform peri care and apply a perineal pad in a back-to-front direction."**

   _____   "I will drink cranberry and prune juices to make my urine more acidic."

   _____   "I will drink large amounts of fluids to flush the bacteria from my urinary tract."

   X   **"I will not nurse my baby until I have finished taking the antibiotic."**

   _____   "I will take Tylenol for any discomfort."

Acidification of urine inhibits bacterial multiplication. Increased fluids can help to flush the bacteria from the urinary tract. Acetaminophen (Tylenol) is given to reduce discomfort and pain associated with a urinary tract infection. Breastfeeding does not have to be delayed until the course of antibiotics is completed. Perineal cleansing and pad application should be done front-to-back, not back-to-front.

 NCLEX® Connection: Health Promotion and Maintenance, Ante/Intra/Postpartum and Newborn Care

4. A nurse is caring for a client who has mastitis. Which of the following is the typical causative agent of mastitis?

A. *Staphylococcus aureus*

B. *Chlamydia trachomatis*

C. *Klebsiella pneumonia*

D. *Clostridium perfringens*

Staphylococcus aureus, Escherichia coli, and streptococcus are usually the infecting agents that enter the breast due to sore or cracked nipples, which results in mastitis.

 NCLEX® Connection: Health Promotion and Maintenance, Ante/Intra/Postpartum and Newborn Care

UNIT 3	POSTPARTUM NURSING CARE
Section	Complications of the Postpartum Period
Chapter 22	Postpartum Depression

Overview

- Postpartum blues can occur in approximately 50 to 70% of women during the first few days after birth and generally continues for up to 10 days. It is characterized by tearfulness, insomnia, lack of appetite, and feeling of letdown. A mother may experience an intense fear and/or anxiety, anger, and inability to cope with the slightest problems and become despondent. Postpartum blues typically resolves in 10 days without interventions.

- Postpartum depression occurs within 6 months of delivery and is characterized by persistent feelings of sadness and intense mood swings. It occurs in 10 to 15% of new mothers and usually does not resolve without intervention. It is similar to nonpostpartum mood disorders.

- Postpartum psychosis develops within the first 2 to 3 weeks of the postpartum period. Clients who have a history of bipolar disorder are at a higher risk. The symptoms are severe and may include confusion, disorientation, hallucinations, delusions, obsessive behaviors, paranoia, and the client may attempt to harm herself or her infant.

  ○ A nurse should monitor the client for suicidal or delusional thoughts. The infant should be monitored for failure to thrive secondary to an inability of the mother to provide care for her newborn.

Risk Factors

- Hormonal changes with a rapid decline in estrogen and progesterone levels

- Postpartum physical discomfort and/or pain

- Individual socioeconomic factors

- Decreased social support system

- Anxiety about assuming new role as a mother

- Unplanned or unwanted pregnancy

- History of previous depressive episode

- Low self-esteem

- History of domestic violence

Assessment

- Subjective Data
  - Postpartum blues
    - Feelings of sadness
    - Lack of appetite
    - Sleep pattern disturbances
    - Feeling of inadequacies
    - Intense mood swings
  - Postpartum depression
    - Feelings of guilt and inadequacies
    - Irritability
    - Anxiety
    - Fatigue persisting beyond a reasonable amount of time
    - Feeling of loss
    - Lack of appetite
    - Persistent feelings of sadness
    - Intense mood swings
    - Sleep pattern disturbances
  - Postpartum psychosis
    - Pronounced sadness
    - Disorientation
    - Confusion
    - Paranoia
- Objective Data
  - Physical assessment findings
    - Postpartum blues
      - Crying
    - Postpartum depression
      - Crying
      - Weight loss
      - Flat affect

- Postpartum psychosis
  - Behaviors indicating hallucinations or delusional thoughts of self harm or harming the infant

Collaborative Care

- Nursing Care

  - Monitor interactions between the mother and her infant. Encourage bonding activities.

  - Monitor client's mood and affect.

  - Reinforce with the client that feeling down in the postpartum period is normal and self-limiting. Encourage the mother to notify her primary care provider if the condition persists.

  - Encourage the client to communicate feelings, validate and address personal conflicts, and reinforce personal power and autonomy.

  - Reinforce with the client the importance of compliance with any prescribed antidepressant medication regimen.

  - Contact a community resource to schedule a follow-up visit after discharge for women who are at high risk for postpartum depression.

- Medications

  - Antidepressants may be prescribed by the primary care provider if indicated based on the client's condition.

- Care after Discharge

  - Advise the client to get plenty of rest and to nap when the infant sleeps.

  - Reinforce the importance of the client taking time out for herself.

  - Schedule a follow-up visit prior to the traditional 6-week postpartum visit for clients who are at risk for developing postpartum depression.

  - Provide information about community resources such as La Leche League or community mental health centers.

  - Encourage the client to seek counseling and make referrals to social agencies as indicated.

- Desired Client Outcomes

  - The client will report no signs or symptoms of depression.

  - The client will demonstrate healthy interactions with the infant.

CHAPTER 22: POSTPARTUM DEPRESSION

 Application Exercises

1. A nurse is assessing a postpartum client who is exhibiting signs of tearfulness, insomnia, lack of appetite, and a feeling of letdown. The nurse knows these signs and symptoms are characteristics of

    A. postpartum fatigue.

    B. postpartum psychosis.

    C. the letting-go phase.

    D. postpartum depression.

2. Identify contributing factors of postpartum depression. (Select all that apply.)

    _____ Fatigue from the work of labor and birth

    _____ Disappointment in the characteristics of the infant

    _____ Individual or family socioeconomic factors

    _____ Anxiety about assuming a new role as a mother

    _____ Rapid decline in estrogen and progesterone

    _____ Postpartum physical discomfort and/or pain

3. A nurse is caring for a postpartum client who delivered her third infant 2 days ago. The nurse recognizes that which of the following symptoms are suggestive of postpartum depression? (Select all that apply.)

    _____ Fatigue

    _____ Insomnia

    _____ Euphoria

    _____ Flat affect

    _____ Crying

CHAPTER 22: POSTPARTUM DEPRESSION

(A) Application Exercises Answer Key

1. A nurse is assessing a postpartum client who is exhibiting signs of tearfulness, insomnia, lack of appetite, and a feeling of letdown. The nurse knows these signs and symptoms are characteristics of

    A. postpartum fatigue.

    B. postpartum psychosis.

    C. the letting-go phase.

    D. postpartum depression.

Postpartum depression in the mother is characterized by tearfulness, insomnia, lack of appetite, and feeling letdown. Postpartum fatigue results from the work of labor. It is normally self-limiting. The letting-go phase is the phase in which the mother assumes her position at home and her new maternal role, focusing on the forward movement of the family unit. The client who has postpartum psychosis will exhibit pronounced feelings of sadness, confusion, disorientation, hallucinations, delusions, and paranoia, and may attempt to harm herself or her infant.

(N) NCLEX® Connection: Physiological Adaptation, Alterations in Body Systems

2. Identify contributing factors of postpartum depression. (Select all that apply.)

    __X__   **Fatigue from the work of labor and birth**

    _____   Disappointment in the characteristics of the infant

    __X__   **Individual or family socioeconomic factors**

    __X__   **Anxiety about assuming a new role as a mother**

    __X__   **Rapid decline in estrogen and progesterone**

    __X__   **Postpartum physical discomfort and/or pain**

There are several factors that contribute to postpartum depression including maternal fatigue from the work of labor and birth, socioeconomic factors, maternal anxiety about assuming a new role, the rapid decline in maternal estrogen and progesterone levels with the expulsion of the placenta, and postpartum physical discomfort and/or pain. Disappointment in the characteristics of the infant would be an indication of impaired mother-infant bonding.

(N) NCLEX® Connection: Physiological Adaptation, Alterations in Body Systems

3. A nurse is caring for a postpartum client who delivered her third infant 2 days ago. The nurse recognizes that which of the following symptoms are suggestive of postpartum depression? (Select all that apply.)

X	**Fatigue**
X	**Insomnia**
	Euphoria
X	**Flat affect**
X	**Crying**

Symptoms of fatigue, insomnia, flat affect, and bouts of crying are symptoms that are commonly seen in postpartum clients who are experiencing depression. Euphoria is not associated with postpartum depression.

Ⓝ NCLEX® Connection: Health Promotion and Maintenance, Developmental Stages and Transitions

UNIT 4: NEWBORN NURSING CARE

- Low-Risk Newborn
- Complications of the Newborn

NCLEX® CONNECTIONS

When reviewing the chapters in this unit, keep in mind the relevant sections of the NCLEX® outline, in particular:

CLIENT NEEDS: HEALTH PROMOTION AND MAINTENANCE

Relevant topics/tasks include:
- Ante/Intra/Postpartum and Newborn Care
  - Provide newborn care and education.
- Health and Wellness
  - Apply knowledge of nutrition to assessing the client's weight.
- Techniques of Physical Assessment
  - Apply knowledge of nursing procedures and psychomotor skills to techniques of physical assessment.

CLIENT NEEDS: BASIC CARE AND COMFORT

Relevant topics/tasks include:
- Nonpharmacological Comfort Interventions
  - Apply knowledge of pathophysiology to nonpharmacological comfort/palliative care interventions.

CLIENT NEEDS: REDUCTION OF RISK POTENTIAL

Relevant topics/tasks include:
- Changes/Abnormalities in Vital Signs
  - Apply knowledge of client pathophysiology when measuring vital signs.
- Laboratory Values
  - Identify laboratory values for ABGs, BUN, cholesterol, glucose, hematocrit, hemoglobin, glycosylated hemoglobin, platelets, potassium, sodium, WBC, creatinine, PT, PTT and APTT, INR.
- System Specific Assessment
  - Assess the client for signs of hypoglycemia or hyperglycemia.

UNIT 4	NEWBORN NURSING CARE
Section	Low-Risk Newborn
Chapter 23	Newborn Assessment

Overview

- Understanding physiologic responses of a newborn to birth and physical assessment findings are imperative for providing nursing care following the birth of a newborn. Apgar scoring, physical examination of the newborn, New Ballard Scale (gestational age assessment), normal newborn vital signs and measurements, classifications of a newborn by gestational age and weight, diagnostic and therapeutic procedures, and complications of a newborn will be addressed in this chapter.

Physiologic Response of Newborn to Birth

- Adjustments to extrauterine life occur as a newborn's respiratory and circulatory systems are required to rapidly adjust to life outside of the uterus.

- The establishment of respiratory function with the cutting of the umbilical cord is the most critical extrauterine adjustment as air inflates the lungs with the first breath.

- Circulatory changes after birth occur with the expulsion of the placenta and the cutting of the umbilical cord as a newborn begins breathing independently. The three shunts, ductus arteriosus, ductus venosus, and foramen ovale, functionally close during a newborn's transition to extrauterine life with the flow of oxygenated blood in the lungs and readjustment of atrial blood pressure in the heart.

Physical Assessment of Newborn Following Birth

- APGAR scoring and a brief physical exam is done immediately following birth to rule out abnormalities. An APGAR score is assigned based on a quick review of systems that is completed at 1 and 5 min of life. This allows the nurse to rapidly assess extrauterine adaptation and intervene with appropriate nursing actions.

  - 0 to 3 indicates severe distress

  - 4 to 6 indicates moderate distress

  - 7 to 10 indicates no distress

SCORE	0	1	2
Heart rate	Absent	< 100	> 100
Respiratory rate	Absent	Slow, weak cry	Good cry
Muscle tone	Flaccid	Some flexion	Well-flexed
Reflex irritability	None	Grimace	Cry
Color	Blue, pale	Pink body, cyanotic hands and feet (acrocyanosis)	Completely pink

 View Media Supplement: Apgar Scoring (Video)

- o Appropriate equipment for newborn assessment
    - Bulb syringe – used for the suctioning of excess mucus from the newborn's mouth and nose
    - Stethoscope with a pediatric head – used to evaluate the newborn's heart rate, breath sounds, and bowel sounds
    - Axillary thermometer – used to monitor the newborn's temperature and helps to avoid hypothermia; rectal temperatures are avoided because they can injure the delicate rectal mucosa; a rectal temperature may be done initially to evaluate for anal abnormalities
    - Blood pressure cuff 2.5 cm wide – (can use palpation or electronic method) for evaluation of the newborn's blood pressure; blood pressure may be done in all four extremities if evaluating the newborn for cardiac problems
    - Scale with paper in place – scale should be at 0 before weighing the newborn; weight should include pounds, ounces, and grams
    - Tape measure with centimeters – newborn should be measured from crown to heel of foot for length; measure the newborn's head circumference at greatest diameter (occipital to frontal); measure the newborn's chest circumference beginning at the nipple line and abdominal circumference above the umbilicus
    - Clean gloves – used for examining the newborn until he is given his first bath
- The nurse will perform a quick initial assessment to review the newborn's systems and to observe for any abnormalities.
    - o External assessment – skin color, peeling, birthmarks, foot creases, breast tissue, nasal patency, and meconium staining (may indicate fetal hypoxia)
    - o Chest – point of maximal impulse location, ease of breathing, auscultation for heart rate and quality of tones and respirations for crackles, wheezes, and equality of bilateral breath sounds
    - o Abdomen – rounded abdomen and umbilical cord for one vein and two arteries

- Neurologic – muscle tone and reflex reaction (Moro reflex); palpation for the presence and size of fontanels and sutures; assessment of fontanels for fullness or bulge

- Other observations – inspection for gross structural malformations

- A gestational age assessment is performed within 2 to 12 hr of birth. Neonatal morbidity and mortality are related to gestational age and birth weight. This assessment involves taking measurements of the newborn and the use of the New Ballard Scale. This scale provides an estimation of gestational age and a baseline to assess growth and development.

  - The normal ranges of physical measurements

    - Weight – 2,500 to 4,000 g (Weigh the newborn at the same time daily.)

    - Length – 45 to 55 cm (18 to 22 in)

    - Head circumference – 32 to 36.8 cm (12.6 to 14.5 in)

    - Chest circumference – 30 to 33 cm (12 to 13 in)

  - New Ballard Scale – a newborn maturity rating scale that assesses neuromuscular and physical maturity. Each individual assessment parameter displays at least six ranges of development along a continuum. Each range of development within an assessment is assigned a number value from -1 to 5. The totals are added to give a maturity rating in weeks gestation (a score of 35 indicates 38 weeks of gestation).

 View Media Supplement: Gestational Age Assessment (Video)

  - Neuromuscular maturity assesses:

    - Posture ranging from fully extended to fully flexed (0 to 4).

    - Square window formation with the neonate's wrist (-1 to 4).

    - Arm recoil, where the neonate's arm is passively extended and spontaneously returns to flexion (0 to 4).

    - Popliteal angle, which is the degree of the angle to which the newborn's knees can extend (-1 to 5).

    - Scarf sign, which is crossing the neonate's arm over the chest (-1 to 4).

    - Heel to ear, which is how far the neonate's heels reach to her ears (-1 to 4).

  - Physical maturity assesses:

    - Skin texture, ranging from sticky and transparent, to leathery, cracked, and wrinkled (-1 to 5).

    - Lanugo presence and amount, ranging from none, sparse, abundant, thinning, bald, or mostly bald (-1 to 4).

    - Plantar surface creases, ranging from < 40 to 50 mm, to creases over the entire sole (-1 to 4).

    - Breast tissue amount, ranging from imperceptible, to full areola with a 5 to 10 mm bud (-1 to 4).

□ Eyes and ears for amount of eye opening and ear cartilage present (-1 to 4).

□ Genitalia development, ranging from flat smooth scrotum to pendulous testes with deep rugae for males (-1 to 4), and prominent clitoris with flat labia to the labia majora covering the labia minora and clitoris for females (-1 to 4).

○ Following the physical assessment of the newborn, classification of the newborn by gestational age and birth weight is then determined.

- Appropriate for gestational age (AGA) – weight is between the 10th and 90th percentile

- Small for gestational age (SGA) – weight is below the 10th percentile

- Large for gestational age (LGA) – weight is above the 90th percentile

- Low birth weight (LBW) – a weight of 2,500 g or less at birth

- Intrauterine growth restriction (IUGR) – growth rate does not meet expected norms

- Term – birth between the beginning of week 38 and prior to the end of 42 weeks of gestation

- Preterm or premature – born prior to the completion of 37 weeks of gestation

- Postterm (postdate) – born after the completion of 42 weeks of gestation

- Postmature – born after the completion of 42 weeks of gestation with signs of placental insufficiency

• A more extensive physical exam is performed on the neonate within 24 hr of birth. Vital signs are then obtained. A head-to-toe assessment should be performed. Neurological and behavioral assessments are completed by eliciting reflexes and observing the responses of the newborn. Laboratory data is also monitored.

• Vital signs are normally checked in the following sequence: respirations, heart rate, blood pressure, and temperature. The nurse should observe the newborn's respiratory rate first before the newborn becomes active or agitated with the stethoscope, thermometer, and/or the blood pressure cuff.

○ Respiratory rate increases from 30 to 60/min with short periods of apnea (less than 15 seconds) occurring most frequently during the rapid eye movement sleep cycle. Periods of apnea lasting longer than 15 seconds need to be evaluated. Crackles and wheezing are symptoms of fluid or infection in the lungs. Grunting and nasal flaring are signs of respiratory distress.

○ Heart rate should be 100 to 160/min with brief fluctuations above and below this range depending on activity level (crying, sleeping). Apical pulse rate should be obtained for a full minute, preferably when the newborn is sleeping. The pediatric stethoscope head should be placed on the fourth or fifth intercostal space at the left midclavicular line over the apex of the newborn's heart. Heart murmurs should be documented and reported.

○ Blood pressure should be 60 to 80 mm Hg systolic and 40 to 50 mm Hg diastolic.

○   Temperature should be 36.5 to 37.2° C (97.7 to 98.9° F) axillary. The newborn is at risk for hypothermia and hyperthermia until thermoregulation (ability to produce heat and maintain normal body temperature) stabilizes. If the newborn becomes chilled (cold stress), oxygen demands can increase and acidosis can occur.

● Physical exam from head to toe

○   Posture

■   The newborn should be lying in a curled-up position with his arms and legs in moderate flexion.

■   The newborn should be resistant to extension of his extremities.

○   Skin

■   The newborn's skin color should be pink or acrocyanotic with no jaundice present on the first day. Secondary to increased bilirubin, jaundice may appear on the third day of life, but then decrease spontaneously.

■   The newborn's skin turgor should be good, showing that the newborn is well-hydrated. The skin should spring back immediately when pinched.

■   Texture should be dry, soft, and smooth showing good hydration. Cracks in hands and feet may be present. In full-term newborns, desquamation (peeling) occurs a few days after birth.

■   Vernix caseosa (protective, thick, cheesy covering) amounts vary, with more present in the newborn's creases and skin folds.

■   Lanugo (fine downy hair) varies in newborns regarding the amount present. It is usually found on the newborn's pinnas, forehead, and shoulders.

■   Normal deviations

□   Milia (small raised white spots on the nose, chin, and forehead) may be present. These spots disappear spontaneously without treatment (parents should not squeeze the spots).

□   Mongolian spots (bluish purple spots of pigmentation) are commonly noted on the newborn's shoulders, back, and buttocks. These spots are frequently present on newborns who have dark skin. Be sure the parents are aware of Mongolian spots and notify health care providers of the location and presence of them.

□   Telangiectatic nevi (stork bites) are flat pink or red marks that easily blanch and are found on the newborn's back of the neck, nose, upper eyelids, and middle of the forehead. They usually fade by the second year of life.

□   Nevus flammeus (port wine stain) is a capillary angioma below the surface of the skin that is purple or red, varies in size and shape, is commonly seen on the face, and does not blanch or disappear.

□   Erythema toxicum (erythema neonatorum) is a pink rash that appears suddenly anywhere on the body of a term newborn during the first 3 weeks. This is frequently referred to as newborn rash. No treatment is required.

○ Head

- The newborn's head should be 2 to 3 cm larger than his chest circumference. If his head circumference is greater than or equal to 4 cm larger than his chest circumference, this can be an indication of hydrocephalus (excessive cerebral fluid within the brain cavity surrounding the brain). If his head circumference is less than or equal to 32 cm, this can be an indication of microcephaly (abnormally small head).

- The newborn's anterior fontanel should be palpated and approximately 5 cm on average and diamond shaped. The posterior fontanel is smaller and triangle shaped. Both fontanels should be soft and flat. The fontanels may bulge when the newborn cries, coughs, or vomits and flat when the newborn is quiet. Bulging fontanels may indicate increased intracranial pressure, infection, or hemorrhage. Depressed fontanels may indicate dehydration.

- The sutures of the newborn should be palpable, separated, and may be overlapping (molding), a normal occurrence resulting from head compression during labor.

- Caput succedaneum (localized swelling of the soft tissues of the scalp caused by pressure on the head during labor) is a normal finding that may be palpated as a soft edematous mass and may cross over the suture line. Caput succedaneum usually resolves in 3 to 4 days and does not require treatment.

- Cephalohematoma is a collection of blood between the periosteum and the skull bone that it covers. It does not cross the suture line. It results from trauma during birth such as pressure of the fetal head against the maternal pelvis in a prolonged difficult labor or forceps delivery. It appears in the first 1 to 2 days after birth and simultaneously resolves in 2 to 3 weeks.

(M) **View Media Supplement:**
- Caput Succedaneum (Image)   • Cephalohematoma (Image)

○ Eyes

- Assess the newborn's eyes for symmetry in size and shape.

- Each of the newborn's eyes and the space between them should equal one-third of the total distance between the outer canthus of both eyes to rule out chromosomal abnormalities such as Down syndrome.

- The eyes of newborns are normally blue or gray.

- Permanent eye color is established within 3 to 12 months.

- Lacrimal glands are immature in a newborn, resulting in tearless crying.

- Subconjunctival hemorrhages may result from pressure during birth.

- Pupillary and red reflex are present in newborns.

- Eyeball movement will demonstrate random, jerky movements.

- Ears
  - When examining the placement of the newborn's ears, draw an imaginary line through the inner to the outer canthus of the newborn's eye. The eye should be even with the upper tip of the pinna of the newborn's ear. Ears that are low set can indicate a chromosome abnormality such as Down syndrome or a renal disorder.
  - Cartilage should be firm and well-formed. Lack of cartilage indicates prematurity.
  - The newborn should respond to voices and other sounds.
  - Inspect the newborn's ears for skin tags.
- Nose
  - The newborn's nose should be midline, flat, and broad with lack of a bridge.
  - Some mucus should be present, but with no drainage.
  - Newborns are obligate nose breathers and do not develop the response of opening the mouth with a nasal obstruction until 3 weeks after birth; therefore, a nasal blockage may result in flaring of the nares, cyanosis, or asphyxia.
  - The newborn should sneeze to clear his nose.
- Mouth
  - Assess the newborn for palate closure and strength of sucking.
  - The lip movements of the newborn should be symmetrical.
  - Saliva should be scant. Excessive saliva may indicate a tracheoesophageal fistula.
  - Epstein pearls (small white cysts found on the gums and at the junction of the soft and hard palates) are normal in newborns. They result from the accumulation of epithelial cells and disappear a few weeks after birth.
  - The newborn's tongue should move freely, be symmetrical in shape, and not protrude (a protruding tongue may be a sign of Down syndrome).
  - The newborn's soft and hard palate should be intact.
  - The newborn's gums and tongue should be pink. Gray-white patches on the tongue and gums can indicate thrush, a fungal infection caused by *Candida albicans*, sometimes acquired from the mother's vaginal secretions.
- Neck
  - The newborn's neck should be short, thick, surrounded by skin folds, and exhibit no webbing.
  - The newborn's neck should move freely from side to side and up and down.
  - Absence of head control may indicate prematurity or Down syndrome.
- Chest
  - The chest of the newborn should be barrel-shaped.
  - Respirations are primarily diaphragmatic in newborns.

- Clavicles should be intact.

- The newborn should experience no retractions.

- The newborn's nipples should be prominent, well-formed, and symmetrical.

- The newborn's breast nodule should be approximately 6 mm.

o Abdomen

- The umbilical cord will have two arteries and one vein.

- The cord should be odorless and exhibit no intestinal structures.

- The newborn's abdomen should be round, dome-shaped, and nondistended.

- Bowel sounds should be present 1 to 2 hr following birth.

o Anogenital

- The newborn's anus should be present, patent, and not covered by a membrane.

- The genitalia of a male newborn should include rugae on the scrotum.

- Testes should have descended into scrotum.

- Male urinary meatus is located at penile tip.

- The genitalia of a female should include labia majora covering the labia minora and clitoris. Female genitalia are usually edematous.

- Vaginal blood-tinged discharge may occur in female newborns, which is caused by maternal pregnancy hormones. This is a normal finding.

- A hymenal tag should be present.

- Urine should be passed within 24 hr after birth. Uric acid crystals will produce a rust color in the urine the first couple of days of life.

- Meconium should be passed within 24 hr after birth.

o Extremities

- A newborn should be assessed for full range, symmetry of motion, and spontaneous movements.

- Extremities should be flexed.

- Check for bowed legs and flat feet, which should be present because the lateral muscles are more developed than the medial muscles.

- No click should be heard when abducting the hips of a newborn.

- The newborn's gluteal folds should be symmetrical.

- The newborn's soles should be well-lined over two-thirds of his feet.

- The newborn's nail beds should be pink and there should be no extra digits present.

o Spine

- The newborn's spine should be straight, flat, midline and easily flexed.

    o   Reflexes

REFLEX	EXPECTED FINDING	EXPECTED AGE
Sucking and rooting reflex	• This reflex is elicited by stroking the newborn's cheek or edge of his mouth. When this is done, the newborn turns his head toward the side that is touched and starts to suck.	Birth to 4 months
Palmar grasp	• This reflex is elicited by placing an object in the newborn's palm. The newborn will grasp the object.	Birth to 6 months
Plantar grasp	• This reflex is elicited by touching the sole of the newborn's foot. The newborn responds by curling his toes downward.	Birth to 8 months
Moro reflex (startle)	• This reflex is elicited by striking a flat surface that the newborn is lying on, or allowing the head and trunk of the newborn in a semisitting position to fall backward to an angle of at least 30°. The newborn's arms and legs symmetrically extend and then abduct while his fingers spread to form a "C".	Birth to 4 months
Tonic neck reflex (fencer position)	• The newborn will extend his arm and leg on the side when his head is turned to that side with flexion of his arm and leg of the opposite side. • The newborn will turn his head to one side. The newborn will respond by extending his arm and leg on that side, and flex his arm and leg on the opposite side.	Birth to 3 to 4 months

REFLEX	EXPECTED FINDING	EXPECTED AGE
Babinski's reflex	• This reflex is elicited by stroking the outer edge of the newborn's sole of his foot, moving up toward his toes. His toes will fan upward and out.	Birth to 1 year
Stepping	• This reflex is elicited by holding the newborn upright with his feet touching a flat surface. The newborn will respond with stepping movements.	Birth to 4 weeks

    o Senses

- Vision – the newborn should be able to focus on objects 9 to 12 inches away from his face. This is approximately the distance from the mother's face when the newborn is breastfeeding. The newborn's eyes are sensitive to light; therefore, newborns prefer dim lighting. Pupils are reactive to light and the blink reflex is easily stimulated. The newborn can track high contrast objects and prefers bright colors and patterns.

- Hearing – similar to that of an adult once the amniotic fluid drains from the ears. Newborns exhibit selective listening to the familiar voices and rhythms of intrauterine life. The newborn turns toward the general direction of a sound.

- Touch – the newborn should respond to tactile messages of pain and touch. The mouth is the most sensitive to touch in the newborn.

- Taste – the newborn can taste and prefers sweets over salty, sour, or bitter.

- Smell – newborns have a highly developed sense of smell, prefer sweet smells, and can recognize the smell of their mother.

- Provide education to the mother and family about the neonate's appearance, and give reassurance about normal findings that the family may be concerned about (e.g., milia, Epstein's pearls, caput succedaneum).

Diagnostic and Therapeutic Procedures Following Birth

- Cord blood is collected from the newborn at birth. Laboratory tests are conducted on the blood to determine ABO blood type and Rh-status if the mother's blood type is "O" or she is Rh-negative. A CBC may be done in the nursery by a capillary stick to evaluate for anemia, polycythemia, infection, or clotting problems. A glucose level may be done to evaluate for hypoglycemia.

NORMAL LABORATORY VALUES	
Hgb	• 14 to 24 g/dL
Hct	• 44 to 64%
RBC count	• 4,800 to 7,100,000/mm^3
Leukocytes	• 9,000 to 30,000/mm^3
Platelets	• 150,000 to 300,000/mm^3
Glucose	• 40 to 60 mg/dL
Bilirubin	• 0 to 6 mg/dL on day 1 • 8 mg/dL or less on day 2 • 12 mg/dL or less on day 3

Complications

- Airway obstruction related to mucus

  o If excess mucus exists, the newborn's mouth and nose should be suctioned with a bulb syringe. Gentle percussion over the newborn's chest can help loosen secretions.

- Hypothermia

  o Monitor for an axillary newborn temperature of less than 36.5° C (97.7° F).

  o If temperature is unstable, place the newborn in a radiant warmer and maintain skin temperature at approximately 36.5° C (97.7° F).

  o Assess the newborn's axillary temperature every hour until it becomes stable.

  o All exams and assessments should be performed on the newborn under a radiant warmer.

- Inadequate oxygen supply related to obstructed airway, poorly functioning cardiopulmonary system, or hypothermia

  o Monitor the newborn's respirations and skin color for cyanosis.

  o Stabilize the newborn's body temperature or clear airway as indicated, administer oxygen, and if needed, prepare for resuscitation.

CHAPTER 23: NEWBORN ASSESSMENT

(A) Application Exercises

1. A nurse is caring for a newborn who was born at 38 weeks of gestation, weighs 3,200 g, and is in the 60th percentile for weight. Based on the weight and gestational age of this newborn, the nurse should classify this neonate as

    A. low birth weight.

    B. appropriate for gestational age.

    C. small for gestational age.

    D. large for gestational age.

2. During newborn assessment, a nurse observes small white nodules on the roof of the newborn's mouth. This finding is a characteristic of which of the following conditions?

    A. Mongolian spots

    B. Milia spots

    C. Erythema toxicum

    D. Epstein's pearls

3. A nurse is caring for a newborn following a spontaneous vaginal delivery. Five minutes after birth, the newborn's heart rate is 90/min. Which of the following Apgar heart rate scores should the newborn receive?

    A. 0

    B. 1

    C. 2

    D. 3

4. A nurse is assessing the reflexes of a newborn. In checking for the Moro reflex, the nurse should perform which of the following?

    A. Make a loud noise such as clapping hands together over the newborn's crib.

    B. Stimulate the pads of the newborn's hands with stroking or massage.

    C. Stimulate the soles of the newborn's feet on the outer lateral surface of each foot.

    D. Hold the newborn in a semi-sitting position, then allow the newborn's head and trunk to fall backward.

5. Which of the following signs pertaining to respirations indicate that a newborn is having no difficulty adapting to extrauterine life? (Select all that apply.)

_____ Expiratory grunting

_____ Respirations of 46/min

_____ Inspiratory nasal flaring

_____ Apnea for 10-second periods

_____ Obligatory nose breathing

_____ Respirations of 26/min

_____ Crackles and wheezing

6. A nurse is preparing to bathe a newborn and notices a bluish marking across the newborn's lower back. The nurse should understand that this mark is

A. frequently seen in newborns who have dark skin.

B. abnormal and may indicate hyperbilirubinemia.

C. may be a forceps mark from an operative delivery.

D. a sign of prolonged birth or trauma during delivery.

CHAPTER 23: NEWBORN ASSESSMENT

 Application Exercises Answer Key

1. A nurse is caring for a newborn who was born at 38 weeks of gestation, weighs 3,200 g, and is in the 60th percentile for weight. Based on the weight and gestational age of this newborn, the nurse should classify this neonate as

    A. low birth weight.

    B. appropriate for gestational age.

    C. small for gestational age.

    D. large for gestational age.

    This newborn is classified as appropriate for gestational age because her weight is between the 10th and 90th percentile. A newborn who has a low birth weight would weigh less than 2,500 g; a newborn who is small for gestational age would weigh below the 10th percentile; and a newborn who is large for gestational age would weigh above the 90th percentile.

 NCLEX® Connection: Health Promotion and Maintenance, Ante/Intra/Postpartum and Newborn Care

2. During newborn assessment, a nurse observes small white nodules on the roof of the newborn's mouth. This finding is a characteristic of which of the following conditions?

    A. Mongolian spots

    B. Milia spots

    C. Erythema toxicum

    D. Epstein's pearls

    Epstein's pearls are small white nodules that appear on the roof a newborn's mouth. Mongolian spots are dark areas observed in dark-skinned newborns, and erythema toxicum is a transient maculopapular rash seen in newborns. Milia are small white bumps that occur on the nose due to clogged sebaceous glands.

 NCLEX® Connection: Health Promotion and Maintenance, Ante/Intra/Postpartum and Newborn Care

3. A nurse is caring for a newborn following a spontaneous vaginal delivery. Five minutes after birth, the newborn's heart rate is 90/min. Which of the following Apgar heart rate scores should the newborn receive?

    A. 0

    B. 1

    C. 2

    D. 3

    The 5-min heart rate score should be 1 since the heart rate is less than 100/min.

 NCLEX® Connection: Health Promotion and Maintenance, Ante/Intra/Postpartum and Newborn Care

4. A nurse is assessing the reflexes of a newborn. In checking for the Moro reflex, the nurse should perform which of the following?

    A. Make a loud noise such as clapping hands together over the newborn's crib.

    B. Stimulate the pads of the newborn's hands with stroking or massage.

    C. Stimulate the soles of the newborn's feet on the outer lateral surface of each foot.

    D. Hold the newborn in a semi-sitting position, then allow the newborn's head and trunk to fall backward.

The Moro reflex is elicited by holding the newborn in a semi-sitting position and then allowing the head and trunk to fall backward. Clapping hands will elicit the startle reflex. Stimulating the pads of the newborn's hands will elicit the grasp reflex. Stimulating the outer lateral portion of the newborn's soles will elicit a Babinski's reflex.

 NCLEX® Connection: Health Promotion and Maintenance, Ante/Intra/Postpartum and Newborn Care

5. Which of the following signs pertaining to respirations indicate that a newborn is having no difficulty adapting to extrauterine life? (Select all that apply.)

    _____ Expiratory grunting

    __X__ **Respirations of 46/min**

    _____ Inspiratory nasal flaring

    __X__ **Apnea for 10-second periods**

    __X__ **Obligatory nose breathing**

    _____ Respirations of 26/min

    _____ Crackles and wheezing

Normal respiratory rate for a newborn increases from 30 to 60/min with short periods of apnea (less than 15 seconds) occurring most frequently during the rapid eye movement (REM) sleep cycle. Periods of apnea lasting less than 15 seconds are normal. Newborns are obligatory nose breathers. Grunting and nasal flaring are signs of respiratory distress. Crackles and wheezing are symptoms of fluid or infection in the lungs.

 NCLEX® Connection: Health Promotion and Maintenance, Ante/Intra/Postpartum and Newborn Care

6. A nurse is preparing to bathe a newborn and notices a bluish marking across the newborn's lower back. The nurse should understand that this mark is

A. frequently seen in newborns who have dark skin.

B. abnormal and may indicate hyperbilirubinemia.

C. may be a forceps mark from an operative delivery.

D. a sign of prolonged birth or trauma during delivery.

Mongolian spots are commonly found over the lumbosacral area of newborns who have dark skin and are of African-American, Asian, or Native-American origin. Hyperbilirubinemia would be present as jaundice. Forceps marks would most likely present as a cephalohematoma, and birth trauma would be present as ecchymosis.

Ⓝ NCLEX® Connection: Health Promotion and Maintenance, Ante/Intra/Postpartum and Newborn Care

UNIT 4	NEWBORN NURSING CARE
Section	Low-Risk Newborn
Chapter 24	Nursing Care of the Newborn

 Overview

- Newborn care consists of stabilization and/or resuscitation. This may include establishing a patent airway, maintaining adequate oxygenation, and thermoregulation for the maintenance of body temperature. A physical assessment will be done every 8 hr or as needed (physical examination, measurements, and monitoring laboratory studies). Nursing interventions and family teaching (umbilical cord care, prophylactic measures, newborn screening, newborn feedings and bathing, and facilitating parent-newborn attachment) are integrated into a newborn's plan of care.

Assessment

- Physical Assessment

  ○ The newborn's vital signs should be checked on admission/birth and every 30 min x 2, every 1 hr x 2, and then every 8 hr.

  ○ The newborn's weight, length, and head and chest circumference should be assessed at birth. Weight should be checked daily.

  ○ Inspect the newborn's umbilical cord for two arteries and one vein. Observe for any bleeding from the cord, and ensure that the cord is clamped securely to prevent hemorrhage.

  ○ In the first 6 to 8 hr of life as the newborn's body systems stabilize and pass through periods of adjustment, observe for periods of reactivity in the newborn.

    ■ First period of reactivity – The newborn is alert and exhibits exploring activity, makes sucking sounds, and has a rapid heartbeat and respiratory rate. Heart rate may be as high as 160 to 180/min, but will stabilize at a baseline of 100 to 120/min that lasts 15 to 30 min after birth.

    ■ Period of relative inactivity – The newborn will become quiet and begin rest and sleep. The newborn's heart rate and respirations will decrease, and this period will last from 30 min to 2 hr after birth.

    ■ Second period of reactivity – The newborn reawakens, becomes responsive again, and often gags and chokes on mucus that has accumulated in his mouth. This period usually occurs 2 to 8 hr after birth and may last 10 min to several hours.

  ○ Using the facility's preferred pain assessment tool, conduct a pain assessment on the newborn each shift and following painful procedures.

- Laboratory Tests

  o Hgb and Hct, if ordered

  o Glucose for hypoglycemia, per facility policy or order

  o Metabolic screening

    ■ Newborn genetic screening is mandated in all states. A capillary heel stick should be done 24 hr following birth. For results to be accurate, the newborn must receive formula or breast milk for at least 24 hr. If the newborn is discharged before 24 hr of age, the test should be repeated in 1 to 2 weeks.

    ■ All states require testing for phenylketonuria (PKU). PKU is a defect in protein metabolism in which the accumulation of the amino acid phenylalanine can result in mental retardation (treatment in the first 2 months of life can prevent retardation).

  o Other genetic testing that may be done includes: galactosemia, cystic fibrosis, maple syrup urine disease, hypothyroidism, and sickle cell disease.

  o Collecting blood samples

    ■ Heel stick blood samples are obtained by the nurse.

    ■ Heel sticks are best done by warming the newborn's heel first to increase circulation.

    ■ Cleanse the newborn's heel with alcohol and allow for drying.

    ■ A spring-activated lancet is used so that the skin incision is made quickly and painlessly.

    ■ The outer aspect of the heel should be used, and the lancet should go no deeper than 2.4 mm to prevent necrotizing osteochondritis resulting from penetration of bone with the lancet.

    ■ Cover the five circular areas with blood drawn from the heel of the newborn and drop onto a filter paper.

    ■ Apply pressure with dry gauze (do not use alcohol as it will cause bleeding to continue) until bleeding stops and cover with an adhesive bandage.

    ■ Cuddle and comfort the newborn when the procedure is completed to reassure the newborn and promote feelings of safety.

- Diagnostic Procedures

  o Newborn hearing screening is required in 46 states, 2 territories and the District of Columbia. Newborns are being screened in the nursery so that deafness can be detected and treated early.

Collaborative Care

- Nursing Care

  o Stabilize and/or give resuscitation to the newborn.

○ Monitor the newborn for signs and symptoms of respiratory complications.

  ■ Bradypnea – respirations less than 25/min

  ■ Tachypnea – respirations greater than 60/min

  ■ Abnormal breath sounds – expiratory grunting, crackles, and wheezes

  ■ Respiratory distress – nasal flaring, retractions, grunting, and labored breathing

○ Interventions for stabilization and resuscitation of airway

  ■ The newborn is able to clear most secretions in air passages by the cough reflex. Routine suctioning of the mouth and nasal passages with a bulb syringe is done to remove excess mucus in the respiratory tract.

  ■ Newborns delivered by cesarean birth are more susceptible to fluid remaining in the lungs than newborns who were delivered vaginally.

  ■ The newborn's nasal passages are suctioned one nostril at a time.

  ■ If bulb suctioning is unsuccessful, mechanical suction and/or back blows and chest thrusts may need to be used as well as the institution of emergency procedures.

  ■ The bulb syringe should be kept with the newborn and the newborn's family should be instructed on how to use it. Family members should be asked to perform a demonstration to show that they understand bulb syringe techniques.

○ Identification is applied to the newborn immediately after birth by the nurse. It is an important safety measure to prevent the newborn from being given to the wrong parents, switched, or abducted.

  ■ The mother, newborn, and significant other are identified by plastic identification wristbands with permanent locks that must be cut to be removed. Identification bands should include the newborn's name, sex, date, time of birth and mother's hospital number. The newborn should have one placed on the ankle and one on the wrist. In addition, the newborn's footprints and mother's thumb prints are taken. The above information is also included with the footprint sheet.

  ■ Each time the newborn is taken to the parents, the identification band should be verified against his mother's identification band.

  ■ All facility staff who assist in caring for the newborn are required to wear picture identification badges.

  ■ The newborn is not to be given to anyone who does not have a picture identification badge that distinguishes that person as a staff member of the facility maternal-newborn unit.

  ■ Many facilities have locked maternal-newborn units that require staff to permit entrance or exit. Some facilities have a sensor device on the ID band or umbilical cord clamp that sounds an alarm if the newborn is removed from the facility.

○ Thermoregulation provides a neutral thermal environment that helps a newborn maintain a normal core temperature with minimal oxygen consumption and caloric expenditure. A newborn has a relatively large surface-to-weight ratio, reduced metabolism per unit area, blood vessels closer to the surface, and small amounts of insulation. The newborn keeps warm by metabolizing brown fat, which is unique to newborns, but only within a very narrow temperature range. Becoming chilled (cold stress) can increase the newborn's oxygen demands and rapidly use up brown fat reserves. Therefore, monitoring temperature regulation is important.

- Monitor for signs and symptoms of hypothermia in the newborn.

  □ Axillary temperature of less than 36.5° C (97.7° F)

  □ Cyanosis

  □ Increased respiratory rate

- Interventions to maintain thermoregulation

  □ Core temperature varies within newborns, but it should be kept around 36.5° C (97.7° F). Heat can be lost by four mechanisms. Below is a summary of those mechanisms and how to avoid loss of heat.

    ▸ Conduction – loss of body heat resulting from direct contact with a cooler surface. The nurse should preheat a radiant warmer, warm a stethoscope and other instruments, and pad a scale with paper before weighing the newborn. The newborn should also be placed directly on the mother's abdomen and covered with a warm blanket.

    ▸ Convection – flow of heat from the body surface to cooler environmental air. The nurse should place the newborn's bassinet out of the direct line of a fan or air conditioning vent, swaddle the newborn in a blanket, and keep the newborn's head covered. Any procedure that must be done with the newborn uncovered should be performed under a radiant heat source.

    ▸ Evaporation – loss of heat as surface liquid is converted to vapor. The nurse should gently rub the newborn dry with a warm sterile blanket (adhering to standard precautions) immediately after delivery. If thermoregulation is unstable, postpone the initial bath until the newborn's skin temperature is 36.5° C (97.7° F). When bathing the newborn, expose only one body part at a time, washing and drying thoroughly.

    ▸ Radiation – loss of heat from the body surface to a cooler solid surface that is close to, but not in direct contact. The nurse should keep the newborn and examining tables away from windows and air conditioners.

  □ The newborn's temperature stabilizes at 37° C (98.6° F) within 4 hr after birth if chilling is prevented.

o   Bathing of the newborn can begin once the newborn's temperature has stabilized to at least 36.5° C (97.7° F). A complete sponge bath should be given within the first 1 to 2 hr after birth under a radiant heat source to prevent heat loss. If necessary, the first bath will be postponed until thermoregulation stabilizes.

  ■   Gloves should be worn until the newborn's first bath to avoid exposure to body secretions.

o   Feedings may be started immediately following birth.

  ■   Breastfeeding is initiated as soon as possible after birth and promotes maternal-newborn bonding.

  ■   Formula feeding is usually started at about 2 to 4 hr of age. A few sips of sterile water may be given to assess sucking and swallowing reflexes and assure that there are no anomalies such as a tracheoesophageal fistula prior to starting formula feeding.

    □   The newborn is fed on demand, which is normally every 3 to 4 hr for bottle-fed newborns and more frequently for breastfed newborns.

    □   Monitor and document feedings per facility protocol.

o   Sleep-wake states are variations of consciousness in the newborn consisting of six states along a continuum comprised of: deep sleep, light sleep, drowsy, quiet alert, active alert, and extreme irritability (crying).

  ■   Newborns sleep approximately 17 hr a day, an average of 4 hr at a time. It is important that newborns are positioned supine, "back to sleep," to decrease the incidence of sudden infant death syndrome.

o   Closely monitor the newborn's elimination habits.

  ■   Newborns should void once within 24 hr of birth. They should void 6 to 10 times a day after 4 days of life.

  ■   Meconium should be passed within the first 24 hr after birth. The newborn will then continue to stool 3 to 4 times a day depending on whether he is being breast or bottle fed.

  ■   The stools of newborns who are breastfed may appear yellow and seedy. These stools are lighter in color and looser than the stools of newborns who are formula fed.

o   Monitor and document the newborn's output.

  ■   Keep the perineal area of the newborn clean and dry. The ammonia in the urine is very irritating to the skin and can cause a diaper rash.

  ■   After each diaper change, the newborn's perineal area should be washed with clear water or water with a mild soap. Diaper wipes with alcohol should be avoided. Pat dry and apply triple antibiotic ointment, petroleum jelly, or zinc oxide, depending on facility protocol.

- ○ Infection control is essential in preventing cross contamination from newborn to newborn and between newborns and staff. All newborns are at risk for infection during the first few months of life because of immature immune systems.

  - Newborns should have their own bassinet equipped with a thermometer, diapers, T-shirts, and bathing supplies.

  - All personnel caring for a newborn should scrub with antimicrobial soap from elbows to finger tips before entering the nursery. In between care of the newborn, the nurse should follow good hand hygiene. Cover gowns or special uniforms are used to avoid direct contact with clothes.

  - ○ Family education and promotion of parent-newborn attachment

    - Provide family education while performing all nursing care. Encourage family involvement, allowing the mother and family to perform newborn care with direct supervision and support by the nurse.

    - Encourage mothers and family to hold the newborn so that they can experience eye-to-eye contact and interaction.

- • Medications

  - ○ Erythromycin (Romycin)

    - Prophylactic eye care is the mandatory instillation of antibiotic ointment into the newborn's eyes to prevent ophthalmia neonatorum. Infections can be transmitted during descent through the birth canal. Ophthalmia neonatorum is caused by *Neisseria gonorrhoeae* or *Chlamydia trachomatis* and can cause blindness in the newborn.

    - Nursing Considerations and Client Education

      - ☐ Erythromycin is the medication of choice.

      - ☐ Use a single-dose unit to avoid cross-contamination between newborns.

      - ☐ Apply a 1 to 2 cm ribbon of erythromycin ointment to the lower conjunctival sac of each of the newborn's eyes, starting from the inner canthus and moving outward.

      - ☐ A possible adverse reaction is chemical conjunctivitis, which may cause redness, swelling, drainage, and temporarily blurred vision for 24 to 48 hr. This is a normal response to the medication. Reassure the newborn's parents that this will resolve on its own.

      - ☐ Application may be delayed for 1 hr after birth to facilitate parent-newborn bonding and eye contact during the first period of newborn reactivity.

  - ○ Vitamin K (Aquamephyton)

    - This vitamin injection is administered to prevent hemorrhagic disorders. Vitamin K is not produced in the gastrointestinal tract of the newborn until around day 8. Vitamin K is produced in the colon by bacteria that forms once formula or breast milk is introduced into the gut of the newborn.

- Nursing Considerations and Client Education
    - Administer 0.5 to 1 mg intramuscularly into the vastus lateralis (where muscle development is adequate) within 1 hr after birth.
  - Hepatitis B vaccination
    - This vaccine provides protection for the newborn against hepatitis B.
    - Nursing Considerations and Client Education
      - This vaccine is recommended to be given to all newborns.
      - For newborns born to healthy women, recommended dosage schedule is at birth, 1 month, and 6 months.
      - Consent must be obtained prior to administering the vaccination.
      - For women infected with hepatitis B, hepatitis B immuno globulin (HBIG) along with the hepatitis B vaccine is given within 12 hr of birth. The hepatitis B vaccine is given alone at 1, 2, and 12 months.
      - It is important not to give the vitamin K and the hepatitis B injections in the same thigh. Sites should be alternated.
  - Triple Dye
    - Topical antimicrobial may be used for umbilical cord care.
    - Nursing Considerations
      - Care for the cord as prescribed by the primary care provider. This may include applying triple dye to the umbilical stump or cleansing with neutral pH cleanser and sterile water, as recommended by the Association of Women's Health, Obstetrics and Neonatal Nurses. The cord should be kept clean and dry to prevent infection.
- Client Outcomes
  - The newborn adapts to extrauterine life.

Complications

- Cold stress (complication of ineffective thermoregulation) can lead to hypoxia, acidosis, and hypoglycemia. Newborns with respiratory distress are at a higher risk for hypothermia.
  - Nursing Actions
    - Monitor the newborn for signs and symptoms of cold stress (cyanotic trunk, depressed respirations).
    - To prevent cold stress, avoid heat loss by any of the heat loss mechanisms. If cold stress does occur, the newborn should be warmed slowly over a period of 2 to 4 hr. Correct the hypoxia by administering oxygen. Correct the acidosis and hypoglycemia.

- Hypoglycemia frequently occurs in the first few hours of life secondary to the use of energy to establish respirations and maintain body heat. Newborns of mothers who have diabetes mellitus, are small or large for gestational age, are less than 37 weeks of gestation, or greater than 42 weeks of gestation, are at risk for hypoglycemia and should have a blood glucose drawn within the first 2 hr of life. Follow facility protocols regarding frequency of assessing blood glucose levels.

  ○ Nursing Actions

    ▪ Monitor for signs of jitteriness, twitching, a weak, high-pitched cry, irregular respiratory effort, cyanosis, lethargy, eye rolling, seizures, and a blood glucose level less than 40 mg/dL by heel stick.

    ▪ Give newborn formula immediately or have the mother breastfeed to elevate the newborn's blood glucose. Brain damage can result if brain cells are completely depleted of glucose.

- Hemorrhage (complication of improper cord care) can occur if the cord clamp is not tight enough.

  ○ Nursing Actions

    ▪ Monitor the newborn to assure that the clamp is tight and if seepage of blood is noted. Then, a second clamp should be applied.

    ▪ If the cord continues to bleed, notify the primary care provider immediately.

CHAPTER 24: NURSING CARE OF THE NEWBORN

 Application Exercises

1. A nurse is preparing to administer prophylactic eye ointment into the eyes of a newborn to treat ophthalmia neonatorum. Which of the following medications should the nurse anticipate administering?

    A. Ofloxacin (Floxin)

    B. Nystatin (Mycostatin)

    C. Erythromycin (Romycin)

    D. Ceftriaxone (Rocephin)

2. A nurse is caring for a newborn who was born to a mother who is infected with hepatitis B. What treatment should this newborn receive?

3. A newborn was not dried completely after delivery. The nurse understands that which of the following mechanisms causes the newborn to lose heat?

    A. Conduction

    B. Convection

    C. Evaporation

    D. Radiation

4. When performing nursing care for a newborn after birth, which of the following nursing interventions is the highest priority?

    A. Initiating breastfeeding

    B. Performing the initial bath

    C. Giving a vitamin K injection

    D. Covering the newborn's head with a cap

5. A nurse is preparing to administer a vitamin K (Aquamephyton) injection to a newborn. Which of the following is an appropriate response by the nurse to the newborn's mother regarding why this medication is given?

    A. "Vitamin K assists with blood clotting."

    B. "Vitamin K assists the bowel in maturing."

    C. "Vitamin K is a preventative vaccination."

    D. "Vitamin K provides immunity."

6. Which of the following actions should a nurse take when bringing a newborn to a mother for breastfeeding for security purposes?

    A. Ask the mother to state her full name.

    B. Look at the name on the newborn's bassinet.

    C. Match the mother's identification band with the newborn's.

    D. Compare names on the bassinet and room number.

CHAPTER 24: NURSING CARE OF THE NEWBORN

 Application Exercises Answer Key

1. A nurse is preparing to administer prophylactic eye ointment into the eyes of a newborn to treat ophthalmia neonatorum. Which of the following medications should the nurse anticipate administering?

    A. Ofloxacin (Floxin)

    B. Nystatin (Mycostatin)

    C. Erythromycin (Romycin)

    D. Ceftriaxone (Rocephin)

    The medication of choice for ophthalmia neonatorum is erythromycin ophthalmic ointment 0.5%. This antibiotic provides prophylaxis against *Neisseria gonorrhoeae* and *Chlamydia trachomatis*. Ofloxacin is an antibiotic also, but is not used for ophthalmia neonatorum. Nystatin is used for *Candida albicans* in oral yeast infections. Ceftriaxone is an antibiotic, but it is not used for ophthalmia neonatorum.

    NCLEX® Connection: Health Promotion and Maintenance, Ante/Intra/Postpartum and Newborn Care

2. A nurse is caring for a newborn who was born to a mother who is infected with hepatitis B. What treatment should this newborn receive?

    If a newborn is born to a mother who is infected with hepatitis B, the newborn should receive the hepatitis B and the hepatitis B immuno globulin (HBIG) vaccines. Both should be administered within 12 hr of birth. The hepatitis B vaccine induces protective antibodies in newborns who receive the recommended three doses. HBIG provides a high titer of antibody to hepatitis B surface antigen. The vaccine provides prophylaxis against infection of newborns born to mothers who carry or are infected with hepatitis B.

    NCLEX® Connection: Health Promotion and Maintenance, Ante/Intra/Postpartum and Newborn Care

3. A newborn was not dried completely after delivery. The nurse understands that which of the following mechanisms causes the newborn to lose heat?

    A. Conduction

    B. Convection

    C. Evaporation

    D. Radiation

Evaporation is the loss of heat that occurs when a liquid is converted to a vapor. In a newborn, heat loss by evaporation occurs as a result of vaporization of the moisture from the skin. Conduction is the loss of heat from the body surface area to cooler surfaces that the newborn may be in contact with. Convection is the flow of heat from the body surface area to cooler air. Radiation is the loss of heat to a cooler surface that is not in direct contact with the newborn.

NCLEX® Connection: Health Promotion and Maintenance, Ante/Intra/Postpartum and Newborn Care

4. When performing nursing care for a newborn after birth, which of the following nursing interventions is the highest priority?

    A. Initiating breastfeeding

    B. Performing the initial bath

    C. Giving a vitamin K injection

    D. Covering the newborn's head with a cap

The greatest risk to the newborn is cold stress. Therefore the highest priority intervention is to prevent heat loss. Covering a newborn's head with a cap prevents cold stress due to excessive evaporative heat loss. Initiating breastfeeding is important following birth, but it is not the priority. Initial baths aren't given until the newborn's temperature is stable. Vitamin K can be given immediately after birth, but it is not as high of a priority as the immediate stabilization of body temperature.

NCLEX® Connection: Health Promotion and Maintenance, Ante/Intra/Postpartum and Newborn Care

5. A nurse is preparing to administer a vitamin K (Aquamephyton) injection to a newborn. Which of the following is an appropriate response by the nurse to the newborn's mother regarding why this medication is given?

    A. "Vitamin K assists with blood clotting."

    B. "Vitamin K assists the bowel in maturing."

    C. "Vitamin K is a preventative vaccination."

    D. "Vitamin K provides immunity."

Vitamin K is deficient in a newborn because the colon is sterile. For vitamin K to be produced, there must be bacteria available. Once a newborn receives the first feeding, the bacteria will be produced. Until that point, a newborn is at risk of hemorrhagic disease. Vitamin K is required to activate clotting factors II, VII, IX, and X. Vitamin K does not assist the bowel to mature. Vitamin K is not part of the vaccinations that are administered. Vitamin K does not provide immunity.

Ⓝ **NCLEX® Connection: Health Promotion and Maintenance, Ante/Intra/Postpartum and Newborn Care**

6. Which of the following actions should a nurse take when bringing a newborn to a mother for breastfeeding for security purposes?

    A. Ask the mother to state her full name.

    B. Look at the name on the newborn's bassinet.

    C. Match the mother's identification band with the newborn's.

    D. Compare names on the bassinet and room number.

The mother, newborn, and significant other are identified by plastic identification wristbands with permanent locks that must be cut to be removed. Identification bands should include the newborn's name, sex, date, and time of birth. Each time a newborn is taken to the parents, the identification band should be verified against the mother's identification band.

Ⓝ **NCLEX® Connection: Safety and Infection Control, Security Plan**

UNIT 4	NEWBORN NURSING CARE
Section	Low-Risk Newborn

Chapter 25	Newborn Nutrition

 Overview

- Acquiring an understanding of the nutritional needs of newborns (breastfeeding, bottle feeding) is essential. The factors, complications, and interventions will be explored in this chapter.

Nutritional Needs for the Newborn

- Desirable growth and development in the newborn is enhanced by good nutrition. Feeding the newborn provides an opportunity for parents to meet the newborn's nutritional needs as well as an opportunity for them to bond with the newborn. Whether the mother chooses to breast or bottle feed, nurses should provide education and support.

- Normal newborn weight loss immediately after birth and weight gain with growth and development should be as follows:

NEWBORN WEIGHT LOSS/GAIN
• Loss of 5 to 10% immediately after birth (regain 10 to 14 days after birth)
• Gain of 110 to 200 g/week for first 3 months

- Healthy newborns need a fluid intake of 100 to 140 mL/kg/24 hr. Newborns do not need to be given water supplemented because they receive enough water from either breast milk or formula.

- Adequate caloric intake is essential to provide energy for growth, digestion, metabolic needs, and activity. For the first 3 months, the newborn requires 110 kcal/kg/day. From 3 to 6 months, the requirement decreases to 100 kcal/kg/day. Both breast milk and formula provide 20 kcal/oz.

- Carbohydrates should make up 40 to 50% of the newborn's total caloric intake. The most abundant carbohydrate in breast milk or formula is lactose.

- At least 15% of calories must come from fat (triglycerides). The fat in breast milk is easier to digest than the fat in cow's milk.

- For adequate growth and development to take place, a newborn must receive 2.25 to 4 g/kg of protein per day.

- All vitamins are contained in breast milk, but must be added to formulas. Vitamin D may be deficient in breast milk, so supplementation may be necessary. Supplementation is recommended for newborns who are breastfed and whose mothers are vegetarians and exclude meat, fish, and dairy products.

- The mineral content of commercial newborn formula and breast milk is adequate with the exception of iron and fluoride.

  o Iron is low in all forms of milk, but it is absorbed better from breast milk. Newborns who only breastfed for the first 6 months maintain adequate Hgb levels and do not need any additional iron supplementation. After 6 months of age, all newborns need to be fed iron-fortified cereal and other foods rich in iron. Newborns who are formula fed should receive iron-fortified newborn formula until 12 months of age. Mothers who breastfeed their newborns are encouraged to do so for the newborn's first 12 months of life.

  o Fluoride levels in breast milk and formulas are low. A fluoride supplement should be given to newborns not receiving fluoridated water after 6 months of age.

- Solids are not introduced until 6 months of age. If introduced too early, food allergies may develop.

Breastfeeding

- Breastfeeding is the optimal source of nutrition for newborns. Breastfeeding is recommended exclusively for the first 6 months of age by the American Academy of Pediatrics. Newborns should be breastfed every 2 to 3 hr. Parents should awaken the newborn to feed at least every 3 hr during the day and at least every 4 hr during the night until the newborn is feeding well and gaining weight adequately. Breastfeeding should occur 8 to 12 times within a 24-hr window. Then, a feed-on-demand schedule may be followed.

- Colostrum is secreted from the mother's breasts during postpartum days 1 to 3. It contains the IgA immunoglobulin that provides passive immunity to the newborn.

- Nursing interventions can help a new mother be successful in breastfeeding.

- Advantages of breastfeeding – Parents should be presented with factual information about the nutritional and immunological needs of their newborn. The nurse should present information about both breastfeeding and bottle feeding in a nonjudgmental manner. The optimal time to provide newborn nutritional information is during pregnancy, so the parents will have made a decision prior to hospital admission.

  o Benefits of breastfeeding

    ▪ Reduces the risk of infection by providing IgA antibodies, lysozymes, leukocytes, macrophages, and lactoferrin that prevents infections.

    ▪ Promotes rapid brain growth due to large amounts of lactose.

    ▪ Provides protein and nitrogen for neurological cell building.

    ▪ Contains electrolytes and minerals.

- Breastmilk is easy for the newborn to digest.

- Breastfeeding is convenient and inexpensive.

- It improves the newborn's ability to regulate calcium and phosphorus levels.

- Sucking associated with breastfeeding reduces dental problems.

- Colostrum provides IgA antibodies.

- Nursing Interventions to Promote Successful Breastfeeding

  - Explain breastfeeding techniques to the mother. Have the mother wash her hands, get comfortable, and have fluids to drink during breastfeeding.

  - Offer the newborn the breast immediately after birth and frequently thereafter.

  - Explain the let-down reflex (stimulation of maternal nipple releases oxytocin that causes the letdown of milk).

  - Reassure the mother that uterine cramps are normal during breastfeeding, resulting from oxytocin.

  - Express a few drops of colostrum or milk and spread it over the nipple to lubricate the nipple and entice the newborn.

  - Show the mother the proper latch-on position. Have her support the breast in one hand with the thumb on top and four fingers underneath. With the newborn's mouth in front of the nipple, the newborn can be stimulated to open his mouth by tickling his lower lip with the tip of the nipple. The mother pulls the newborn to the nipple with his mouth covering part of the areola as well as the nipple.

 View Media Supplement: Breastfeeding Techniques (Images)

  - Explain to the mother that when her newborn is latched on correctly, his nose, cheeks, and chin will all be touching her breast.

  - Demonstrate the four basic breastfeeding positions: football, cradle or modified cradle, across the lap, and side-lying.

  - Encourage the mother to breastfeed at least 15 to 20 min/breast to ensure that her newborn receives adequate fat and protein in rich hind milk.

  - Avoid educating mothers regarding the duration of newborn feedings. Clients should be instructed to evaluate when the newborn has completed the feeding, including slowing of newborn suckling, a softened breast, or sleeping.

  - Explain to the mother that newborns will nurse on demand.

  - Show the mother how to insert a finger in the side of the newborn's mouth to break the suction from the nipple prior to removing the newborn from the breast to prevent nipple trauma.

  - Show the mother how to burp the newborn when she alternates breasts. The newborn should be burped either over the shoulder or in an upright position with his chin supported. The mother should gently pat the newborn on his back to elicit a burp.

- o Tell the mother to begin the newborn's next feeding with the breast she stopped feeding him with in the previous feeding.

- o Tell the mother how to tell if her newborn is receiving adequate feeding (gaining weight, voiding 6 to 8 diapers a day, and contentedness between feedings).

- o Explain to the mother that the newborn may have loose, pale, and/or yellow stools during breastfeeding, and that this is normal.

- o Tell the mother how to avoid nipple confusion in the newborn by not offering supplemental formula feeding or pacifier. Supplementation can be provided using a small feeding or syringe feeding, if needed.

- o Tell the mother to always place her newborn on his back after feedings.

- Nursing Interventions to Promote Successful Storage of Breast Milk Obtained by a Breast Pump

  - o Inform the mother that breast milk can still be provided to the newborn during periods of separation by using a breast pump.

    - Breast pumps can be manual, electric, or battery-operated and pumped directly into a bottle or freezer bag.

    - One or both breasts can be pumped, and suction is adjustable for comfort.

  - o Teach the parents that breast milk must be stored according to guidelines for proper containers, labeling, refrigerating, and freezing.

    - Breast milk may be stored at room temperature for 4 to 6 hr. It may be refrigerated in sterile bottles for use within 8 days, or may be frozen in sterile containers for 3 to 6 months. Breast milk may be stored in a deep freezer for 6 to 12 months.

    - Thawing the milk in the refrigerator for 24 hr is the best way to preserve the immunoglobulins present in it. It can also be thawed by holding the container under running lukewarm water or placing it in a container of lukewarm water. The bottle should be rotated often, but not shaken when thawing in this manner.

    - Thawing by microwave is contraindicated, because it destroys some of the immune factors and lysozymes contained in the milk. Microwave thawing also leads to the development of uneven hot spots in the milk because of uneven heating, which can burn the newborn.

    - Do not refreeze thawed milk.

    - Used portions of breast milk must be discarded.

    - Avoid consuming alcohol and limit caffeine.

    - Do not take medications unless prescribed by a provider.

Bottle feeding

- Formula feeding can be a successful and adequate source of nutrition if the mother chooses not to breastfeed. The newborn should be fed every 3 to 4 hr. Parents should awaken the newborn to feed at least every 3 hr during the day and at least every 4 hr during the night until the newborn is feeding well and gaining weight adequately. Then, a feed-on-demand schedule may be followed.

- Nursing Interventions to Promote Successful Bottle Feeding

    o Teach the parents how to prepare formula, bottles, and nipples.

    o Teach the parents about the different forms of formula (ready-to-feed, concentrated, and powder) and how to prepare each correctly.

    o Bottles can be put in the dishwasher or washed by hand in hot soapy water using a good bottle and nipple brush.

    o Teach parents to wipe the lid clean on the concentrated can before opening it.

    o Instruct parents to use tap water to mix concentrated or powder formula. If the water source is questionable, tap water should be boiled first.

    o Instruct parents that prepared formula can be refrigerated for up to 48 hr.

    o Teach the parents to check the flow of formula from the bottle to assure it is not coming out too slow or too fast.

    o Show the parents how to cradle the newborn in their arms in a semi-upright position. The newborn should not be placed in the supine position during bottle feeding because of the danger of aspiration. Newborns who bottle feed do best when held close and at a 45° angle.

    o Instruct the mother how to place the nipple on top of the newborn's tongue.

    o Keep the nipple filled with formula to prevent the newborn from swallowing air.

    o Always hold the bottle and never prop it.

    o Newborns should be burped several times during a feeding, usually after each ½ to 1 oz of formula or breastmilk.

    o Place the newborn in a supine position after feedings.

    o Tell the parents to discard any unused formula remaining in the bottle when the newborn is finished feeding due to the possibility of bacterial contamination.

    o Teach the parents how to tell if their newborn is being adequately fed (gaining weight, voiding 6 to 8 diapers per day, and satisfaction between feedings).

Risk Factors for Impaired Newborn Nutrition

- Risk factors for failure to thrive (newborn) can be related to ineffective feeding patterns of the newborn or inadequate breastfeeding by the mother.

- Newborn factor
  - Inadequate breastfeeding
  - Illness
  - Infection
  - Malabsorption
  - Other circumstances that increase newborn's energy needs
- Maternal factor
  - Inadequate emptying of the breast
  - Inappropriate timing of feeding
  - Inadequate breast tissue
  - Pain with feeding
  - Maternal hemorrhage
  - Illness
  - Infections

Monitoring Newborn for Adequate Growth

- Monitor the newborn for adequate growth and weight gain.

  - Weights are done daily in the newborn nursery and then usually at 2 days of age after discharge for newborns who are breastfed and 6 weeks of age for newborns who are formula fed. Growth is followed by placing the newborn's weight on a growth chart. Adequate growth should be within the 10th to 90th percentile. Poor weight gain would be below 10% and too much weight gain would be above 90%.

  - The newborn's length and head circumference are also monitored closely.

- Assessment of newborn nutrition begins during pregnancy and continues after birth by assessing the parents' attitudes and choices about their newborn's feeding. Breastfeeding is the preferred method. However, if the mother chooses not to breastfeed, she must not be made to feel guilty.

  - Newborn
    - Maturity level
    - History of labor and delivery
    - Birth trauma
    - Maternal risk factors
    - Congenital defects
    - Physical stability
    - State of alertness
    - Presence of bowel sounds

- o Mother
  - Previous experience with breastfeeding
  - Knowledge about breastfeeding
  - Cultural factors
  - Feelings about breastfeeding
  - Physical features of breasts
  - Physical/psychological readiness
  - Support of family and significant others
- Assess the mother's ability to feed her newborn, whether by breast or bottle.
- Calculate the newborn's 24-hr I&O, if indicated, to assure adequate nutrition.

Intervening for Newborn Nutrition

- Provide the client with education about feeding-readiness cues exhibited by newborns and encourage the mother to begin feeding her newborn upon cues rather than waiting until the newborn is crying. Cues include:
  - o Hand-to-mouth or hand-to-hand movements.
  - o Sucking motions.
  - o Rooting.
  - o Mouthing.

Complications for Newborn Nutrition

- There may be special considerations when a newborn has difficulty receiving adequate nutrition. Nursing interventions can often help these newborns receive adequate nutrition.
  - o Newborns who are sleepy
    - Unwrap the newborn.
    - Change the newborn's diaper.
    - Hold the newborn upright and turn him from side to side.
    - Talk to the newborn.
    - Massage the newborn's back, and rub his hands and feet.
    - Apply a cool cloth to the newborn's face.
  - o Newborns who are fussy
    - Swaddle the newborn.
    - Hold the newborn close, move, and rock him gently.
    - Reduce the newborn's environmental stimuli.
    - Place the newborn skin to skin.

- Failure to thrive is slow weight gain. A newborn usually falls below the 5th percentile on the growth chart.

  o Newborns who are breastfeeding

    ▪ Evaluate positioning and latch-on during breastfeeding.

    ▪ Massage the breast during feeding.

    ▪ Determine feeding patterns and length of feedings.

    ▪ If the newborn is spitting up, the newborn may have an allergy to dairy products. Determine the maternal intake of dairy products. The mother may need to eliminate dairy from her diet. Instruct her to consume other food sources high in calcium or calcium supplements.

  o Newborns who are formula feeding

    ▪ Evaluate how much and how often the newborn is feeding.

    ▪ If the newborn is spitting up or vomiting he may have an allergy or intolerance to cow-milk based formula and may require a switch to a soy-based formula.

CHAPTER 25: NEWBORN NUTRITION

Ⓐ Application Exercises

Scenario: A newborn weighs 3.2 kg (7 lb) at birth. The mother plans to breastfeed.

1. Why is it important that the newborn breastfeed and receive colostrum?

2. The mother asks the nurse, "How can I tell if my baby is receiving enough to eat?" What should the nurse tell the mother?

3. How often should the newborn be burped during breastfeeding?

4. A nurse is giving instructions to a mother about how to breastfeed her newborn. Which of the following actions by the mother indicates the need for additional teaching?

   A. The mother expresses a few drops of colostrum and places it on her nipple.

   B. The mother inserts a finger in the side of the newborn's mouth before removing the nipple from the newborn's mouth.

   C. The mother gently strokes the newborn's lips with her nipple when she is ready to breastfeed.

   D. The mother places a breast shield over her nipple before placing the nipple in the newborn's mouth.

5. A nurse is teaching a group of new parents about proper techniques for bottle feeding. Which of the following instructions should the nurse provide?

   A. Burp the newborn at the end of the feeding.

   B. Hold the newborn close in a supine position.

   C. Keep the nipple full of formula throughout the feeding.

   D. Refrigerate any unused formula.

6. Four hours after admission to the nursery a newborn is taken to his mother for his first feeding. The mother wants to bottle feed. The nurse reviews basic principles of bottle feeding with the mother. Which of the following observations by the nurse indicates that the mother needs additional teaching?

   A. The mother burps the newborn after each $1/_2$ oz of formula he consumes.

   B. The mother discards unused formula after feeding.

   C. The mother places the nipple on the tongue of the newborn.

   D. The mother places the newborn in a supine position during feeding.

7. A mother asks why it is important to keep the nipple full of formula when bottle feeding. The nurse explains that the nipple is always full of formula to

    A. prevent damaging the newborn's gums.

    B. keep the newborn from getting too tired.

    C. keep the newborn from regurgitating the formula.

    D. prevent the newborn from swallowing air when sucking.

8. What percentage of a newborn's birth weight is expected to be lost during the first 24 hr?

CHAPTER 25: NEWBORN NUTRITION

 Application Exercises Answer Key

Scenario: A newborn weighs 3.2 kg (7 lb) at birth. The mother plans to breastfeed.

1. Why is it important that the newborn breastfeed and receive colostrum?

Colostrum is secreted during days 1 to 3 and contains the IgA immunoglobulin that provides passive immunity to the newborn.

 NCLEX® Connection: Health Promotion and Maintenance, Ante/Intra/Postpartum and Newborn Care

2. The mother asks the nurse, "How can I tell if my baby is receiving enough to eat?" What should the nurse tell the mother?

A newborn is receiving adequate nutrition if he is content between feedings, gains weight, and has 6 to 8 wet diapers/day.

 NCLEX® Connection: Health Promotion and Maintenance, Ante/Intra/Postpartum and Newborn Care

3. How often should the newborn be burped during breastfeeding?

A newborn should be burped when alternating breasts.

 NCLEX® Connection: Health Promotion and Maintenance, Ante/Intra/Postpartum and Newborn Care

4. A nurse is giving instructions to a mother about how to breastfeed her newborn. Which of the following actions by the mother indicates the need for additional teaching?

A. The mother expresses a few drops of colostrum and places it on her nipple.

B. The mother inserts a finger in the side of the newborn's mouth before removing the nipple from the newborn's mouth.

C. The mother gently strokes the newborn's lips with her nipple when she is ready to breastfeed.

D. The mother places a breast shield over her nipple before placing the nipple in the newborn's mouth.

A breast shield is not routinely used for breastfeeding. A breast shield is worn when the nipples are flat or inverted, or occasionally when they are sore and cracked. All the other techniques are appropriate for breastfeeding.

 NCLEX® Connection: Health Promotion and Maintenance, Ante/Intra/Postpartum and Newborn Care

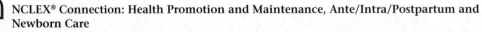

5. A nurse is teaching a group of new parents about proper techniques for bottle feeding. Which of the following instructions should the nurse provide?

    A. Burp the newborn at the end of the feeding.

    B. Hold the newborn close in a supine position.

    C. Keep the nipple full of formula throughout the feeding.

    D. Refrigerate any unused formula.

The nipple should always be kept full of formula to prevent the newborn from sucking in air during the feeding. The newborn should be burped after each ½ oz, and he should be cradled in a semi-upright position. Any unused formula should be discarded due to the possibility of bacterial contamination.

 NCLEX® Connection: Health Promotion and Maintenance, Ante/Intra/Postpartum and Newborn Care

6. Four hours after admission to the nursery a newborn is taken to his mother for his first feeding. The mother wants to bottle feed. The nurse reviews basic principles of bottle feeding with the mother. Which of the following observations by the nurse indicates that the mother needs additional teaching?

    A. The mother burps the newborn after each $1/2$ oz of formula he consumes.

    B. The mother discards unused formula after feeding.

    C. The mother places the nipple on the tongue of the newborn.

    D. The mother places the newborn in a supine position during feeding.

The newborn should not be placed in the supine position because of the danger of aspiration. Newborns who are bottle feeding do best when they are held close and at a 45° angle. All other techniques are correct for bottle feeding the newborn.

 NCLEX® Connection: Health Promotion and Maintenance, Ante/Intra/Postpartum and Newborn Care

7. A mother asks why it is important to keep the nipple full of formula when bottle feeding. The nurse explains that the nipple is always full of formula to

    A. prevent damaging the newborn's gums.

    B. keep the newborn from getting too tired.

    C. keep the newborn from regurgitating the formula.

    D. prevent the newborn from swallowing air when sucking.

Positioning the bottle so the nipple remains full of formula throughout the feeding prevents the newborn from swallowing air. Keeping the nipple full of formula does not prevent damage to the newborn's gums nor will it prevent regurgitation. There is no indication that this technique prevents fatigue in the newborn either.

 NCLEX® Connection: Health Promotion and Maintenance, Ante/Intra/Postpartum and Newborn Care

8. What percentage of a newborn's birth weight is expected to be lost during the first 24 hr?

5 to 10%

The normal weight loss after birth is 5 to 10%. All newborns should lose some weight after birth due to fluid loss.

Ⓝ NCLEX® Connection: Health Promotion and Maintenance, Ante/Intra/Postpartum and Newborn Care

UNIT 4	NEWBORN NURSING CARE
Section	Low-Risk Newborn

Chapter 26 Nursing Care and Discharge Teaching

ⓐ Overview

- Discharge teaching and newborn care including bathing, umbilical cord care, circumcision, car seat safety, environmental safety, newborn behaviors, feeding, elimination and signs of illness to report to the primary care provider will be discussed in this chapter.

- Prior to discharge, a nurse should provide anticipatory guidance to prepare new parents to care for their newborn at home. Mothers and newborns are normally discharged once the newborn is 6 to 48 hr old. Serious complications can result if improper discharge instructions are not given to the parents prior to taking the newborn home.

- A nurse should inquire about the family's current experience and knowledge regarding newborn care, anticipate the learning needs of the parent's, and assess their readiness for learning to provide education about newborn care.

- Parents should be made aware of some general guidelines about newborn behavior and care. These guidelines include causes of crying in the newborn, quieting techniques, sleeping patterns, hunger cues, and feeding, bathing, and clothing the newborn.

- Parents need to be aware of the importance of well-newborn checkups, immunization schedules, and when to call the primary care provider for signs of illness.

- Providing a safe protective environment at home should be stressed to new parents and should include instruction about proper car seat usage, which is a very important part of the discharge instruction process.

- Assessment of the family's readiness to care for the newborn at home

  - Previous newborn experience and knowledge

  - Parent-newborn attachment

  - Adjustment to the parental role

  - Social support

  - Educational needs

  - Sibling rivalry issues

  - Readiness of the parents to have their home and lifestyle altered to accommodate their newborn

  - Parents' ability to verbalize and demonstrate newborn care following teaching

Interventions for Home Care of the Newborn

- Through verbal discussion, pamphlets, and demonstration, the nurse should provide education to the client and family regarding newborn behavior, quieting techniques, newborn care, signs of newborn well-being and illness, and issues of newborn safety.

- Crying

  ○ Inform the parents that newborns cry when they are hungry, need to be burped, are overstimulated, wet, cold, hot, tired, or bored. Assure the mother that in time, she will learn what her newborn's cry means. The mother should be instructed not to feed her newborn every time he cries. Overfeeding can lead to stomach aches and diarrhea. It is okay to let a newborn cry for short periods of time.

- Quieting Techniques

  ○ Swaddling

  ○ Close skin contact

  ○ Nonnutritive sucking

  ○ Rhythmic noises to simulate utero sounds

  ○ Movement (a car ride, vibrating chair, infant swing, rocking newborn)

  ○ Placing the newborn on his stomach across a holder's lap while bouncing legs

  ○ En face

  ○ Stimulation

- Sleep-Wake Cycle

  ○ Reinforce to the parents that placing the newborn in the supine position for sleeping greatly decreases the risk of sudden infant death syndrome.

  ○ Most newborns sleep 16 out of every 24 hr the first week at home and sleep 2 to 3 hr at a time.

  ○ Many parents believe that adding solid food to the newborn's diet will help with sleep patterns. The parents should be instructed not to add cereal to the newborn's formula or feed the newborn solid foods until 4 to 6 months of age. During the first 6 months of life, the American Academy of Pediatrics recommends only breastfeeding. Most newborns will sleep through the night without a feeding by 4 to 5 months of age. The primary care provider will instruct the parents when to add solid food to the newborn's diet.

  ○ Keep the newborn's environment quiet and dark at night.

  ○ The newborn should never sleep in the parents' bed (suffocation).

  ○ Most newborns get their days and nights mixed up. Provide basic suggestions for helping the parents develop a predictable routine. Bring the newborn out into the center of the action in the afternoon, and keep him there for the rest of the evening. Bathe him right before bedtime so that he feels soothed. Give him his last feeding around 11 p.m. and then place him into a crib or bassinet.

    ○   For nighttime feedings and diaper changes, keep a small night light on to avoid having to turn on bright lights. Speak softly and handle the newborn gently so that he goes back to sleep easily.

- Oral and Nasal Suctioning

  ○ Teach the parents to use a bulb syringe to suction any excess mucus from the newborn's nose and mouth.

  ○ Parents should suction the newborn's mouth first and then the nose, one nostril at a time.

  ○ The bulb should be compressed before inserting it into the newborn's mouth or nose.

  ○ When suctioning the newborn's mouth, always insert the bulb on the sides of his mouth, not in the middle, and do not touch the back of the throat to avoid eliciting the newborn's gag reflex.

- Positioning and Holding of Newborn (Support Head)

  ○ Teach the parents that the newborn has minimal head control. His head must be supported whenever he is lifted, especially since his head is larger than the rest of his body.

  ○ Four basic ways to hold the newborn:

    ■ Cradle hold – cradle the newborn's head in the bend of the elbow. This permits eye-to-eye contact (good for feeding).

    ■ Upright position – hold the newborn upright and face him toward the holder while supporting his head, upper back, and buttocks (good for burping).

    ■ Football hold – support half of the newborn's body in the holder's forearm with the newborn's head and neck resting in the palm of the hand (good for shampooing and breastfeeding).

    ■ Colic hold – place the newborn facedown along the holder's forearm with the hand firmly between the newborn's legs. The newborn's cheek should be by the holder's elbow on the outside. The newborn should be able to see the ground, and the holder's arm should be close to their body, using it to brace and steady the newborn (good for quieting a newborn who is fussy).

- Bathing

  ○ After the initial bath, the newborn's face, diaper area, and skin folds are cleansed daily. Complete bathing is performed 2 to 3 times a week.

  ○ Bathing by immersion is not done until the newborn's umbilical cord has fallen off and the circumcision has healed on males. Wash the area around the cord, taking care not to get the cord wet. Move from the cleanest to dirtiest part of the newborn's body, beginning with his eyes, face, and head; and proceed to the chest, arms, and legs; and wash the groin area last.

  ○ Provide parent teaching about bathing of the newborn (bathing should go from clean to dirty areas).

- o Teach the parents proper newborn bathing techniques by a demonstration. Have the parents return the demonstration. The newborn's face and perineal area should be cleansed daily. Completely bathe the newborn 2 to 3 times a week using mild soap.

- o Bathing should take place before a feeding to prevent spitting up or vomiting.

- o Organize all equipment so that the newborn is not left unattended in the water (safety). Never leave the newborn alone in the tub or sink.

- o Make sure the hot water heater is set at 49° C (120.2° F) or less. The room should be warm and bath water should be 36.6° to 37.2° C (98° to 99° F). Test the water for comfort on inner wrist prior to bathing the newborn.

- o Avoid drafts or chilling of the newborn. Expose only the body part being bathed (convection) and dry the newborn thoroughly (evaporation).

- o The newborn's eyes should be cleaned using a clean portion of the wash cloth. Clear water should be used to clean each eye, moving from the inner to the outer canthus.

- o Each area of the newborn's body should be washed, rinsed, and dried, with no soap left on the skin.

- o Soap used should be mild and not contain hexachlorophene.

- o Wrap the newborn in a towel and swaddle him in a football hold to shampoo his head.

- o Rinse shampoo from the newborn's head and dry to avoid chilling.

- o In male newborns, to cleanse an uncircumcised penis, wash with soap and water and rinse the penis. The foreskin should not be forced back or constriction may result.

- o In female newborns, wash the vulva by wiping from front to back to prevent contamination of the vagina or urethra from rectal bacteria.

- o Do not use lotions, oils, or powders, because they can alter a newborn's skin and provide a medium for bacterial growth or cause an allergic reaction.

- o Inform the parents that powder should be avoided because it can cause respiratory problems if inhaled by the newborn.

- Feeding/Elimination

  - o The newborn is offered the breast immediately after birth and frequently thereafter. Feedings should be 8 to 12 times in a 24-hour period. Feeding for a newborn who is breastfeeding should be on demand or every 2 to 3 hr. Newborns who are formula fed should also be fed on demand or every 3 to 4 hr. Newborns who are breastfed will average 15 to 20 min per breast and 30 to 40 min for the total feeding.

  - o The newborn should nurse up to 15 to 20 min per breast. However, educating clients regarding duration of feedings should be avoided. Clients should be instructed to evaluate when the newborn has completed the feeding, which may be indicated by slowing of the newborn's suckling, softened breast, or the newborn falls asleep. Do not offer the newborn any other fluids unless medically indicated.

  - o The mother's milk supply is equal to the demand of the newborn.

- o Eventually, the newborn will empty a breast within 5 to 10 min, but may need to continue to suck to meet comfort needs.

- o Frequent feedings (every 2 hr may be indicated) and manual expression of milk to initiate flow may be needed.

- o Burping between breasts prevents gas build-up in the newborn and decreases the risk of the newborn vomiting.

- o Newborns who are formula fed should be burped every 15 to 30 mL.

- o Most newborns spit up a little after feedings. Keep the newborn upright and quiet for a few minutes after feedings.

- o Newborns should have 6 to 8 wet diapers a day with adequate feedings and may have 3 to 4 stools per day.

- o Newborns should sleep on their back.

- Cord Care

  - o Before discharge, the cord clamp is removed.

  - o Cord infection (complication of improper cord care) can result if the cord is not kept clean and dry.

    - ■ Monitor for symptoms of a cord that is moist and red, has a foul odor, or has purulent drainage.

  - o Notify the primary care provider immediately if signs and symptoms of cord infection are present.

    - ■ Keep the cord dry and keep the top of the diaper folded underneath it.

    - ■ Avoid submerging the newborn in water until the cord falls off around 10 to 14 days after birth.

    - ■ Sponge baths should only be given until the cord falls off.

    - ■ Any foul smelling, purulent drainage, or redness at the cord site should be reported to the primary care provider.

- Circumcision Care

  - o Circumcision is the surgical removal of the foreskin of the penis.

    - ■ Circumcision is a personal choice made by the newborn's family for reasons of hygiene, religious conviction (Jewish male on eighth day after birth, tradition, culture, social norms). Parents should make a well-informed decision.

    - ■ Contraindications for circumcision include newborns born with the congenital anomalies of hypospadias (abnormal positioning of urethra on ventral undersurface of the penis) and epispadias (urethral canal terminates on dorsum of penis) because the prepuce skin may be needed when the plastic surgeon repairs the defect. Familiar history of bleeding disorders is also a contraindication.

- Circumcision should not be done immediately following birth because the newborn's level of vitamin K, which prevents hemorrhage, is at a low point and the newborn would be at risk for bleeding.

- Another major reason circumcision is not done immediately after birth is because of the danger of cold stress.

- The American Academy of Pediatrics does not recommend routine circumcision.

- Advocates of circumcision state that circumcision promotes a penis with clean glans, minimizes the risk of phimosis later in life, and reduces the risk of penile cancer and cervical cancer in sexual partners.

○ Diagnostic and therapeutic procedures and management

- Anesthesia is now mandatory for all circumcisions. Types of anesthesia include a ring block, dorsal-penile nerve block, and topical anesthetic (eutectic mixture of local anesthetics). Oral sucrose, oral acetaminophen and nonpharmacologic methods, such as swaddling and nonnutritive sucking, may be employed prior to the procedure.

- There are several surgical methods for removing the foreskin including the Yellen, Mogen, and Gomco clamps, and Plastibell.

  □ The primary care provider applies the Yellen, Mogen, or Gomco clamp to the penis, loosens the foreskin, and inserts the cone under the foreskin to provide a cutting surface for removal of the foreskin and to protect the penis.

  □ The wound is covered with sterile petroleum gauze to prevent infection and control bleeding.

○ Plastibell procedure

- The primary care provider slides the Plastibell device between the foreskin and the glans of the penis.

- The provider ties a suture tightly around the foreskin at the coronal edge of the glans. This applies pressure, as the excess foreskin is removed from the penis.

- After 5 to 7 days, the Plastibell drops off, leaving a clean, well-healed excision.

- No petroleum is used for circumcision with the Plastibell.

○ Nursing assessments

- Preprocedure – The newborn should be assessed for:

  □ A history of bleeding tendencies in the family (hemophilia and clotting disorders).

  □ Hypospadias or epispadias.

  □ Ambiguous genitalia (when the newborn has genitalia that may include both male and female characteristics).

  □ An illness or an infection.

- Postprocedure – The newborn should be assessed for:
    - Bleeding every 15 min for the first hour and then every hour for at least 12 hr.
    - The first voiding.
  - Nursing interventions
    - Preprocedure – parent teaching
      - A signed consent form should be on the newborn's chart prior to the procedure.
      - Explain to the parents that the newborn will not be able to be bottle feed for up to 4 hr prior to the procedure to prevent vomiting and aspiration based on the preferences of the primary care provider. Newborns who are breastfed may nurse up until the procedure.
      - Explain the procedure to the parents and assure them that an anesthetic will be administered to minimize pain.
      - Explain that the newborn will need to be restrained on a special board during the procedure.
    - Gather and prepare supplies.
    - Assist with procedure by:
      - Placing the newborn on the restraining board and restraining the newborn's arms and legs. Do not leave the newborn unattended. Have bulb syringe readily available.
      - Assisting the primary care provider as needed and comforting the newborn as needed.
      - Documenting in the nurse's notes – circumcision type, date, and time; parent teaching provided; any excessive bleeding; and time newborn urinates before discharge.
  - Postprocedure care
    - Remove the newborn from the restraining board.
    - Check the newborn for bleeding.
    - Fan fold diapers to prevent pressure on the circumcised area.
  - Postprocedure parent teaching
    - Teach the parents to keep the area clean. Change the newborn's diaper at least every 4 hr and clean the penis with warm water with each diaper change. With clamp procedures, apply petroleum jelly with each diaper change for at least 24 hr after the circumcision to keep the diaper from adhering to the penis. The diaper should be fan folded to prevent pressure on the circumcised area.
    - Avoid wrapping the penis in tight gauze, which can impair circulation to the glans.

- A tub bath should not be given until the circumcision is completely healed. Until then, warm water should be trickled gently over the penis.

- Notify the primary care provider if there is any redness, discharge, swelling, strong odor, tenderness, decrease in urination, or excessive crying from the newborn.

- Tell the parents that a film of yellowish mucus may form over the glans by day 2 and it is important not to wash it off.

- Teach the parents to avoid using premoistened towelettes to clean the penis because they contain alcohol.

- Inform the parents that the newborn may be fussy or may sleep for several hours after the circumcision.

- Inform the parents that the circumcision will heal completely within a couple of weeks.

○ Complications and nursing management

- Hemorrhage

□ Monitor the newborn for bleeding.

□ Provide gentle pressure on the penis using 4 x 4 gauze. Gelfoam powder or a sponge may be applied to stop bleeding. If bleeding persists, notify the primary care provider that a blood vessel may need to be ligated. Have a nurse continue to hold pressure until the primary care provider arrives while another nurse prepares the circumcision tray and suture material.

- Cold stress/hypoglycemia

□ Monitor the newborn for excessive loss of heat resulting in increased respirations and lowered body temperature.

□ Provide a heat source during the procedure (heat lamp or radiant warmer) and swaddle and feed the newborn as soon as the procedure is over.

- Other complications

□ Report any frank bleeding, foul-smelling drainage, or lack of voiding immediately to the primary care provider.

□ Advise the parents to monitor for other complications (infection, urethral fistula, delayed healing and scarring, fibrous bands that will likely not be seen until after discharge if they occur).

□ Provide adequate discharge instructions to the parents about signs and symptoms to observe for and how to report them to the primary care provider.

- Diapering

○ To avoid diaper rash, the newborn's diaper area should be kept clean and dry. Diapers should be changed frequently, and the perineal area cleaned with warm water or wipes and dried thoroughly to prevent skin breakdown.

- Clothing

  - Instruct the parents about how to properly clothe their newborn. The best clothing is soft and made of cotton. Clothes should be washed separately with mild detergent and hot water. Dress lightly for indoors and on hot days. Too many layers of clothing or blankets can make the newborn too hot. On cold days, cover the newborn's head when outdoors. A general rule is to dress the newborn as the parents would dress themselves.

- Swaddling

  - Parents should be shown how to swaddle their newborn. Swaddling the newborn snuggly in a receiving blanket helps the newborn to feel more secure. Swaddling brings the newborn's extremities in closer to his trunk, which is similar to the intrauterine position.

- Safety

  - Never leave the newborn unattended with pets or other small children.

  - Keep small objects (coins) out of the reach of newborns (choking hazard).

  - Never leave the newborn alone on a bed, couch, or table. Newborns move enough to reach the edge and fall off.

  - Never place the newborn on his stomach to sleep during the first few months of life. The back-lying position is the position of choice.

  - Never provide a newborn with a soft surface to sleep on (pillows and waterbed). The newborn's mattress should be firm. Never put pillows, large floppy toys, or loose plastic sheeting in a crib. The newborn can suffocate.

  - Do not tie anything around the newborn's neck.

  - Monitor the safety of the newborn's crib. The space between the mattress and sides of the crib should be less than 2 fingerbreadths.

  - The slats on the crib should be no more than 2.5 inches apart.

  - The newborn's crib or playpen should be away from window blinds and drapery cords. Newborns can become strangled in them.

  - The bassinet or crib should be placed on an inner wall, not next to a window, to prevent cold stress by radiation.

  - If an infant carrier is placed on a high place, such as a table, always be within arm's reach.

  - Smoke detectors should be on every floor of a home and should be checked monthly to assure that they are working. Batteries should be changed yearly. (Change batteries when daylight savings time occurs or on a child's birthday).

  - Eliminate potential fire hazards. Keep a crib and playpen away from heaters, radiators, and heat vents. Linens could catch fire if they come into contact with heat sources.

  - Control the temperature and humidity of the newborn's environment by providing adequate ventilation.

- o   Avoid exposing the newborn to cigarette smoke in a home or elsewhere. Second-hand exposure increases the newborn's risk of developing respiratory illnesses.

- o   Never leave the newborn alone during bath time.

- o   All visitors should wash their hands before touching the newborn.

- o   Any individual with an infection should be kept away from the newborn.

- o   Carefully handle the newborn. Do not throw the newborn up in the air or swing him by his extremities.

- o   Provide community resources to clients who may need additional and ongoing assessment and instruction on newborn care (adolescent parents).

- • Car Seat Safety

  - o   Use an approved rear-facing car seat in the back seat, preferably in the middle, (away from air bags and side impact) to transport the newborn. Newborns should be in rear-facing car seats for the first year of life and until they weigh 9.1 kg (20 lb). It is recommended to have the infant ride rear facing until he has reached the weight limit allowed for the car seat as long as the top of his head is below the top of the seat back. In addition, a five-point harness or T-shield should be part of the convertible restraint. Do not use a used or second-hand car seat.

- • Newborn-Wellness Checkups

  - o   Parents should be advised that their newborn will require well-newborn checkups at 2 to 6 weeks of age, and then every 2 months until 6 months of age. Newborns who are breastfed usually have a weight check around 2 days after discharge.

  - o   The schedule for immunizations should be reviewed with the parents. The nurse should stress the importance of receiving these immunizations on a schedule for the newborn to be protected against diphtheria, tetanus, pertussis, hepatitis B, *Haemophilus influenzae*, polio, measles, mumps, rubella, influenza, rotavirus, pneumococcal, and varicella.

- • Signs of Illness to Report

  - o   Parents should be instructed regarding the signs of illness and to report them immediately.

    - ▪   A fever above 38° C (100.4° F) or a temperature below 36.6° C (97.9° F)

    - ▪   Poor feeding or little interest in food

    - ▪   Forceful vomiting or frequent vomiting

    - ▪   Decreased urination

    - ▪   Diarrhea or decreased bowel movements

    - ▪   Labored breathing with flared nostrils or an absence of breathing for greater than 15 seconds

    - ▪   Jaundice

    - ▪   Cyanosis

    - ▪   Lethargy

- ▪ Inconsolable crying
- ▪ Difficulty waking
- ▪ Bleeding or purulent drainage around umbilical cord or circumcision
- ▪ Drainage developing in eyes.
- • Parents should be instructed in relieving airway obstruction.

Complications Related to Newborn Home Care

- • Complications stemming from improper understanding of discharge instructions may include:

    - ○ An infected cord or circumcision from improper cord care or tub bathing too soon.

    - ○ Falls, suffocation, strangulation, burns resulting in injuries, fractures, aspiration, or even death due to improper safety precautions.

    - ○ Respiratory infections due to passive smoke or inhaled powders.

    - ○ Improper or no use of a car seat resulting in injuries or death.

    - ○ Serious infections due to lack of noncompliance with immunization schedule.

CHAPTER 26: NURSING CARE AND DISCHARGE TEACHING

 Application Exercises

1. What is the single most important nursing measure that should be done to prevent newborn infection?

2. When teaching parent's about how to care for their newborn's umbilical cord, a nurse should include which of the following nursing interventions?

    A. Cover the cord with petroleum jelly after bathing.

    B. Wash the cord with soap and water each day during a tub bath.

    C. Apply hydrogen peroxide to the cord with each diaper change.

    D. Keep the cord dry and clean with the diaper folded below it.

3. A parent has been given instructions about care of a newborn following circumcision. Which of the following statements made by the parent indicates a need for further clarification?

    A. "His circumcision will heal completely within a couple of weeks."

    B. "I do not need to remove the yellow exudate that will form."

    C. "I will clean his penis with each diaper change."

    D. "I will give him a tub bath within a couple of days."

4. Twenty-four hours after delivery, and just prior to discharge, a newborn is about to undergo a circumcision. He has not been fed for several hours and is restrained on a circumcision board. The procedure will be done using a Gomco clamp. The nurse will provide care for the newborn after the circumcision and prior to discharge. Identify the priority nursing intervention that should be included in the newborn's postcircumcision care.

5. A nurse is aware that which of the following is a contraindication for circumcising a male newborn? (Select all that apply.)

    _____ Hypospadias

    _____ Hydrocele

    _____ Familiar history of hemophilia

    _____ Hyperbilirubinemia

    _____ Epispadias

6. A newborn has just been circumcised using a Gomco procedure. Which of the following nursing interventions is part of the initial care for this newborn?

    A. Apply alcohol to the site.

    B. Keep the newborn in the prone position.

    C. Apply petroleum gauze to the site for 24 hr.

    D. Avoid changing the newborn's diaper unless absolutely needed.

7. When providing teaching about car seat safety to the parents of a newborn, the nurse should instruct the parents to restrain the newborn in a car seat in the

    A. front seat in a semi-reclined, rear-facing position.

    B. front seat in a semi-reclined, forward-facing position.

    C. back seat in a semi-reclined, rear-facing position.

    D. back seat in a semi-reclined, forward-facing position.

8. Which of the following statements made by the parent of a newborn indicates a good understanding of how to use a bulb syringe to suction excess mucus from the newborn's airway?

    A. "My baby's mouth should be suctioned before her nose.

    B. "My baby's nose should be suctioned before her mouth."

    C. "The bulb syringe should reach to the back of the my baby's mouth."

    D. "The bulb syringe should be compressed after it is placed in the my baby's mouth or nose."

CHAPTER 26: NURSING CARE AND DISCHARGE TEACHING

 Application Exercises Answer Key

1. What is the single most important nursing measure that should be done to prevent newborn infection?

> **Hand hygiene is the single most important nursing intervention to prevent infection. The nurse must engage in a 3- to 5-min scrub from elbow to finger tips before entering the nursery and thereafter. Hands should be washed before and after contact with the newborn.**

 NCLEX® Connection: Physiological Adaptation, Alterations in Body Systems

2. When teaching parent's about how to care for their newborn's umbilical cord, a nurse should include which of the following nursing interventions?

> A. Cover the cord with petroleum jelly after bathing.
>
> B. Wash the cord with soap and water each day during a tub bath.
>
> C. Apply hydrogen peroxide to the cord with each diaper change.
>
> **D. Keep the cord dry and clean with the diaper folded below it.**

> **Keeping the newborn's cord dry and clean helps reduce infection and hastens drying. Folding the diaper below the cord prevents urine from the diaper penetrating the cord site. Petroleum jelly prevents the cord from drying and encourages infection. Newborns aren't given tub baths or completely immersed in water until the cord completely falls off. Triple dye and alcohol, not hydrogen peroxide, are applied to the cord site.**

 NCLEX® Connection: Health Promotion and Maintenance, Ante/Intra/Postpartum and Newborn Care

3. A parent has been given instructions about care of a newborn following circumcision. Which of the following statements made by the parent indicates a need for further clarification?

> A. "His circumcision will heal completely within a couple of weeks."
>
> B. "I do not need to remove the yellow exudate that will form."
>
> C. "I will clean his penis with each diaper change."
>
> **D. "I will give him a tub bath within a couple of days."**

> **A tub bath should not be given until the circumcision is completely healed. All of the other answers show that the parent has a good understanding of the teaching.**

 NCLEX® Connection: Reduction of Risk Potential, Potential for Complications of Diagnostic Tests/Treatments/Procedures

4. Twenty-four hours after delivery, and just prior to discharge, a newborn is about to undergo a circumcision. He has not been fed for several hours and is restrained on a circumcision board. The procedure will be done using a Gomco clamp. The nurse will provide care for the newborn after the circumcision and prior to discharge. Identify the priority nursing intervention that should be included in the newborn's postcircumcision care.

> **Observe the newborn for bleeding by conducting checks every 15 min for 1 hr and then every hour for at least 12 hr.**

 NCLEX® Connection: Reduction of Risk Potential, Potential for Complications of Diagnostic Tests/Treatments/Procedures

5. A nurse is aware that which of the following is a contraindication for circumcising a male newborn? (Select all that apply.)

X	**Hypospadias**
	Hydrocele
X	**Familiar history of hemophilia**
	Hyperbilirubinemia
X	**Epispadias**

> **In hypospadias and epispadias, the urethra is located somewhere other than the tip of the urethra, and the foreskin is needed for plastic surgery to repair the defect. Familiar history of bleeding disorders, hypospadias, and epispadias are all contraindications for circumcision of a newborn. Hydrocele and hyperbilirubinemia are not contraindications.**

 NCLEX® Connection: Reduction of Risk Potential, Potential for Complications of Diagnostic Tests/Treatments/Procedures

6. A newborn has just been circumcised using a Gomco procedure. Which of the following nursing interventions is part of the initial care for this newborn?

A. Apply alcohol to the site.

B. Keep the newborn in the prone position.

C. Apply petroleum gauze to the site for 24 hr.

D. Avoid changing the newborn's diaper unless absolutely needed.

> **Petroleum gauze is applied to the site for 24 hr to prevent the skin edges from sticking to the diaper. Newborns should never be placed prone for any reason. Diapers are changed more frequently to inspect the site. Alcohol is contraindicated for circumcision care due to the fresh wound.**

 NCLEX® Connection: Reduction of Risk Potential, Potential for Complications of Diagnostic Tests/ Treatments/ Procedures

7. When providing teaching about car seat safety to the parents of a newborn, the nurse should instruct the parents to restrain the newborn in a car seat in the

    A. front seat in a semi-reclined, rear-facing position.

    B. front seat in a semi-reclined, forward-facing position.

    C. back seat in a semi-reclined, rear-facing position.

    D. back seat in a semi-reclined, forward-facing position.

Infants who weigh up to 9.1 kg (20 lb) should be restrained in a car seat in a semi-reclined, rear-facing position in the back seat of the car. The other options are not appropriate positions for the infant safety seat.

 NCLEX® Connection: Safety and Infection Control, Accident Prevention

8. Which of the following statements made by the parent of a newborn indicates a good understanding of how to use a bulb syringe to suction excess mucus from the newborn's airway?

    A. "My baby's mouth should be suctioned before her nose.

    B. "My baby's nose should be suctioned before her mouth."

    C. "The bulb syringe should reach to the back of the my baby's mouth."

    D. "The bulb syringe should be compressed after it is placed in the my baby's mouth or nose."

When suctioning the newborn with a bulb-syringe, the bulb should be compressed before it is placed in the newborn's mouth or nose. The newborn's mouth should be suctioned before the nose to prevent aspiration during the gasp response. Also, the back of the newborn's throat should not be touched when suctioning the mouth because the gag reflex may be stimulated. The bulb syringe should be compressed before inserting it into the newborn's mouth.

 NCLEX® Connection: Health Promotion and Maintenance, Ante/Intra/Postpartum and Newborn Care

UNIT 4	NEWBORN NURSING CARE
Section	Complications of the Newborn
Chapter 27	Assessment and Management of Newborn Complications

Overview

- This chapter highlights the assessment and management of newborn complications. Assessment, risk factors, collaborative care and desired client outcomes will be discussed. It is essential for a nurse to immediately identify complications and implement appropriate interventions. Ongoing emotional support to a client and significant other is also imperative to the plan of care.

- The following complications including neonatal substance withdrawal, hypoglycemia, respiratory distress syndrome (RDS)/asphyxia/meconium aspiration, preterm newborn, small for gestational age (SGA) newborn, large for gestational age (LGA)/macrosomic newborn, postterm newborn, neonatal infection/sepsis (sepsis neonatorum), birth trauma or injury, hyperbilirubinemia, and congenital anomalies will be detailed in this chapter.

NEONATAL SUBSTANCE WITHDRAWAL

Overview

- Maternal substance abuse during pregnancy consists of any use of alcohol or drugs. Intrauterine drug exposure can cause anomalies, neurobehavioral changes, and signs of withdrawal in the neonate. These changes depend on a specific drug or combination of drugs used, dosage, route of administration, metabolism and excretion by the mother and her fetus, timing of drug exposure, and the length of drug exposure.

- Substance withdrawal in the newborn occurs when the mother uses drugs that have addictive properties during pregnancy. This includes illegal drugs, alcohol, tobacco, and prescription drugs.

- Fetal alcohol syndrome (FAS) results from the chronic or periodic intake of alcohol during pregnancy. Alcohol is considered teratogenic, so the daily intake of alcohol increases the risk of FAS.

- Newborns with FAS are at risk for specific congenital physical defects, along with long-term complications that include:

    o Feeding problems.

    o Central nervous system dysfunction (mental retardation, cerebral palsy).

    o Behavioral difficulties such as hyperactivity.

    o Language abnormalities.

      ○   Future substance abuse.

      ○   Delayed growth and development.

      ○   Poor maternal-newborn bonding.

Risk Factors

- Mother using substances prior to knowing she is pregnant

- Maternal substance abuse and addiction

Assessment

- Objective Data

      ○   Physical assessment findings

          ■   Monitor the neonate for signs and symptoms of abstinence syndrome (withdrawal) and increased wakefulness using the neonatal abstinence scoring system that assesses for and scores the following:

               □   CNS – increased wakefulness, a high-pitched, shrill cry, incessant crying, irritability, tremors, hyperactive with an increased Moro reflex, increased deep-tendon reflexes, increased muscle tone, abrasions and/or excoriations on the face and knees, and convulsions.

               □   Metabolic, vasomotor, and respiratory findings – nasal congestion with flaring, frequent yawning, skin mottling, tachypnea greater than 60/min, sweating, and a temperature greater than 37.2° C (99° F).

               □   Gastrointestinal – poor feeding, regurgitation (projectile vomiting), diarrhea, and excessive, uncoordinated, and constant sucking.

          ■   Opiate withdrawal

               □   Can last for 2 to 3 weeks

               □   Signs and symptoms of neonatal abstinence syndrome – rapid changes in mood, hypersensitivity to noise and external stimuli, dehydration, and poor weight gain

          ■   Heroin withdrawal

               □   Signs and symptoms of neonatal abstinence syndrome – low birth weight and SGA, decreased Moro reflexes (rather than increased), and hypothermia or hyperthermia.

          ■   Methadone withdrawal

               □   Signs and symptoms of neonatal abstinence syndrome – an increased incidence of seizures, sleep pattern disturbances, higher birth weights, and higher risk of sudden infant death syndrome

          ■   Marijuana withdrawal

               □   Signs and symptoms – preterm birth and meconium staining.

- Amphetamine withdrawal
  - □ Signs and symptoms – preterm or SGA, drowsiness, jitteriness, sleep pattern disturbances, respiratory distress, frequent infections, poor weight gain, emotional disturbances, and delayed growth and development
- Fetal alcohol syndrome
  - □ Signs and symptoms
    - ▸ Facial anomalies include eyes with epicanthal folds, strabismus, and ptosis; mouth with a poor suck, small teeth, and cleft lip or palate
    - ▸ Deafness
    - ▸ Abnormal palmar creases and irregular hair
    - ▸ Many vital organ anomalies, such as heart defects, including atrial and ventricular septal defects, tetralogy of Fallot, and patent-ductus arteriosus
    - ▸ Developmental delays and neurologic abnormalities
    - ▸ Prenatal and postnatal growth retardation
    - ▸ Sleep disturbances
- Tobacco
  - □ Signs and symptoms – prematurity, low birth weight, increased risk for sudden infant death syndrome, increased risk for bronchitis, pneumonia, and developmental delays

Collaborative Care

- Nursing Care
  - o Nursing care for maternal substance abuse and neonatal effects or withdrawal include the following in addition to normal newborn care.
    - Perform a neonatal abstinence scoring system assessment, as ordered by the provider.
    - Elicit and assess the newborn's reflexes.
    - Monitor the newborn's ability to feed and digest intake.
    - Monitor the newborn's fluids and electrolytes such as skin turgor, mucous membranes, fontanels, and I&O.
    - Observe the infant's behavior.
- Laboratory Tests
  - o Blood tests should be done to differentiate between neonatal drug withdrawal and central nervous system irritability.
    - CBC
    - Blood glucose

- Calcium
- Magnesium
- TSH, T_4, T_3
- Drug screen of urine or meconium to reveal the agent abused by the mother
- Hair analysis

- Diagnostic Procedures

  ○ Chest x-ray for FAS to rule out congenital heart defects

- Medications

  ○ Phenobarbital (Solfoton)

    - Classification

      □ Anticonvulsant

    - Intended effect

      □ It is prescribed to decrease CNS irritability and control seizures for neonates who have alcohol or opioid addiction.

    - Nursing considerations

      □ Assess IV site frequently.

      □ Check for any medication incompatibilities.

      □ Reduce external stimuli.

      □ Swaddle the newborn to reduce self-stimulation and protect the skin from abrasions.

      □ Administer frequent, small feedings of high-calorie formula – may need gavage feedings.

      □ Elevate the infant's head during and following feedings, and burp the infant to reduce vomiting and aspiration.

      □ Trying various nipples to compensate for a poor suck reflex.

      □ Have suction available to reduce the risk for aspiration.

      □ For newborns who are addicted to cocaine, avoid eye contact and use vertical rocking and a pacifier.

      □ Prevent infection.

      □ Initiate a consult with child protective services.

      □ Consult lactation services to evaluate if breastfeeding is contraindicated or desired.

- Health Promotion and Disease Prevention

  ○ Client education

    - Refer the mother to a drug and/or alcohol treatment center.

- Client outcomes

    ○ The newborn will adapt to extrauterine life without injury.

    ○ The newborn will not exhibit signs of seizures.

    ○ The newborn will take and retain feedings.

HYPOGLYCEMIA

Overview

- Hypoglycemia is a serum glucose level of less than 40 mg/dL. Routine assessment of all newborns, especially newborns who are LGA and SGA, should include observing for symptoms of hypoglycemia.

- Hypoglycemia – differs for a newborn who is preterm or term. Hypoglycemia occurring in the first 3 days of life in the term newborn is defined as a blood glucose level of < 40 mg/dL. In the preterm newborn, hypoglycemia is defined as a blood glucose level of < 25 mg/dL.

- Untreated hypoglycemia can result in seizures, brain damage, and/or death.

Risk Factors

- Maternal diabetes mellitus

- Preterm infant

- LGA or SGA

- Stress at birth, such as cold stress and asphyxia

- Maternal epidural anesthesia

Assessment

- Objective Data

    ○ Physical assessment findings

        ▪ Poor feeding

        ▪ Jitteriness/tremors

        ▪ Hypothermia

        ▪ Diaphoresis

        ▪ Weak shrill cry

        ▪ Lethargy

        ▪ Flaccid muscle tone

        ▪ Seizures/coma

- Irregular respirations

- Cyanosis

- Apnea

  o Laboratory tests and diagnostic procedures

- Two consecutive plasma glucose levels less than 40 mg/dL in a newborn who is term, and less than 25 mg/dL in a newborn who is preterm

Collaborative Care

- Nursing Care

  o Obtain blood per heel stick for glucose monitoring.

  o Provide frequent oral and/or gavage feedings or continuous parenteral nutrition early after birth to treat hypoglycemia.

  o Monitor the neonate's blood glucose level closely per facility protocol.

  o Monitor IV if the neonate's unable to orally feed.

- Client Outcomes

  o The newborn will exhibit blood glucose levels within the normal range.

RESPIRATORY DISTRESS SYNDROME (RDS)/ASPHYXIA/MECONIUM ASPIRATION

Overview

- Respiratory distress syndrome (RDS) occurs as a result of surfactant deficiency in the lungs and is characterized by poor gas exchange and ventilatory failure.

- Surfactant is a phospholipid that assists in alveoli expansion. Surfactant keeps alveoli from collapsing and allows gas exchange to occur.

- Atelectasis (collapsing of a portion of lung) increases the work of breathing. As a result, respiratory acidosis and hypoxemia can develop.

- Birth weight alone is not an indicator of fetal lung maturity.

- Complications from RDS are related to oxygen therapy and mechanical ventilation.

  o Pneumothorax

  o Pneumomediastinum

  o Retinopathy of prematurity

  o Bronchopulmonary dysplasia

  o Infection

  o Intraventricular hemorrhage

Risk Factors

- ○ Preterm gestation
- ○ Perinatal asphyxia (meconium staining, cord prolapse, and nuchal cord)
- ○ Maternal diabetes mellitus
- ○ Premature rupture of membranes
- ○ Maternal use of barbiturates or narcotics close to birth
- ○ Maternal hypotension
- ○ Cesarean birth without labor
- ○ Hydrops fetalis (massive edema of the fetus caused by hyperbilirubinemia)
- ○ Maternal bleeding during the third trimester

Assessment

- • Objective Data
  - ○ Physical assessment findings
    - ■ Tachypnea (respiratory rate greater than 60/min)
    - ■ Nasal flaring
    - ■ Expiratory grunting
    - ■ Intercostal and substernal retractions
    - ■ Labored breathing
    - ■ Fine rales on auscultation
    - ■ Cyanosis
    - ■ Unresponsiveness, flaccidity, and apnea with decreased breath sounds (signs and symptoms of worsened RDS)
  - ○ Laboratory tests
    - ■ Culture-and-sensitivity of the blood, urine, and cerebrospinal fluid
    - ■ Blood glucose and serum calcium
  - ○ Diagnostic procedures
    - ■ ABGs reveal hypercapnia (excess of carbon dioxide in the blood) and respiratory or mixed acidosis.
    - ■ Chest x-ray

Collaborative Care

- Nursing Care

  o Suction the infant's mouth, trachea, and nose as needed.

  o Maintain thermoregulation.

  o Provide mouth and skin care.

  o Correct respiratory acidosis with ventilatory support.

  o Correct metabolic acidosis by administering sodium bicarbonate.

  o Maintain adequate oxygenation, prevent lactic acidosis, and avoid the toxic effects of oxygen.

  o Decrease stimuli.

- Medications

  o Beractant (Survanta)

  o Classification

    ■ Lung surfactant

  o Intended effect

    ■ It is prescribed for newborns who are premature and have RDS. It restores surfactant and improves respiratory compliance.

  o Nursing considerations

    ■ Perform a respiratory assessment including ABGs, respiratory rhythm, and rate and color before and after administration of agent.

    ■ Provide suction to the newborn prior to administration of the medication.

    ■ Assess endotracheal tube placement.

    ■ Avoid suctioning of the endotracheal tube for 1 hr after administration of the medication.

- Client Outcomes

  o The newborn will display adequate oxygenation as evidenced by respiratory rate and blood gas levels within normal range.

- Miscellaneous

  o Factors that can accelerate lung maturation in the fetus while in utero include increased gestational age, intrauterine stress, exogenous steroid use, and ruptured membranes.

PRETERM NEWBORN

Overview

- A preterm newborn's birth occurs after 20 weeks of gestation and before 37 weeks of gestation. This may occur once the cervix has dilated to 4 cm.

- Preterm newborns are at risk for a variety of complications due to immature organ systems. The degree of complications depends on gestational age. There is a decreased risk for complications the closer the newborn is to 40 weeks of gestation.

  o Respiratory distress syndrome – decreased surfactant in the alveoli occurs, regardless of a newborn's birth weight

  o Bronchopulmonary dysplasia – causes the lungs to become stiff and noncompliant, requiring an infant to receive mechanical ventilation and oxygen, and it is sometimes difficult to remove the infant from ventilation and oxygen after initial placement

  o Aspiration – a result of an infant who is premature not having an intact gag reflex or the ability to effectively suck or swallow

  o Apnea of prematurity – a result of immature neurological and chemical mechanisms

  o Intraventricular hemorrhage – bleeding in or around the ventricles of the brain.

  o Retinopathy of prematurity – disease caused by abnormal growth of retinal blood vessels and is a complication associated with oxygen administration to the neonate, and it can cause mild to severe eye and vision problems

  o Patent ductus arteriosus – occurs when the ductus arteriosus reopens after birth due to neonatal hypoxia.

  o Necrotizing enterocolitis (NEC) – an inflammatory disease of the gastrointestinal mucosa due to ischemia, and it results in necrosis and perforation of the bowel (short-gut syndrome may be the result secondary to removal of most or part of the small intestine due to necrosis)

  o Additional complications include infection, hyperbilirubinemia, anemia, hypoglycemia, and delayed growth and development.

    ■ Goals include meeting the infant's growth and development needs and anticipating and managing associated complications such as RDS and sepsis.

    ■ The main priority in treating newborns who are preterm is supporting the cardiac and respiratory systems as needed. Most newborns who are preterm are cared for in a neonatal intensive care unit (NICU). Meticulous care and observation in the NICU is necessary until the newborn can receive oral feedings, maintain body temperature, and weighs approximately 2 kg (4.4 lb).

Risk Factors

- Maternal gestational hypertension

- Multiple pregnancies

- Adolescent pregnancy

- Lack of prenatal care

- Substance abuse

- Smoking

- Previous history of preterm delivery

- Abnormalities of the uterus

- Cervical incompetence

- Premature rupture of the membranes

- Placenta previa

- Premature labor

- Premature rupture of membranes

Assessment

- Objective Data

    o Physical assessment findings

        ■ A Ballard assessment shows a physical and neurological assessment totaling less than 37 weeks of gestation.

        ■ Periodic breathing consists of 5- to 10-second respiratory pauses, followed by 10- to 15-second compensatory rapid respirations.

        ■ Signs of increased respiratory effort and/or respiratory distress include nasal flaring or retractions of the chest wall during inspirations, expiratory grunting, and tachypnea.

        ■ Apnea is a pause in respirations longer than 10 to 15 seconds.

        ■ The newborn has a low birth weight.

        ■ The newborn has minimal subcutaneous fat deposits.

        ■ The newborn's head is large in comparison to his body.

        ■ The newborn has wrinkled features.

        ■ The newborn's skull and rib cage feel soft.

        ■ The newborn's eyes are closed eyes if he is born at 22 to 24 weeks of gestation.

        ■ The newborn has a weak grasp reflex.

        ■ The newborn has an inability to coordinate suck and swallow, and a weak or absent gag, suck, and cough reflex; weak swallow.

        ■ The newborn has hypotonic muscles, decreased level of activity, and a weak cry for more than 24 hr.

        ■ The newborn is lethargic, is experiencing tachycardia, and has poor weight gain.

- Signs of infection
  - ☐ Observe the newborn for signs of dehydration or overhydration (resulting from IV nutrition and fluid administration).
  - ☐ Dehydration
    - ▸ Urine output less than 1 mL/kg/hr
    - ▸ Urine-specific gravity more than 1.015
    - ▸ Weight loss
    - ▸ Dry mucous membranes
    - ▸ Poor skin turgor
    - ▸ Depressed fontanel
  - ☐ Overhydration
    - ▸ Urine output greater than 3 mL/kg/hr
    - ▸ Urine-specific gravity less than 1.001
    - ▸ Edema
    - ▸ Increased weight gain
    - ▸ Rales
    - ▸ Intake greater than output
- Laboratory tests
  - CBC shows decreased Hgb and Hct as a result of the slow production of RBCs
  - Urinalysis and specific gravity
  - Increased PT and aPTT time with an increased tendency to bleed
  - Serum glucose
  - Calcium
  - Bilirubin
  - ABGs
- Diagnostic procedures
  - Chest x-ray
  - Head ultrasounds
  - Echocardiography
  - Eye exams

Collaborative Care

- Nursing Care

  o Perform rapid initial assessment.

  o Perform resuscitative measures if needed.

  o Monitor the infant's vital signs.

  o Assess the infant's ability to consume and digest nutrients. Before a newborn who is immature can feed by breast or nipple, the infant must have an intact gag reflex and be able to suck and swallow to prevent aspiration.

  o Monitor the infant's I&O, and daily weight.

  o Monitor the newborn for bleeding from puncture sites and the gastrointestinal tract.

  o Ensure and maintain thermoregulation in a newborn who is premature by using a radiant heat warmer.

  o Administer respiratory support measures such as surfactant and/or oxygen administration.

  o Administer parental or enteral nutrition and fluids as prescribed (most premature newborns who are less than 34 weeks of gestation will receive fluids either by IV and/or gavage feedings). Provide for nonnutritive sucking, such as using a pacifier while gavage feeding.

  o Minimize the newborn's stimulation. Cluster nursing care. Touch the newborn very smoothly and lightly. Keep lighting dim and noise levels reduced.

  o Position the infant in neutral flexion with his extremities close to his body to conserve body heat. Prone and side-lying positions are preferred to supine with body containment using blanket rolls and swaddling, but only in the nursery.

  o Protect the newborn against infection by enforcing hand hygiene and gowning procedures. Also, equipment should not be shared with other newborns.

- Medications

  o Betamethasone (Celestone)

- Classification

  o Glucocorticoids

- Intended Effect

  o It is administered for a 24-hr period prior to delivery to promote fetal lung development and increase surfactant in an attempt to prevent RDS.

- Health Promotion and Disease Prevention

  o Client education

    ▪ Keep parents informed and educated about the care of their preterm newborn.

- Client Outcomes

  ○ The infant adapts to extrauterine life as evidenced by taking and retaining feedings.

  ○ The infant maintains body temperature.

  ○ The infant is free of signs of infection.

SMALL FOR GESTATIONAL AGE NEWBORN (SGA)

Overview

- Small for gestational age (SGA) describes an infant whose birth weight is at or below the 10th percentile.

- Common complications of infants who are SGA are perinatal asphyxia, meconium aspiration, hypoglycemia, polycythemia, and instability of body temperature.

Risk Factors

- Congenital or chromosomal anomalies

- Maternal infections, disease, or malnutrition

- Gestational hypertension and/or diabetes mellitus

- Smoking, drug, or alcohol use

- Multiple gestations

- Placental factors (small placenta, placenta previa, decreased placental perfusion)

- Fetal congenital infections such as rubella or toxoplasmosis

Assessment

- Objective Data

  ○ Physical assessment findings

    - Weight below 10th percentile

    - Normal skull, but reduced body dimensions

    - Hair is sparse on scalp

    - Wide skull sutures from inadequate bone growth

    - Dry, loose skin

    - Decreased subcutaneous fat

    - Decreased muscle mass, particularly over the cheeks and buttocks

    - Thin, dry, yellow, and dull umbilical cord rather than gray, glistening, and moist

    - Drawn abdomen rather than well-rounded

- Signs of respiratory distress and hypoxia
- Wide-eyed and alert, which is attributed to prolonged fetal hypoxia
- Hypotonia
- Signs of meconium aspiration
- Signs of hypoglycemia
- Signs of hypothermia
  - Laboratory tests
    - Blood glucose level for hypoglycemia
    - CBC will show polycythemia resulting from fetal hypoxia and intrauterine stress
    - ABGs may be prescribed due to chronic hypoxia in utero due to placental insufficiency
  - Diagnostic procedures
    - Chest x-ray to rule out meconium aspiration syndrome

Collaborative Care

- Nursing Care
  - Support respiratory efforts and suction the newborn as necessary to maintain an open airway.
  - Provide a neutral thermal environment for the newborn (isolette or radiant heat warmer) to prevent cold stress.
  - Initiate early feedings (An infant who is SGA will require feedings that are more frequent).
  - Administer parenteral nutrition if necessary.
  - Maintain adequate hydration.
  - Conserve the newborn's energy level.
  - Prevent skin breakdown.
  - Protect the newborn from infection.
- Health Promotion and Disease Prevention
  - Client education
    - Provide support to the newborn's parents and extended family, and encourage them to participate in caring for the newborn care.
- Client Outcomes
    - The newborn adapts to extrauterine life.
    - The newborn takes and retains feedings.
    - The newborn maintains a blood glucose level within normal limits.

LARGE FOR GESTATIONAL AGE NEWBORN (LGA)/MACROSOMIC

Overview

- Large for gestational age (LGA) occurs in neonates who weigh above the 90th percentile or more than 4,000 g (8 lb, 12 oz).

- Neonates who are LGA may be preterm, postterm, or full-term. LGA does not necessarily mean postmature.

- Infants who are macrosomic are at risk for birth injuries (shoulder dystocia, clavicle fracture or a cesarean birth, asphyxia, hypoglycemia, polycythemia and Erb-Duchenne paralysis due to birth trauma).

- Uncontrolled hyperglycemia during pregnancy (leading risk factor for LGA) can lead to congenital defects with the most common being congenital heart defects, tracheoesophageal fistula, and CNS anomalies.

Risk Factors

- Infants who are postterm

- Maternal diabetes mellitus during pregnancy (high glucose levels stimulate continued insulin production by the fetus)

- Fetal cardiovascular disorder of transposition of the great vessels

- Genetic factors

- Obesity

- A mother who is multiparous

Assessment

- Objective Data

  - Physical assessment findings

    - Weight above 90th percentile (4,000 g)

    - Plump and full-faced (cushingoid appearance) from increased subcutaneous fat

    - Signs of hypoxia including tachypnea, retractions, cyanosis, nasal flaring, and grunting

    - Birth trauma (e.g., fractures, intracranial hemorrhage, and CNS injury)

    - Sluggishness, hypotonic muscles, and hypoactivity

    - Tremors from hypocalcemia

    - Signs of hypoglycemia

    - Signs of respiratory distress from immature lungs or meconium aspiration

○ Laboratory tests

- Blood glucose levels to monitor closely for hypoglycemia (less than 40 mg/dL)

- ABGs may be prescribed due to chronic hypoxia in utero secondary to placental insufficiency

- CBC shows polycythemia (Hct greater than 65%) from in utero hypoxia

- Hyperbilirubinemia resulting from polycythemia as excessive RBCs break down after birth

- Hypocalcemia may result in response to a long and difficult birth

○ Diagnostic procedures

- Cesarean birth if necessary

- Chest x-ray to rule out meconium aspiration syndrome

Collaborative Care

- Nursing Care Prior to Delivery

  ○ Prepare the client for a possible vacuum-assisted birth.

  ○ Prepare to place the client in McRoberts' position (lithotomy position with legs flexed to chest to maximize pelvic outlet).

  ○ Prepare to apply suprapubic pressure to aid in the delivery of the anterior shoulder, which is located inferior to the maternal symphysis pubis.

  ○ Assess the neonate for birth trauma such as a broken clavicle or Erb-Duchenne paralysis.

- Nursing Care for an Infant Who is LGA Following Delivery

  ○ Obtain early and frequent heel sticks (glucose testing).

  ○ Initiate early feedings or intravenous therapy to maintain normal glucose levels.

  ○ Provide thermoregulation with isolette care.

  ○ Administer surfactant by endotracheal tube if indicated.

  ○ Identify and treat any birth injuries.

- Client Outcomes

  ○ The newborn adapts to extrauterine life.

  ○ The newborn maintains a blood glucose level within normal limits.

POSTTERM INFANT

Overview

- An infant who is postterm is one who is born after the completion of 42 weeks of gestation. Postmaturity of the infant can be associated with either of the following:

    ○ Dysmaturity from placental degeneration and uteroplacental insufficiency (placenta functions effectively for only 40 weeks) resulting in chronic fetal hypoxia and fetal distress in utero. The fetal response is polycythemia, meconium aspiration, and/or neonatal respiratory problems. Perinatal mortality is higher when a postmature placenta fails to meet increased oxygen demands of the infant during labor.

    ○ Continued growth of the fetus in utero because the placenta continues to function effectively and the infant becomes LGA at birth. This leads to a difficult delivery, cephalopelvic disproportion, as well as high insulin reserves and insufficient glucose reserves at birth. The neonatal response can be birth trauma, perinatal asphyxia, a clavicle fracture, seizures, hypoglycemia, and/or temperature instability (cold stress).

- An infant who is postmature may be either SGA or LGA depending on how well the placenta functions during the last weeks of pregnancy.

- Infants who are postmature have an increased risk for aspirating the meconium passed by the fetus in utero.

- Persistent pulmonary hypertension (persistent fetal circulation) is a complication that can result from meconium aspiration. There is an interference in the transition from fetal to neonatal circulation, and the ductus arteriosus (connecting main pulmonary artery and the aorta) and foramen ovale (shunt between the right and left atria) remain open and fetal pathways of blood flow continue.

Risk Factors

- In most cases, the cause of a pregnancy that extends beyond 40 weeks of gestation is unknown, but there is a higher incidence in first pregnancies and in women who have had a previous postterm pregnancy.

Assessment

- Objective Data

    ○ Physical assessment findings

        ▪ Wasted appearance, thin with loose skin, having lost some of the subcutaneous fat

        ▪ Peeling, cracked, and dry skin; leathery from decrease protection of vernix and amniotic fluid

        ▪ Long, thin body

        ▪ Meconium staining of fingernails and umbilical cord

        ▪ Hair and nails may be long

- May demonstrate more alertness similar to a 2-week-old newborn
- May have difficulty establishing respirations secondary to meconium aspiration
- Signs and symptoms of hypoglycemia due to insufficient stores of glycogen
- Signs and symptoms of cold stress
- Neurological symptoms that become apparent with the development of fine motor skills
- Macrosomia

- Laboratory Tests

  ○ Blood glucose levels to monitor for hypoglycemia

  ○ ABGs secondary to chronic hypoxia in utero due to placental insufficiency

  ○ CBC may show polycythemia from decreased oxygenation in utero

  ○ Hct elevated from polycythemia and dehydration

- Diagnostic Procedures

  ○ Cesarean birth

  ○ Chest x-ray to rule out meconium aspiration syndrome

Collaborative Care

- Nursing Care

  ○ Monitor the newborn's vital signs.

  ○ Administer and monitor the newborn's IV fluids.

  ○ Use mechanical ventilation if necessary.

  ○ Administer oxygen as prescribed.

  ○ Prepare and/or assist with exchange transfusion if hematocrit is high.

  ○ Provide thermoregulation in an isolette to avoid cold stress.

  ○ Provide early feedings to avoid hypoglycemia.

  ○ Identify and treat any birth injuries.

- Client Outcomes

  ○ Infant adapts to extrauterine life.

  ○ The newborn maintains a blood glucose level within normal limits.

NEONATAL INFECTION/SEPSIS (SEPSIS NEONATORUM)

Overview

- Infection may be contracted by the newborn before, during, or after delivery. Newborns are more susceptible to microorganisms because of their limited immunity and inability to localize infection. The infection can spread rapidly into the bloodstream.

- Neonatal sepsis is the presence of microorganisms or their toxins in the blood or tissues of the infant during the first month after birth. Signs of sepsis are subtle and may resemble other diseases; the nurse often notices them during routine care of the infant.

- Organisms frequently responsible for neonatal infections include: *Staphylococcus aureus, S. epidermidis, Escherichia coli, Haemophilus influenzae*, and streptococcus ß-hemolytic, Group B.

- Prevention of infection and neonatal sepsis starts perinatally with maternal screening for infections, prophylactic interventions, and the use of sterile and aseptic techniques during delivery. Prophylactic antibiotic treatment of the eyes of all newborns and appropriate umbilical cord care also help to prevent neonatal infection and sepsis.

Risk Factors

- Premature rupture of the membranes

- TORCH (toxoplasmosis, rubella, cytomegalovirus, and herpes)

- Chorioamnionitis

- Premature birth

- Low birth weight

- Substance abuse

- Maternal urinary-tract infection

- Meconium

- HIV transmitted from the mother to the newborn perinatally through the placenta and postnatally through the breast milk

Assessment

- Objective Data

  - Physical assessment findings

    - Temperature instability

    - Suspicious drainage (eyes, umbilical stump)

    - Poor feeding pattern, such as a weak suck or decreased intake

    - Vomiting and diarrhea

- Poor weight gain

- Abdominal distention, large residual if feeding by gavage

- Apnea, sternal retractions, grunting, and nasal flaring

- Decreased oxygen saturation

- Color changes such as pallor, jaundice, and petechiae

- Tachycardia or bradycardia

- Tachypnea

- Low blood pressure

- Irritability and seizure activity

- Poor muscle tone and lethargic

    o Laboratory tests

    - CBC

    - Blood, urine, and cerebrospinal fluid cultures and sensitivities

    - Positive blood cultures, usually polymicrobial (more than one pathogen) indicates the presence of infection/sepsis

        □ Chemical profile shows a fluid and electrolyte imbalance.

Collaborative Care

- Nursing Care

    o Assess infection risks (review maternal record).

    o Monitor the newborn for signs of opportunistic infection.

    o Monitor the newborn's vital signs continuously.

    o Monitor the newborn's I&O and daily weight.

    o Monitor the newborn's fluid and electrolyte status.

    o Monitor the newborn's visitors for infection.

    o Obtain specimens (blood, urine, stool) to assist in identifying the causative organism.

    o Initiate and maintain IV therapy as prescribed to administer electrolyte replacements, fluids, and medications.

    o Administer medications as prescribed (broad-spectrum antibiotics prior to cultures being obtained).

- Medications

    o Ampicillin (Principen)

- Classifications

    o Antibiotic

- Intended Effect

    o It is a broad-spectrum antibiotic that is bactericidal.

- Nursing Considerations

    o Obtain cultures prior to administration of antibiotics.

        ■ Gentamicin sulfate (Garamycin)

- Classification

    o Aminoglycoside antibiotic

- Intended Effect

    o It is a bactericidal that causes cell death

- Nursing Considerations

    o Obtain cultures prior to administration of antibiotics.

    o Monitor the newborn's peak and trough levels as prescribed.

- Nursing Considerations

    o Initiate and maintain respiratory support as needed.

    o Provide newborn care to maintain temperature.

    o Maintain standard precautions.

    o Clean and sterilize all equipment to be used.

- Health Promotion and Disease Prevention

    o Discharge instructions

        □ Provide the family with education about infection control, which includes:

            ‣ Instructing them how to use clean bottles and nipples for each feeding.

            ‣ Discarding any unused formula.

            ‣ Supervising hand hygiene.

        ■ Provide emotional support to the family.

- Client Outcomes

    o The infant will remain free of infection and neonatal injury.

BIRTH TRAUMA OR INJURY

 Overview

- Birth injury occurs during childbirth resulting in physical injury to a newborn. Most injuries are minor and resolve rapidly. Other injuries may require some intervention. A few are serious enough to be fatal.

- Types of birth injuries

  ○ Skull (linear fracture, depressed fracture)

  ○ Scalp (caput succedaneum)

  ○ Intracranial (epidural or subdural hematoma, cerebral contusion)

  ○ Spinal cord (spinal cord transaction or injury, vertebral artery injury)

  ○ Plexus (brachial plexus injury, Klumpke's palsy)

  ○ Cranial and peripheral nerve (radial nerve palsy, diaphragmatic paralysis)

Risk Factors

- Fetal macrosomia

- Abnormal or difficult presentations

- Prolonged labor

- Precipitous labor

- Cephalopelvic disproportion

- Multifetal gestation

- Congenital abnormalities

- Internal FHR monitoring

- Forceps or vacuum extraction

- External version

- Cesarean birth

Assessment

- Objective Data

  ○ Physical assessment findings

    ■ Irritability, seizures within the first 72 hr, and a decreased level of consciousness are all signs of a subarachnoid hemorrhage.

    ■ Facial flattening and unresponsiveness to grimace that accompanies crying or stimulation, as well as eyes remaining open, are all symptoms to assess for facial paralysis.

- A weak or hoarse cry is characteristic of laryngeal nerve palsy from excessive traction on the neck.

- Flaccid muscle tone may signal joint dislocations and separation during birth.

- Flaccid muscle tone of the extremities suggests nerve-plexus injuries or long bone fractures.

- Limited motion of an arm, crepitus over a clavicle, and absence of the Moro reflex on the affected side are symptoms of clavicular fractures.

- A flaccid arm with the elbow extended and the hand rotated inward, absence of the Moro reflex on the affected side, sensory loss over the lateral aspect of the arm, and intact grasp reflex are all symptoms of Erb-Duchenne paralysis (brachial paralysis).

- Localized discoloration, ecchymosis, petechiae, and edema over the presenting part are seen with soft-tissue injuries.

   ○ Diagnostic Procedures

- Birth injuries are normally diagnosed by a CT scan, x-ray of suspected area of fracture, or neurological exam to determine paralysis of nerves.

Collaborative Care

- Nursing Care

   ○ Review maternal history to look for factors that may predispose the newborn to injuries.

   ○ Review Apgar scoring that might indicate a possibility of birth injury.

   ○ Perform frequent head-to-toe physical assessments.

   ○ Obtain vital signs and temperature.

   ○ Administer treatment to the newborn based on the injury and according to the primary care provider's prescriptions.

- Health Promotion and Disease Prevention

   ○ Discharge instructions

- Educate the infant's parents and family regarding the injury and the management of the injury.

- Promote parent-newborn bonding.

- Client Outcomes

   ○ The newborn immediately receives appropriate interventions and condition is stabilized.

HYPERBILIRUBINEMIA

 Overview

- Hyperbilirubinemia is an elevation of serum bilirubin levels resulting in jaundice. Jaundice normally appears in the head (especially the sclera and mucous membranes), and then progresses down the thorax, abdomen, and extremities.

- Jaundice can be either physiologic or pathologic

  o Physiologic jaundice is considered benign (resulting from normal newborn physiology of increased bilirubin production due to the shortened lifespan and breakdown of fetal RBCs and liver immaturity). The infant with physiological jaundice has no other symptoms and shows signs of jaundice after 24 hr of age.

  o Pathologic jaundice is a result of an underlying disease. Pathologic jaundice appears before 24 hr of age or is persistent after day 7. In the term infant, bilirubin levels increase more than 0.5 mg/dL/hr, peaks at greater than 13 mg/dL, or is associated with anemia and hepatosplenomegaly. Pathologic jaundice is usually caused by a blood group incompatibility or an infection, but may be the result of RBC disorders.

- Kernicterus (bilirubin encephalopathy) can result from untreated hyperbilirubinemia with bilirubin levels at or higher than 25 mg/dL. It is a neurological syndrome caused by bilirubin depositing in brain cells. Survivors may develop cerebral palsy, epilepsy, or mental retardation. They may have minor effects such as learning disorders or perceptual-motor disabilities.

Risk Factors

- Increased RBC production or breakdown

- Rh- or ABO-incompatibility

- Decreased liver function

- Ineffective breastfeeding

- Sibling with diagnosed jaundice

- Certain medications (maternal ingestion of aspirin, tranquilizers, and sulfonamides)

- Hypoglycemia

- Hypothermia

- Anoxia

- Prematurity

Assessment

- Objective Data
  - Physical assessment findings
    - Note yellowish tint to skin, sclera, and mucous membranes.
    - To verify jaundice, press the infant's skin on the cheek or abdomen lightly with one finger. Then, release pressure and observe the infant's skin color for yellowish tint as the skin is blanched.
    - Note the time of jaundice onset to distinguish between physiologic and pathologic jaundice.
    - Assess the underlying cause by reviewing the maternal prenatal, family, and newborn history.
    - Signs of hypoxia, hypothermia, hypoglycemia, and metabolic acidosis can occur as a result of hyperbilirubinemia and may increase the risk of brain damage.
    - Signs and symptoms of kernicterus.
      - Very yellowish or orange skin
      - Lethargy
      - Hypotonic
      - Poor suck reflex
      - Increased sleepiness
      - If untreated, the infant will become hypertonic with backward arching of the neck and trunk
      - High-pitched cry
      - Fever
  - Laboratory tests
    - An elevated serum bilirubin level may occur (direct and indirect bilirubin). Monitor the infant's bilirubin levels every 4 hr until the level returns to normal.
    - Assess maternal and newborn blood type to determine if there is a presence of ABO-incapability. This occurs if the newborn has blood type A, B or AB, and the mother is type O.
    - Review Hgb and Hct.
    - A direct Coombs' test reveals the presence of antibody-coated (sensitized) Rh-positive RBCs in the newborn.
    - Check electrolyte levels for dehydration from phototherapy.
  - Diagnostic procedures
    - Transcutaneous bilirubin level is a noninvasive method to measure an infant's bilirubin level.

- o   Treatment

    - ■   Phototherapy is the primary treatment for hyperbilirubinemia. It is prescribed if an infant's serum bilirubin is >15 mg/dL prior to 48 hr of age, >18 mg/dL prior to 72 hr of age, and >20 mg/dL at anytime.

Collaborative Care

- •   Nursing Care

    - o   Observe the infant's skin and mucous membranes for signs of jaundice.

    - o   Monitor the infant's vital signs.

    - o   Set up phototherapy if prescribed.

        - ■   Maintain an eye mask over the newborn's eyes for protection of corneas and retinas.

        - ■   Keep the newborn undressed with the exception of a male newborn. A surgical mask should be placed (make like a bikini) over the genitalia to prevent possible testicular damage from heat and light waves. Be sure to remove the metal strip from the mask to prevent burning.

        - ■   Avoid applying lotions or ointments to the infant because they absorb heat and can cause burns.

        - ■   Remove the newborn from phototherapy every 4 hr and unmask the newborn's eyes, checking for signs of inflammation or injury.

        - ■   Reposition the newborn every 2 hr to expose all of the body surfaces to the phototherapy lights and prevent pressure sores.

        - ■   Check the lamp energy with a photometer per unit protocol.

        - ■   Turn off the phototherapy lights before drawing blood for testing.

    - o   Observe the newborn for side effects of phototherapy.

        - ■   Bronze discoloration – not a serious complication

        - ■   Maculopapular skin rash – not a serious complication

        - ■   Development of pressure areas

        - ■   Dehydration (poor skin turgor, dry mucous membranes, decreased urinary output)

        - ■   Elevated temperature

    - o   Monitor elimination and daily weights, watching for signs of dehydration.

    - o   Check the newborn's axillary temperature every 4 hr during phototherapy, because temperature may become elevated.

    - o   Feed the newborn early and frequently – every 3 to 4 hr. This will promote bilirubin excretion in the stools.

    - o   Continue to breastfeed the newborn. Supplementing with formula may be prescribed.

    - o   Maintain adequate fluid intake to prevent dehydration.

- Reassure the parents that most newborns experience some degree of jaundice.

- Explain hyperbilirubinemia, its causes, diagnostic tests, and treatment to parents.

- Explain that the newborn's stool contains some bile that will be loose and green.

- Administer an exchange transfusion for infants who are at risk for kernicterus.

- Discharge Instructions

   - Educate the parents regarding the newborn's plan of care.

- Client Outcomes

   - The newborn will display a serum-bilirubin level within a normal range.

CONGENITAL ANOMALIES

Overview

- Newborns can be born with congenital anomalies involving all systems. Anomalies are often diagnosed prenatally. A nurse should provide emotional support to the parents whose infant is facing procedures or surgeries to correct the defects.

- When congenital anomalies are present at birth, they can involve any of the body systems. Major anomalies causing serious problems include:

   - Congenital heart disease (atrial septal defects, ventricular septal defects, coarctation of the aorta, tetralogy of Fallot, transposition of the great vessels, stenosis, atresia of valves).

   - Neurological defects (neural-tube defects, hydrocephalus, anencephaly, encephalocele, meningocele, or myelomeningocele).

   - Gastrointestinal problems (cleft lip/palate, diaphragmatic hernia, imperforate anus, tracheoesophageal fistula/esophageal atresia, duodenal atresia, omphalocele, gastroschisis, umbilical hernia, or intestinal obstruction).

   - Musculoskeletal deformities (clubfoot, polydactyly, developmental dysplasia of the hip).

   - Genitourinary deformities (hypospadias, epispadias, exstrophy of the bladder).

   - Metabolic disorders (phenylketonuria, galactosemia, hypothyroidism).

   - Chromosomal abnormalities (Down syndrome [trisomy 21], which is the most common trisomic abnormality with 47 chromosomes in each cell).

- Congenital anomalies are generally identified soon after birth by Apgar scoring and a brief assessment indicating the need for further investigation. Once identified, congenital anomalies are treated in a pediatric setting.

Risk Factors

- Risk factors for congenital anomalies include genetic and/or environmental factors.

    o Maternal age greater than 40 years

    o Chromosome abnormalities such as Down syndrome

    o Viral infections such as rubella

    o Excessive body heat exposure during the first trimester (neural tube defects)

    o Medications and substance abuse during pregnancy

    o Radiation exposure

    o Maternal metabolic disorders (phenylketonuria, diabetes mellitus)

    o Poor maternal nutrition such as folic acid deficiency (neural tube defects)

    o Infants who are premature

    o Infants who are SGA

    o Oligohydramnios or polyhydramnios

Assessments

- Monitor the newborn for signs and symptoms of congenital anomalies:

    o Cleft lip/palate – failure of the lip or hard or soft palate to fuse

    o Tracheoesophageal atresia – failure of the esophagus to connect to the stomach, excessive mucous secretions and drooling, periodic cyanotic episodes and choking, abdominal distention after birth, and immediate regurgitation after birth

    o Duodenal atresia – is common in infants who have Down syndrome and is when the first part of the small bowel has not developed properly and is not open and stomach contents are unable to pass; surgical intervention is required

    o Phenylketonuria (PKU) – the inability to metabolize the amino acid phenylalanine; can result in mental retardation if untreated; this will not be evident at birth, but will be identified with neonatal screening

    o Galactosemia – inability to metabolize galactose into glucose; can result in failure to thrive, cataracts, jaundice, cirrhosis of the liver, sepsis, and mental retardation if untreated; this will not be evident at birth, but will be identified with neonatal screening

    o Hypothyroidism – slow metabolism caused by maternal iodine deficiency or maternal antithyroid medications during pregnancy; can result in hypothermia, poor feeding, lethargy, jaundice, and cretinism if untreated

    o Neurologic anomalies (spina bifida) – a neural tube defect in which the vertebral arch fails to close and there may be a protrusion of the meninges and/or spinal cord

- Hydrocephalus – excessive spinal fluid accumulation in the ventricles of the brain causing the head to enlarge and the fontanels to bulge; sun-setting sign is common in which the whites of the eyes are visible above the iris

- Patent ductus arteriosus – a noncyanotic heart defect in which the ductus arteriosus connecting the pulmonary artery and the aorta fails to close after birth; signs and symptoms consist of murmurs, abnormal heart rate or rhythm, breathlessness, and fatigue while feeding

- Tetralogy of Fallot – cyanotic heart defect characterized by a ventricular septal defect, the aorta positioned over the ventricular septal defect, stenosis of the pulmonary valve, and hypertrophy of the right ventricle; distinguished by respiratory difficulties, cyanosis, tachycardia, tachypnea, and diaphoresis

- Down syndrome – oblique palpebral fissures or upward slant of eyes, epicanthal folds, flat facial profile with a depressed nasal bridge and a small nose, protruding tongue, small low-set ears, short broad hands with a fifth finger that has one flexion crease instead of two, a deep crease across the center of the palm frequently referred to as a simian crease, hyperflexibility, and hypotonic muscles

- Nursing assessments of infants who have congenital anomalies

  - Newborn's ability to take in adequate nourishment

  - Newborn's ability to eliminate waste products

  - Vital signs and axillary temperature

  - Infant-parental bonding, observing the parent's response to the diagnosis of a congenital defect, and encouraging the parents to verbalize concerns

Diagnostic and Therapeutic Procedures

- Prenatal screening for congenital anomalies may be done by ultrasound and multiple-marker screening (triple and quad screen).

- Confirmation of a diagnosis depends on the anomaly.

- Prenatal diagnosis or confirmation of congenital anomalies are often made by amniocentesis, chorionic villi sampling, or ultrasound.

- Routine testing of newborns for metabolic disorders (inborn errors of metabolism)

  - A Guthrie test for PKU is done to show elevations of phenylalanine in the blood and urine. It is not reliable until the infant has ingested sufficient amounts of protein.

  - Monitor blood and urine levels of galactose (galactosemia).

  - Measure thyroxine (hypothyroidism).

  - Cytologic studies (karyotyping of chromosomes), such as a buccal smear, uses cells scraped from the mucosa from inside the newborn's mouth.

Collaborative Care

- Nursing Care

  - Nursing interventions for congenital anomalies are dependent upon the type and extent of the anomaly.

    - Neurologic anomalies (spina bifida)

      - Protect the membrane with a sterile covering and plastic to prevent drying.

      - Observe for leakage of the cerebrospinal fluid.

      - Handle the newborn gently by positioning him prone or to the side to prevent trauma.

      - Prevent infection by keeping the area free from contamination by urine and feces.

      - Measure the circumference of the newborn's head to identify hydrocephalus.

      - Assess the newborn for increased intracranial pressure.

    - Hydrocephalus

      - Frequently reposition the infant's head to prevent sores.

      - Measure the infant's head circumference daily.

      - Assess the infant for signs of increased intracranial pressure such as vomiting and a shrill cry.

    - Patent ductus arteriosus

      - Educate the parents about surgical treatment.

    - Tetralogy of Fallot

      - Conserve the infant's energy to reduce the workload on the heart.

      - Administer gavage feedings or give oral feedings with a special nipple.

      - Elevate the infant's head and shoulders to improve respirations and reduce the cardiac workload.

      - Prevent infection.

      - Place the infant in a knee-chest position during respiratory distress.

  - Nursing interventions for congenital anomalies

    - Establish and maintain an adequate respiratory status.

    - Establish and maintain extrauterine circulation.

    - Establish and maintain adequate thermoregulation.

    - Administer medications as prescribed such as thyroid replacement for hypothyroidism.

    - Educate the parents regarding preoperative and postoperative treatment procedures.

- Provide adequate nutrition.

  □ Cleft lip/palate – determine the most effective nipple for feeding. Feed the infant in the upright position to decrease aspiration risk. Feed the infant slowly, and burp him frequently so that he does not swallow air. Cleanse his mouth with water after feedings.

  □ Tracheoesophageal atresia – withhold the newborn's feedings until esophageal patency is determined. Elevate the head of the newborn's crib to prevent gastric juice reflux. Supervise the newborn's first feeding to observe for this anomaly.

  □ Duodenal atresia – withhold the newborn's feedings until surgical repair is done and the infant has begun to pass stools. Administer IV fluids, as prescribed. Monitor the newborn for jaundice.

  □ PKU – special synthetic formula in which phenylalanine is removed or reduced. The mother should restrict meat, dairy products, diet drinks, and protein during pregnancy. Aspartame must be avoided.

  □ Galactosemia – give the infant a soy-based formula because galactose is present in milk. Eliminate lactose and galactose in the newborn's diet. Breastfeeding is also contraindicated.

- Encourage the parents to hold, touch, and talk to their newborn.

- Ensure that the parents provide consistent care to the newborn.

CHAPTER 27: ASSESSMENT AND MANAGEMENT OF NEWBORN COMPLICATIONS

Ⓐ Application Exercises

1. A nurse is called to the birthing room to assist with the assessment of a newborn who was born at 32 weeks of gestation. The newborn's birth weight is 1,100 g. His Apgar scores are 3 at 1 min and 7 at 5 min. He is experiencing nasal flaring, grunting, and intercostal retractions. Which of the following are characteristics that the nurse may see at this birth? (Select all that apply.)

_____ Large head in comparison to body

_____ Lanugo

_____ Long hair

_____ Long nails

_____ Weak grasp reflex

_____ Translucent skin

_____ Plump face

2. Which of the following assessment findings in a newborn who was born at 32 weeks of gestation should indicate that a complication may be developing?

3. Discuss why a preterm infant is at risk for ineffective thermoregulation?

4. A nurse is examining an infant who was just delivered at 41 weeks of gestation. Which of the following characteristics indicates that this infant is postterm?

   A. Abundant lanugo

   B. Flat areola without breast buds

   C. Heels movable fully to the ears

   D. Leathery skin

5. A nurse is caring for a multiparous client who just gave birth to her newborn at 40 weeks of gestation. After prolonged pushing in the second stage, a forceps-assisted birth was necessary. The newborn weighs 9 lb, 8 oz (4,318 g). The newborn has marked caput succedaneum and marked bruising about the face, head, and shoulders. How should the nurse characterize this infant? (Select all that apply.)

   _____ Preterm

   _____ Term

   _____ Postterm

   _____ LGA

   _____ SGA

   _____ AGA

6. A nurse is caring for an infant who has a high bilirubin level and is receiving phototherapy. Which of the following findings in the newborn is the highest priority?

    A. Conjunctivitis

    B. Bronze skin discoloration

    C. Sunken fontanels

    D. Maculopapular skin rash

7. A nurse is caring for an infant who is preterm and has respiratory distress syndrome. Which of the following assessment findings will assist the nurse in evaluating the efficacy of synthetic surfactant?

    A. Oxygen saturation

    B. Body temperature

    C. Bilirubin levels

    D. Heart rate

8. A nurse should consider the possibility of neonatal withdrawal syndrome if a newborn

    A. has decreased muscle tone.

    B. has a continuous high-pitched cry.

    C. sleeps for 2 hr after feeding.

    D. has mild tremors when disturbed.

CHAPTER 27: ASSESSMENT AND MANAGEMENT OF NEWBORN COMPLICATIONS

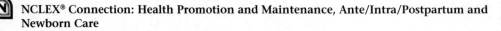 Application Exercises Answer Key

1. A nurse is called to the birthing room to assist with the assessment of a newborn who was born at 32 weeks of gestation. The newborn's birth weight is 1,100 g. His Apgar scores are 3 at 1 min and 7 at 5 min. He is experiencing nasal flaring, grunting, and intercostal retractions. Which of the following are characteristics that the nurse may see at this birth? (Select all that apply.)

__X__	**Large head in comparison to body**
__X__	**Lanugo**
_____	Long hair
_____	Long nails
__X__	**Weak grasp reflex**
__X__	**Translucent skin**
_____	Plump face

Characteristics of an infant who is preterm includes a large head in comparison to the body, lanugo over the body, a weak grasp reflex, and skin that is thin, smooth, shiny, and possibly translucent. Long hair and nails are signs found in an infant who is postterm. A plump face would be seen in a infant who is macrosomic.

 NCLEX® Connection: Health Promotion and Maintenance, Ante/Intra/Postpartum and Newborn Care

2. Which of the following assessment findings in a newborn who was born at 32 weeks of gestation should indicate that a complication may be developing?

Nasal flaring, grunting, and substernal and intercostal retractions indicate that the infant is experiencing respiratory distress.

 NCLEX® Connection: Health Promotion and Maintenance, Ante/Intra/Postpartum and Newborn Care

3. Discuss why a preterm infant is at risk for ineffective thermoregulation?

The infant's low birth weight and gestational age means that the infant has little glycogen stored in his liver and little brown fat available for producing heat. An infant who is preterm lacks subcutaneous fat to insulate his body and his flaccid muscle tone does not allow him to take a flexed position to prevent heat loss.

 NCLEX® Connection: Physiological Adaptation, Alterations in Body Systems

4. A nurse is examining an infant who was just delivered at 41 weeks of gestation. Which of the following characteristics indicates that this infant is postterm?

    A. Abundant lanugo

    B. Flat areola without breast buds

    C. Heels movable fully to the ears

    D. Leathery skin

    Leathery, cracked, and wrinkled skin is seen in a newborn who is postterm due to placental insufficiency. Abundant lanugo, flat areolas without breast buds, and heels that are movable fully to the ears are found in preterm newborns.

 NCLEX® Connection: Physiological Adaptation, Alterations in Body Systems

5. A nurse is caring for a multiparous client who just gave birth to her newborn at 40 weeks of gestation. After prolonged pushing in the second stage, a forceps-assisted birth was necessary. The newborn weighs 9 lb, 8 oz (4,318 g). The newborn has marked caput succedaneum and marked bruising about the face, head, and shoulders. How should the nurse characterize this infant? (Select all that apply.)

_____	Preterm
X	**Term**
_____	Postterm
X	**LGA**
_____	SGA
_____	AGA

    The infant is at term (40 weeks) and LGA (greater than the 90th percentile in weight). Preterm is prior to 37 weeks of gestation and postterm is after the completion of the 42nd week of gestation. An SGA infant is at or below the 10th percentile in weight. An AGA is between the 10th and 90th percentile for weight.

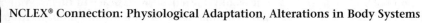 NCLEX® Connection: Health Promotion and Maintenance, Ante/Intra/Postpartum and Newborn Care

6. A nurse is caring for an infant who has a high bilirubin level and is receiving phototherapy. Which of the following findings in the newborn is the highest priority?

    A. Conjunctivitis

    B. Bronze skin discoloration

    C. Sunken fontanels

    D. Maculopapular skin rash

    Infants receiving phototherapy are at greatest risk for dehydration related to loss of water from frequent loose stools due to increased bilirubin excretion. Supplemental oral or IV fluids are given as needed to prevent this complication. Conjunctivitis, bronze skin discoloration, and maculopapular rash are all important findings, but are not the highest priority finding.

NCLEX® Connection: Physiological Adaptation, Alterations in Body Systems

7. A nurse is caring for an infant who is preterm and has respiratory distress syndrome (RDS). Which of the following assessment findings will assist the nurse in evaluating the efficacy of synthetic surfactant?

    A. Oxygen saturation

    B. Body temperature

    C. Bilirubin levels

    D. Heart rate

    Surfactant therapy stabilizes the alveoli and prevents collapse, thereby increasing lung compliance and maintaining or improving oxygen saturation. Surfactant would not have a direct effect on body temperature, thus it would not reflect the efficacy of this treatment. The nurse must provide a neutral thermal environment for this infant and monitor his body temperature continuously. Surfactant does not have a direct effect on bilirubin levels. It is important to monitor the heart rate of any infant who is preterm, as well as any infant who has RDS. However, heart rate is not a reflection of the efficacy of surfactant therapy.

    NCLEX® Connection: Reduction of Risk Potential, Potential for Complications of Diagnostic Tests/Treatments/Procedures

8. A nurse should consider the possibility of neonatal withdrawal syndrome if a newborn

    A. has decreased muscle tone.

    B. has a continuous high-pitched cry.

    C. sleeps for 2 hr after feeding.

    D. has mild tremors when disturbed.

    Symptoms of withdrawal from maternal substance abuse include CNS disturbances such as an excessive or continuous high-pitched cry and a markedly hyperactive Moro reflex. An infant withdrawing from opioids or other substances abused maternally is likely to have an increased muscle tone along with other CNS disturbances. Most newborns sleep for varying amounts of time after feeding. Symptoms of withdrawal from maternal substance abuse include difficulty moving through various sleep stages. This sleep pattern disturbance is related to CNS excitation secondary to drug or alcohol withdrawal. Many newborns have mild tremors when they are disturbed. What distinguishes infants who have neonatal abstinence syndrome from this normal pattern is that they have moderate to severe tremors when they are undisturbed.

    NCLEX® Connection: Health Promotion and Maintenance, Ante/Intra/Postpartum and Newborn Care

References

Dudek, S. G. (2010). *Nutrition essentials for nursing practice* (6th ed.). Philadelphia, PA: Lippincott Williams & Wilkins.

Grodner, M., Long, S., & Walkingshaw, B. C. (2007). *Foundations and clinical applications of nutrition: A nursing approach* (4th ed.). St. Louis, MO: Mosby.

Lehne, R. A. (2010). *Pharmacology for nursing care* (7th ed.). St. Louis, MO: Saunders.

Lowdermilk, D. L., & Perry, S. E. (2007). *Maternity & women's health care* (9th ed.). St. Louis, MO: Mosby.

Pillitteri, A. (2007). *Maternal and child health nursing: Care of the childbearing and childrearing family* (5th ed.). Philadelphia, PA: Lippincott Williams & Wilkins.

Wilson, B. A., Shannon, M. T., & Shields, K. M. (2010). *Pearson nurse's drug guide 2010.* Upper Saddle River, NJ: Prentice-Hall.